Developing and Managing
CARDIAC REHABILITATION
PROGRAMS

Linda K. Hall, PhD

Allegheny General Hospital
Pittsburgh, PA

Editor

Human Kinetics Publishers

Library of Congress Cataloging-in-Publication Data

Developing and managing cardiac rehabilitation programs / Linda K.
  Hall, editor.
      p.   cm.
    Includes bibliographical references and index.
    ISBN 0-87322-358-6
    1. Heart--Diseases--Patients--Rehabilitation.   2. Heart--Diseases-
  -Patients--Services for--Administration.   I. Hall, Linda K.
    [DNLM: 1. Heart Diseases--rehabilitation. 2. Rehabilitation
  Centers--organization & administration.   WG 200 D489]
  RC682.D48   1993
  616.1'203--dc20
  DNLM/DLC
  for Library of Congress   93-1448
                                                            CIP

ISBN: 0-87322-358-6

Developmental Editor: Mary E. Fowler
Assistant Editors: Dawn Roselund, Laura Bofinger
Copyeditor: Julie Anderson
Proofreader: Pam Johnson
Production Director: Ernie Noa
Typesetter: Ruby Zimmerman
Text Design: Keith Blomberg
Text Layout: Tara Welsch, Kimberlie Henris
Cover Design: Jack Davis
Cover Photo: Wilmer Zehr
Interior Photos: Mary Jane Bent
Printer: Braun-Brumfield

Printed in the United States of America

10 9 8 7 6 5 4 3 2 1

Human Kinetics Publishers
Box 5076, Champaign, IL 61825-5076
1-800-747-4457

Canada Office:
Human Kinetics Publishers
P.O. Box 2503, Windsor, ON N8Y 4S2
1-800-465-7301 (in Canada only)

Europe Office:
Human Kinetics Publishers (Europe) Ltd.
P.O. Box IW14
Leeds LS16 6TR
England   0532-781708

Australia Office:
Human Kinetics Publishers
P.O. Box 80
Kingswood 5062
South Australia   374-0433

Contents

Contributors

Linda K. Hall, PhD
Editor

Linda K. Hall is the director of Cardiac and Pulmonary Rehabilitation at Allegheny General Hospital in Pittsburgh, PA, and is one of the leading experts in the field of Cardiac and Pulmonary Rehabilitation. She was the president of the American Association of Cardiovascular and Pulmonary Rehabilitation for 1990 and 1991, and served as senior editor for the 1990 edition of the *Guidelines for Cardiac Rehabilitation*. She has edited three other books on cardiac rehabilitation and has given more than 150 national presentations on cardiac rehabilitation. She directed the Cardiac Rehabilitation unit of the La Crosse exercise program at the University of Wisconsin-La Crosse, La Crosse, WI, for 5 years, and is a member of the American College of Sports Medicine.

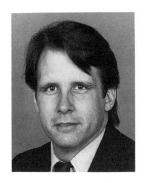

Kathy Berra, BSN, FAACVPR

Kathy Berra is a past president of the American Association of Cardiovascular and Pulmonary Rehabilitation (AACVPR) and has been involved in the field of cardiac and pulmonary rehabilitation for over 20 years. She lectures nationally on many subjects related to cardiac rehabilitation and is widely known for her expertise in community-based programs. Kathy is coauthor of a six-part video series on cardiac rehabilitation sponsored by the American Heart Association and is clinical editor of the *Journal of Cardiopulmonary Rehabilitation*. She has participated in cardiac rehabilitation research and has published extensively. She received the ''Award of Excellence'' from AACVPR in 1991.

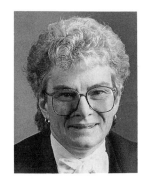

Lance H. Crosby, RN, MS, FAACVPR

Lance H. Crosby has had extensive experience in the rehabilitation of the inpatient during the last 10 years. He currently is clinical coordinator of the Cardiac Rehabilitation Department at Allegheny General Hospital, Pittsburgh, PA, where he directs the country's largest inpatient rehabilitation program, with 15 professional staff who make more than 10,000 inpatient visits annually. Lance has authored a number of papers on inpatient cardiac rehabilitation. He is a fellow of the AACVPR and has been active on several of its committees. Crosby also serves on the review board for the *Journal of Cardiopulmonary Rehabilitation*.

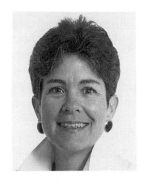

Terri Hornbach, BS

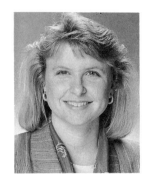

Terri Hornbach is director of public relations at ChoiceCare, greater Cincinnati's largest managed care organization. Before joining Choice-Care, Terri worked in hospital public relations for 8 years, most recently as assistant director of public relations at The Christ Hospital in Cincinnati. There she was instrumental in helping to establish the hospital's image as Cincinnati's "heart hospital." Terri holds a bachelor's degree in mass communications from Miami University (Oxford, OH) and is studying for her master's in business administration. She is a member of the American Society for Health Care Marketing and Public Relations and the Public Relations Society of America. Terri has received more than 25 awards from local, state, and regional associations for her work in health care public relations.

Martha D. Livingston, RN, MS, MBA, FAACVPR

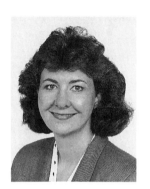

Martha D. Livingston is the director of cardiovascular services at Central DuPage Hospital in Winfield, IL. She has been involved in caring for individuals with known or suspected cardiovascular disease for more than 16 years. She has worked in all aspects of cardiac rehabilitation, from clinical practice, education, and research to administration. Martha lectures extensively and is best known for developing innovative programs and creating a behavior change model that promotes positive outcomes. She has been involved with AACVPR since its inception, serving in several capacities on the board of directors including the office of president. Martha is a fellow of AACVPR and was a contributor to its *Guidelines for Cardiac Rehabilitation Programs* and serves as the finance editor for the *Journal of Cardiopulmonary Rehabilitation*.

Karen E. Luffey, RD

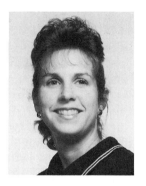

Karen E. Luffey, RD, has designed and administered several weight loss/maintenance programs with cardiopulmonary emphasis. Most recently at Allegheny General Hospital in Pittsburgh, PA, she developed and managed a successful cardiac weight loss/maintenance program with emphasis on individualizing realistic programs for patients. Luffey received her bachelor's degree from West Virginia, completed a dietetic internship program, and was awarded the Irene Wilson Award of Distinction. Luffey resides in Pittsburgh where she teaches, writes, and pursues a career in cardiopulmonary nutrition.

G. Curt Meyer, MS

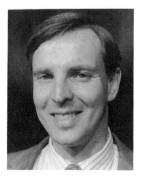

G. Curt Meyer is the chief executive officer for the Wesley Rehabilitation Hospital in Wichita, KS. Before accepting his position in Wichita, Meyer was the director of rehabilitation and wellness services at Lee Memorial Hospital in Fort Myers, FL. Curt has edited three books for Human Kinetics and has contributed to chapters in three others. He has published and presented nationally in the area of third-party reimbursement outcomes and organization and administration of cardiac rehabilitation and wellness programs. He was invited to speak to the Sub-committee on Health of the Committee of Finance in the United States Senate, presenting information relative to the impact of wellness centers on older adults. He has served on the Executive Committee of AACVPR for 5 years and is active in the committees on reimbursement and outcomes.

Cindy Lamendola Rudd, BSN, FAACVPR

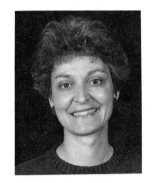

Cindy Lamendola Rudd has been involved in cardiac rehabilitation for more than 15 years. She is the codirector of YMCA Cardiac and Pulmonary Rehabilitation and was instrumental in developing their pulmonary and renal rehabilitation programs. She is a board member and past president of the California Society for Cardiac Rehabilitation and is a fellow and board member of AACVPR. She is well-known for her expertise on special populations and has spoken internationally on this subject.

Ruth E. Townsend, MS

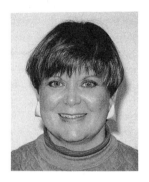

Ruth E. Townsend, MS, is the executive director of CAPRI (Cardiopulmonary Rehabilitation Institute) in Seattle, WA, the largest and most nationally recognized outpatient cardiac maintenance program in the United States. Ruth graduated from the University of Wisconsin, La Crosse, with an MS in adult fitness and cardiac rehabilitation. She was a founding member of the Washington Association of Cardiovascular and Pulmonary Rehabilitation and is currently the organization's vice president and an active member of its conference planning committee. She is a member of the American College of Sports Medicine and the American Association of Cardiovascular and Pulmonary Rehabilitation. Ruth is on the AACVPR Professional Education Committee and has written articles for the association's newsletter, *News and Views*.

Linda J. Walker, PhD, MSW, MPH, ACSW

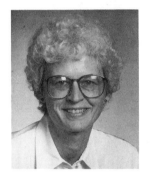

Linda J. Walker is familiar with health care issues and the role of health professionals through her 20 years' experience as a social worker in numerous medical centers. She is a former Peace Corps volunteer and currently a social work supervisor at Allegheny General Hospital in Pittsburgh, PA. Linda has authored or coauthored several publications dealing with developmental disabilities and relocation. She is a member of the National Association of Social Workers and the American Public Health Association.

Preface

Professionals and prospective professionals in cardiac rehabilitation will find *Developing and Managing Cardiac Rehabilitation Programs* a contemporary and comprehensive text for program development and operation. Part I, Program Development, describes cardiac rehabilitation programs, the rehabilitative continuum, and patient populations. In Part II, Program Implementation and Operation, the practical how-to for managing people, programs, and budgets in cardiac rehabilitation is presented.

Developing and Managing Cardiac Rehabilitation Programs will be helpful to master's and doctoral students as well as those who are setting up rehabilitation programs in hospitals or clinical settings. The book also will help those who have been managing cardiac rehabilitation programs for several years to review and evaluate their management techniques.

The contributors to *Developing and Managing Cardiac Rehabilitation Programs* are knowledgeable and prominent leaders in the field, individuals who are developing innovative approaches to managing cardiac rehabilitation programs.

As editor, my objective has been to make this book as practical and relevant to the management of cardiac rehabilitation programs as possible. The contributors have provided you with step-by-step procedures through lists, forms, tables, and charts. This book is not about the theory of managing cardiac rehabilitation programs; it's about the real world of cardiac rehabilitation management.

Linda Hall

Part I

Program Development

In the 1940s and 1950s the cardiac patient faced as much as 8 weeks of bed rest for recovery from a myocardial infarction (MI), commonly referred to as a heart attack. In the late 1980s, the stable myocardial infarction patient or the low-risk bypass surgery patient required as little as 1 day of complete bed rest and as few as 3 or 4 days in the hospital, in some instances.

Here begin the study and description of cardiac rehabilitation as a clinical practice in the care of people suffering from heart disease. The text will examine the different phases and courses of treatment for the cardiac patient as well as for those with the various diagnoses of heart disease who have proven most likely to benefit from cardiac rehabilitation.

Learning Objectives

1. To appreciate the historical development of cardiac rehabilitation in the treatment of the patient recovering from heart disease

2. To gain an understanding of the stated goals of cardiac rehabilitation and of the success in attaining these goals that has been achieved to date

3. To begin to formulate future directions for the role of cardiac rehabilitation in the treatment of heart disease

Key Terms

Cardiac Rehabilitation—The use of exercise, education, and psychological and emotional support to facilitate a patient's recovery from heart disease.

Phase I—Cardiac rehabilitation applied while the patient is in the hospital.

Phase II—Cardiac rehabilitation applied immediately after the patient is discharged from the hospital or within 2 to 3 weeks after discharge.

Phase III/Phase IV—Cardiac rehabilitation applied after the patient's cardiovascular and physiological responses to exercise have stabilized. Phase III is less supervised than Phase II and more supervised than Phase IV.

More change has occurred in the cardiac patient's treatment from the 1950s to the present than took place in the previous 150 years. Up through the 1950s, therapy for the MI patient was strict bed rest for as long as 2 months, with nursing personnel performing or assisting with all activities of daily living (ADL) such as eating, drinking, grooming, bathing, and even position change (Nite & Willis, 1961). Levine and Lown (1952) reported that the reason for the strictly enforced bed rest was to reduce cardiac work load and as a result prevent complications. Mallory, White, and Salcedo-Salgar (1939) identified such complications as ventricular aneurysm formation (ballooning of ventricle wall), cardiac rupture, congestive heart failure (loss of pumping power), reinfarction, dysrhythmias (interruption of normal sinus rhythm), and sudden death. In the 1930s and 1940s several groups studied the effects of bed rest versus activity and successfully demonstrated there were no deleterious effects with the patient's guarded return to normal activity within a few days after the myocardial infarction (Deitrick & Whedon, 1948; Dock, 1944; Harrison, 1944). Even with this scientific evidence demonstrating the efficacy of activity, professionals in the field who were considered to be the authorities continued to recommend a minimum of 4 weeks of bed rest (Irvin & Burgess, 1950).

Levine and Lown (1952) studied activity progression after MI from "armchair" sitting through early mobilization and observed no adverse effects; in fact, early activity reduced some of the harmful effects of strict bed rest. Additionally, increased activity had significant beneficial psychological effects on the patient. Thus the early foundations of rehabilitation were initiated; the stated objectives were to not only return the patient to vocational and economic usefulness but also improve his own personal capacity for living (Benton & Rusk, 1953).

During the 1950s, work led by Hellerstein and associates at the Cleveland Work Classification Clinic made considerable progress in assisting many cardiac patients to return to work (Hellerstein & Ford, 1957; Hellerstein & Goldston, 1954). Hellerstein conceptualized cardiac rehabilitation into the original and current model of three phases: inpatient, immediate outpatient/convalescence, and recovery and return to work (Hellerstein & Goldston, 1954). He also recognized the need for a team approach in enhancing the medical, psychiatric, social, and vocational rehabilitation of the patient.

Although evidence documented the benefits of early activity, there was still resistance to early activity as the standard mode of treatment after myocardial infarction. Newman, Wasserman, and Borden (1956) reported on a 6-week progressive mobilization program that produced definite therapeutic benefits. However, an activity program developed by Cain, Frasher, and Stivelman (1961) was accepted for implementation and the results were published in a refereed journal only with difficulty, because it was believed by some members of the medical profession and reviewers of the paper that the program was too dangerous for the patients (Froelicher & McKirnan, 1981).

The efforts of these people during the 1950s and 1960s became the foundation of modern cardiac rehabilitation. Through the 1960s and into the 1970s many programs were started not only on an inpatient basis (Acker, 1971; Brock, 1973; Naughton, Bruhn, Lategola, & Whitsett, 1969; Tobis & Zohman, 1968; Wenger, 1971) but also as outpatient programs. The use of gradual exercise, graded exercise testing, and electrocardiographic monitoring produced beneficial physiological as well as financial results in the form of earlier discharge from the hospital (Wenger, 1981). In 1979 the median length of stay for a myocardial infarction was 14 days, compared to 1 to 2 months during the 1950s. In 1989 the length of stay for an individual with an uncomplicated course for MI was as short as 3 to 4 days (Topol et al., 1988); however, the national average was 7 to 10 days for most hospital MI programs.

Even today, with the efficacy of cardiac rehabilitation programs scientifically proven relative to reduced hospital length of stay, more rapid return to ADL and work, and increased sense of well-being, cardiac rehabilitation as an integral part of patient care has not yet been universally accepted. And quite often, the person who requires the hard sell about the benefit of cardiac rehabilitation is the physician.

Past, Present, and Future Definitions

Although 30 or more years have elapsed since the beginnings of cardiac rehabilitation, its definition has changed very little. When formed, the definition was very broad and general, which has helped it remain applicable despite changes in patient populations and in the application of therapy due to innovative techniques, documentation, and research.

When Greenland and Chu (1988) reviewed past studies, they found significant differences in the recovery of individuals who went through cardiac rehabilitation programs and those who did not. But the "magnitude of the differences was relatively small" (Greenland & Chu, 1988, p. 652). The authors therefore implied that the patient population that will most benefit from cardiac rehabilitation is the one that is the most severely limited in functional capacity. These severely limited patients comprise the population currently being served by rehabilitation programs.

Past

Traditionally, cardiac rehabilitation has been defined as "the process by which a person is restored to an optimal physical, medical, psychologic, social, emotional, sexual, vocational and economic status" (Hellerstein & Ford, 1968, p. 225).

Originally, cardiac rehabilitation delineated these additional specific objectives: limiting the physiological and psychological effects of cardiovascular disease, reducing the risk of sudden death and reinfarction, controlling the symptoms of cardiac disease medically and surgically, stabilizing or reversing the atherosclerotic process, and enhancing psychosocial and vocational status (Wenger & Fletcher, 1986). The literature, which includes the meta-analyses by O'Connor and associates (1989) and Oldridge, Guyatt, Fischer, and Rimm (1988), reveals mixed findings with regard to these objectives (Greenland & Chu, 1988; Leon et al., 1990; Miller, Taylor, Davidson, Hill, & Krantz, 1990; National Center for Health Services Research and Health Care Technology Assessment, 1987). The literature shows that cardiac rehabilitation services do limit the physiological effects of cardiovascular disease and do improve a person's functional status while increasing the threshold for the onset of chest pain or ischemia. Cardiac rehabilitation also has been shown to significantly reduce the occurrence of sudden death in the 1st year after myocardial infarction; however, cardiac rehabilitation does not have any impact on incidence of reinfarction.

Probably one of the most important reasons that physicians have chosen to refer patients to cardiac rehabilitation in the past is because of the increased medical surveillance and control of symptoms. This is supported and documented by the research. However, control of symptoms through surgical intervention is difficult to measure, because surgery is not within the scope of the cardiac rehabilitation program. Previous studies that have attempted to demonstrate a reversal or stabilization in the level of atheroma in

arteries have been equivocal; however, more current studies demonstrate that stopping and even reversing progression are possible with medical and lifestyle management (Blankenhorn et al., 1987; Ornish et al., 1990). And finally, no definitive studies prove that cardiac rehabilitation limits the psychological effects or enhances the psychosocial and vocational status of those suffering from cardiovascular disease (Miller et al., 1990; National Center for Health Services Research and Health Care Technology Assessment, 1987; O'Connor et al., 1989; Oldridge et al., 1988). There are several reasons for the lack of scientific evidence for psychological changes and vocational status.

Often, the reason given for difficulties with the cardiac rehabilitation research is the lack of standardization of research protocols. In the results cited in the previous paragraph, each center that conducted a study applied the treatment differently; researchers started treatment at different times in the patients' recoveries and did not use a standard length of time involvement or standard exercise or educational protocols. Also clouding the research were crossovers in both directions among the control and the experimental groups, plus the fact that the measurement tools used were not validated on a cardiac population. This was especially true in the psychosocial research.

Present

The traditional definition has evolved slowly to its present state, which is concerned not only with the optimal functioning of the patient after the cardiac event but with a number of cardiovascular conditions present before, as well as during and after, the event. Additionally, inpatient and outpatient programs are designed to assist the patient's family in adjusting to an altered lifestyle. Programs have incorporated information and educational classes for the patient's spouse, family, and significant others. Family support groups, nutrition counseling, smoking cessation programs, and many other educational services are offered to the whole family rather than just the patient. Thus, the definition of cardiac rehabilitation should now read "the process by which the patient and family system are restored to optimal physical, medical, psychological, social, emotional, sexual, vocational, and economic status" (adapted from Hellerstein & Ford, 1968).

The objectives of the earlier years are still enumerated; however, there is an impetus from professional organizations such as the American

Association of Cardiovascular and Pulmonary Rehabilitation (AACVPR) and the Joint Commission on Accreditation of Healthcare Organizations (JCAHO) to individualize patient care with defined and measured outcomes. Additionally, the AACVPR has published national guidelines for cardiac rehabilitation (AACVPR, 1990), which will standardize our practice and allow a more scientific evaluation of the objectives.

Future

Future definitions and objectives of cardiac rehabilitation will evolve and certainly impact program development as the patient population changes. AACVPR has had a significant impact and will have major influence as the organization grows stronger, produces more position statements, and updates guideline publications. As the number and size of state societies increase, the vocal impact on reimbursement legislation will be strongly heard. The United States government and leaders in the health care industry will soon be forced to act upon the current status of health care reimbursement (Coddington, Keen, Moore, & Clarke, 1990). It will be critical for cardiac rehabilitation leaders to play a role in those decisions.

The future holds the potential for a truly dichotomous cardiovascular-diseased population. One half of the dichotomy includes the elderly (the most rapidly growing population in the United States is made up of people over 100 years of age, with 85- and 65-year-olds close behind). The other half of the dichotomy is a younger population, people with severe diseases that will change the course of their lives.

The older population will require highly skilled personnel, because older people will have multiple disease presentations and complications, such as chronic obstructive pulmonary disease (COPD), coronary artery disease (CAD), or renal failure, and as a result will require more care. Although aging cardiac patients are presently receiving this care, the potential for older patients with more complex problems and for larger volumes of patients is even greater in the future.

Even though we already are working with the younger patients, these patients will require more intense lifestyle behavior modification, work evaluation, and retraining because of the potential disability and financial loss they will experience without highly developed intervention and rehabilitation programs. Programs for these patients will have to be creatively and responsibly designed with special attention to financial structure, be-

cause reimbursement may be more difficult than programming.

Further Reading

Any of the materials in the reference list will enhance your knowledge of the field; however, the following are recommended as references and texts. They are for you to read and have access to in order to develop a program or apply cardiac rehabilitation to a patient.

American Association of Cardiovascular and Pulmonary Rehabilitation. (1991). *Guidelines for cardiac rehabilitation programs*. Champaign, IL: Human Kinetics.

American College of Sports Medicine. (1991). *Resource manual for guidelines for exercise testing and prescription*. Philadelphia: Lea & Febiger.

American College of Sports Medicine. (1990). *Guidelines for exercise testing and prescription* (4th ed.). Philadelphia: Lea & Febiger.

References

Acker, J.E. (1971). The cardiac rehabilitation unit: Experiences with a program with early activation. *Circulation*, **44**, (Suppl. 2), 119.

American Association of Cardiovascular and Pulmonary Rehabilitation. (1990). *Guidelines for cardiac rehabilitation*. Champaign, IL: Human Kinetics.

Benton, J.G., & Rusk, H.K. (1953). The patient with cardiovascular disease and rehabilitation: The third phase of medical care. *Circulation*, **8**, 417-425.

Blankenhorn, D.H., Nessim, S.A., Johnson, R.L., Sanmarco, M.E., Azen, S.P., & Cashin-Hemphill, L. (1987). Beneficial effects of combined colestipol-niacin therapy on coronary atherosclerosis and coronary venous bypass grafts. *Journal of the American Medical Association*, **257**, 3233-3240.

Brock, L. (1973). Early ambulation of post-myocardial infarction patients. In J.P. Naughton & H.K. Hellerstein (Eds.). *Exercise testing and exercise training in coronary heart disease* (pp. 315-336). New York: Academic Press.

Cain, H.D., Frasher, W.D., & Stivelman, J. (1961). Graded activity program for safe return to self-care after myocardial infarction. *Journal of the American Medical Association*, **177**(2), 111-115.

Coddington, D.C., Keen, D.J., Moore, D.D., & Clarke, R.L. (1990). *The crisis in health care*. San Francisco: Jossey-Bass.

Deitrick, J.E., & Whedon, G.D. (1948). Effects of mobilization upon various metabolic and physiologic functions of normal men. *American Journal of Medicine, 46*(3), 3-35.

Dock, W. (1944). The evil sequelae of complete bed rest. *Journal of the American Medical Association, 125*(16), 1083-1085.

Froelicher, V.F., & McKirnan, M.D. (1981). Rehabilitation and exercise early after acute myocardial infarction. In J.S. Karliner & G. Gregoratos (Eds.), *Coronary care* (897-917). New York: Churchill Livingstone.

Greenland, P., & Chu, J.S. (1988). Efficacy of cardiac rehabilitation services. *Annals of Internal Medicine, 109*, 650-663.

Harrison, T.R. (1944). Abuse of bed rest as a therapeutic measure for patients with cardiovascular disease. *Journal of the American Medical Association, 25*(16), 1076-1077.

Hellerstein, H.K., & Ford, A.B. (1957). Rehabilitation of the cardiac patient. *Journal of the American Medical Association, 164*(3), 225-231.

Hellerstein, H.K., & Ford, A.B. (1968). Comprehensive care of the coronary patient. Optimal (intensive) care, recovery and reconditioning. An opportunity for the physician. Symposium on coronary heart disease. *American Heart Association Monograph No. 2* (2nd ed.). Dallas: Author.

Hellerstein, H.K., & Goldston, E. (1954). Rehabilitation of patients with heart disease. *Postgraduate Medicine, 15*, 265-278.

Irvin, W.C., & Burgess, A.M. (1950). The abuse of bedrest in the treatment of myocardial infarction. *New England Journal of Medicine, 243*, 486-489.

Leon, A.S., Certo, C., Comoss, P., Franklin, B.A., Froelicher, V., Haskell, W.L., Hellerstein, H.K., Marley, W.P., Pollock, M.L., Ries, A., Froelicher, E.S., & Smith, L.K. (1990). Scientific evidence of the value of cardiac rehabilitation services with emphasis on patients following myocardial infarction: Exercise conditioning component. *Guidelines for cardiac rehabilitation programs.* Champaign, IL: Human Kinetics.

Levine, S.A., Lown, B. (1952). "Armchair" treatment of acute coronary thrombosis. *Journal of the American Medical Association, 148*(16), 1356-1369.

Mallory, G.K., White, P.L., & Salcedo-Salgar, J. (1939). The speed of healing on myocardial infarction: A study of the pathologic anatomy in seventy-two cases. *American Heart Journal, 18*, 647-656.

Miller, N.H., Taylor, C.B., Davidson, D.M., Hill, M.N., & Krantz, D.S. (1990). The efficacy of risk factor intervention and psychosocial aspects of cardiac rehabilitation. *Guidelines for cardiac rehabilitation programs.* Champaign, IL: Human Kinetics.

National Center for Health Services Research and Health Care Technology Assessment. (1987). *Health technology assessment reports, cardiac rehabilitation services* (DHHS Publication No. PHS 88-3427, pp. 1-89). Rockville, MD: U.S. Department of Health and Human Services.

Naughton, J.P., Bruhn, J., Lategola, M.T., & Whitsett, T. (1969). Rehabilitation following myocardial infarction. *American Journal of Medicine, 46*, 725-733.

Newman, L.B., Wasserman, R.R., & Borden, C. (1956). Productive living for those with heart disease: The role of physical medicine and rehabilitation. *Archives of Physical Medicine and Rehabilitation, 37*, 137-149.

Nite, G., & Willis, K. (1961). *The coronary patient: Hospital care and rehabilitation.* New York: Macmillan.

O'Connor, G.T., Buring, J.E., Yusuf, S., Goldhaber, S.Z., Olmstead, E.M., Paffenbarger, R.W., & Hennekens, C.H. (1989). An overview of randomized trials of rehabilitation with exercise after myocardial infarction. *Circulation, 80*, 234-244.

Oldridge, N., Guyatt, G., Fischer, M., & Rimm, A. (1988). Cardiac rehabilitation after myocardial infarction: Combined experience of randomized clinical trials. *Journal of the American Medical Association, 260*, 945.

Ornish, D., Brown, S.E., Scherwitz, L.W., Billings, J.H., Armstrong, W.T., Ports, T.A., McLannahan, S.M., Kirkeeide, R.L., Brand, R.J., & Gould, K.L. (1990). Can lifestyle changes reverse coronary heart disease? *The Lancet, 336*, 129-133.

Tobis, J.S., & Zohman, L.R. (1968). A rehabilitation program for inpatients with recent myocardial infarction. *Archives of Physical Medicine and Rehabilitation, 49*(8), 443-448.

Topol, E.J., Burek, K., O'Neil, W.W., Kewman, D.G., Kander, N.H., Shea, M.J., Schork, M.A., Kirscht, J., Juni, J.E., & Pitt, B. (1988). A randomized controlled trial of hospital discharge three days after myocardial infarction in the era of reperfusion. *New England Journal of Medicine, 318*(17), 1083-1088.

Wenger, N.K. (1971). Physical conditioning after myocardial infarction, an early intervention program. *Circulation, 44*, (Suppl. 2), 119.

Wenger, N.K. (1981). In-hospital rehabilitation after myocardial infarction. In L.S. Cohen, M.B. Mock, & I. Rengaquist (Eds.), *Physical conditioning and cardiovascular rehabilitation*. New York: Wiley.

Wenger, N.K., & Fletcher, G.F. (1986). Rehabilitation of the patient with atherosclerotic coronary heart disease. In J.W. Hurst (Ed.), *The heart* (pp. 1025-1037). New York: McGraw-Hill.

Chapter 1

Issues and Special Populations in Inpatient Rehabilitation

Lance H. Crosby, RN, MS, FAACVPR

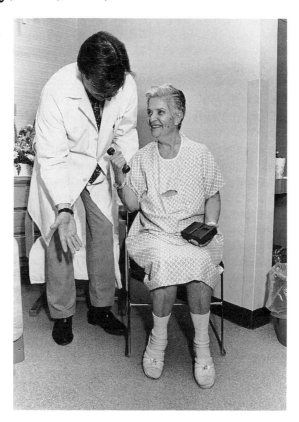

The initial component of a strong cardiac rehabilitation program is a well-structured inpatient program, Phase I, in your hospital, clinic, or other health care continuum. Foundations are laid for a cardiac rehabilitation continuum by the development of a comprehensive patient assessment protocol, job descriptions for therapists, and application of skill as well as applications of exercise therapy. This chapter details these specifics with emphasis on special populations, which are now daily challenges to cardiac rehabilitation therapists.

Learning Objectives

1. To appreciate the need for developing a comprehensive assessment protocol for initiating inpatient cardiac rehabilitation

2. To understand the dimensions of skills required of the cardiac rehabilitation specialist

3. To define the parameters of exercise therapy in an inpatient population

4. To gain insights into applying exercise therapy to selected patient groups in an inpatient setting

---

Inpatient rehabilitation has become a specialized service in the early management of coronary heart disease and other chronic debilitating diseases. The more experience we as practitioners gain, the more we recognize the wide range of challenges provided by the patient. The more we learn, the more we realize what we can accomplish. The types of patients being rehabilitated are more and more complicated and challenging. Today, many patients are mobilized early and exercised who several years ago would not have survived the hospitalization. At large tertiary care hospitals, cardiac rehabilitation personnel are working with patients involved in experimental surgeries, organ transplantation, drug trials, invasive cardiology procedures, and electrophysiology studies. These patients often eventually filter back into the community hospitals. The rehabilitation therapist in this increasingly complex environment has to question whether there are absolute contraindications to exercise. It seems there are always exceptions to the rule of absolutes. Practical experience and an increasing body of scientific knowledge provide mounting evidence to support the importance of activity in most populations facing prolonged physical and emotional debilities.

Cardiac rehabilitation is hardly 3 decades young. The discipline has rightfully prided itself on the multidisciplinary approach to provide an integrated and complete therapy. However, this practice may have inhibited the development of a true singular cardiac rehabilitation professional. This is increasingly apparent as the demand for a specialist in cardiac rehabilitation rather than a generalist is increasing.

The Initial Consultation

The initial consultation results in a written patient evaluation that is provided by all consultants. It is a summary of pertinent information that provides an overview of the patient's medical history. The document is completed with a diagnosis, recommendations, and/or plan.

The initial consultation, whose components appear in Table 1.1, often reflects your professional training and thereby focuses on those areas with which you are most familiar and comfortable. A physical therapist can provide a total patient evaluation but may address the evaluation from a physical therapist's perspective, concentrating on the musculoskeletal system and placing less emphasis on the cardiovascular and pulmonary examination. A nurse may focus on the cardiovascular system, including an exam of the heart and lungs, but may avoid documenting alterations in gait or strength deficits. The exercise physiologist will also have her own unique perspective of patient evaluation. A patient consultation specific to cardiac rehabilitation is not well developed or uniform from institution to institution. The challenge is to develop a patient examination and an evaluation that utilizes the many skills of the rehabilitation specialist. The examination and evaluation should focus on your unique perspective of the patient and should not be a patient summary reviewing other services input.

The purpose of organizing the initial consultation is to integrate many of the professionals working in this field, thereby providing the nurse, physical therapist, and exercise physiologist a

Table 1.1 Components of the Initial Consultation

- Current hospital course: age, gender, diagnosis, pertinent events, lab results, tests, medication, dysrhythmia, and vital signs.
- Significant contributing medical/surgical history: CAD, COPD, diabetes, HTN, PVD, renal disease, orthopedic surgery, and length of and severity of disability.
- Patient interview: learning capabilities/deficits, psychosocial history, work, recreation, risk factors, potential for home rehabilitation, limitations to work, musculoskeletal problems, functional capacity, and adaptation to disease.
- Physical exam: cardiovascular, pulmonary, and musculoskeletal systems, and gait.
- Impression/assessment: description of current physical disability and potential for recovery, learning deficits, risk factor modification, and exercise therapy plans; identification of problems or barriers.

Note. A succinct, practical, and useful evaluation provides a specialized assessment of a patient's functional abilities/limitations, risk factor status, and plan for return to optimum function. CAD = coronary artery disease; COPD = chronic obstructive pulmonary disease; HTN = hypertension; PVD = pulmonary vascular disease.

more uniform method of patient evaluation. This will in turn lead to a concise summary of the pertinent medical facts, pertinent psychosocial history, evaluation of functional abilities, and risk factor assessment that may affect the patient's return to optimal function. A successful evaluation will integrate elements of exercise, cardiopulmonary physiology, anatomy, psychology, and adult learning theory to complete the process necessary for the patient's effective return to a satisfactory lifestyle.

Past History

First, review the patient's past medical history and hospital chart to provide a comprehensive data base. Developing a system for collecting this information is worthwhile. You can limit information to prior hospitalizations and illnesses that may affect exercise therapy or outcomes. Likewise, in reviewing the patient's current hospital stay or ill-

ness, focus on those factors that will influence the patient's rehabilitation plan. Thorough risk factor screening begins in the chart review, which should include the patient's height and weight, changes in health habits, and pertinent family history—limited to cardiovascular disease. Note medications prior to admission with emphasis on those that may directly or indirectly affect the cardiovascular and neuromuscular systems.

The next step is the patient interview. Often, you can conduct this while performing the physical examination. Questions addressing family and social history that may influence health are useful. Direct these questions at ascertaining the patient's cultural background and family structure, who is at home to assist, and whether return to work is an option. Also ascertain the patient's home physical environment including architectural barriers; number of steps; steep grades and driveway; and accessibility to rehabilitation facilities, hospitals, malls, and walk areas that will facilitate home training. Note personal habits such as alcohol and caffeine use as well as personal exercise habits or previous history of exercise and availability of home exercise equipment. Furthermore, determine if the patient has made any successful attempts (especially on his own) to modify his lifestyle.

Assessment of Functional Capacity

Evaluation of functional capacity is a major part of the cardiac rehabilitation patient assessment. Determining the patient's ability to accomplish simple tasks or activities such as climbing steps or walking distance is fundamental. Establishing the rate of decline of exercise capacity is especially important because it predicts the extent of the disability as well as future decline. Through evaluation of a patient's functional capacity it becomes a clear indicator of the patient's ability to adapt to the restrictions of disease.

An excellent tool for the prediction of functional work abilities based on metabolic equivalents (METs) is Goldman's Specific Activity Scale (Goldman, Hashimoto, Cook, & Loscalzo, 1981) (Table 1.2). This is a valid reproducible scale for assessment of functional ability; it uses a series of questions to determine predicted exercise tolerance (Table 1.3). This assessment tool takes only minutes to administer and is more specific than the New York Heart Association Functional Class Scale. For patients who have maintained high

Table 1.2 Summary of Criteria for Specific Activity Scale Classifications

Class I	Patient can perform to completion any activity requiring more than 7 METs
Class II	Patient can perform to completion any activity requiring more than 5 METs but cannot or does not perform to completion activities requiring more than 7 METs
Class III	Patient can perform to completion any activity requiring more than 2 METs but cannot or does not perform to completion any activities requiring more than 5 METs
Class IV	Patient cannot or does not perform to completion activities requiring more than 2 METs

Note. From ''Comparative Reproducibility and Validity of Systems for Assessing Cardiovascular Functional Class: Advantages of a New Specific Activity Scale'' by L. Goldman, B. Hashimoto, F. Cook, and A. Loscalzo, 1981, *Circulation, 64*(6), pp. 1228, 1229. Copyright 1981 by the American Heart Association, Inc. Reprinted by permission of the American Heart Association, Inc.

levels of function prior to their cardiac events, you can use an adaptation of Katch and McArdle's tables (Katch & McArdle, 1988) for energy expenditure of many usual activities to help determine maximal functional ability.

These tables are particularly useful because energy expenditures for the activities are adjusted to body weight. Note how active the patient was in her current or anticipated daily work responsibilities. Often a worker can expend considerable calories during the day, yet therapists often do not regard this as productive activity. The most important concern is the calories used per day, regardless of how they are expended.

In the event that the patient has survived a long, complicated hospitalization resulting in significant weight loss, muscle wasting, altered nutrition, and neuromuscular dysfunction, her current level of function can be accurately described. The Index of Daily Living by Katz, Ford, Moskowitz, Jackson, and Jaffe (1963) is a useful measure of the patient's degree of functional disability or independence and will provide baseline data from which eventual progress can be measured (Table 1.4).

Also, you may document occupation, usual or unusual work requirements, exposure to hazardous environments, and any other physical stresses that may be imposed on the patient on a regular basis.

Musculoskeletal Limitations

A history of musculoskeletal limitations is assessed using the chart and the interview with the patient; limitations may include a prior back injury, limiting arthritis, neuropathies, old fractures, or muscular imbalances that may limit the patient's mobility. In addition, investigate for any evidence of neurological disorders, previous stroke, transient ischemic events, neuropathies, or myopathies. Note whether the patient uses assistive or orthopedic devices such as a cane, a walker, custom shoes, or artificial limbs, and describe the device. These adjunctive devices must be available for inpatient rehabilitation efforts. Even if the patient has been using a device for some time, he should demonstrate competency in its use before rehabilitation sessions begin. Nearly all people will develop energy-efficient methods for transfers and for application of even the most unwieldy equipment, such as an above-the-knee prosthesis. Allowing the patient to develop his own methods often allows for the least taxation of the cardiovascular system.

Physical Examination

A valuable and frequently overlooked component in the initial evaluation is the physical examination. This provides physical contact, which is a useful tool to both you and the patient. If the initial consultation is limited to just a verbal interview, you can miss much information. Physical contact during a physical examination reveals subtle information about the patient, and the patient also learns something about you. This goes a long way toward developing a mutual trust, which can make the patient more relaxed and comfortable. The physical examination need only involve those areas that will be affected by the patient's exercise therapy. This is an excellent opportunity for you to reassure the patient and to demonstrate respect and competence. Unfortunately, many rehabilitation specialists do not possess skills or do not trust their skills for providing a thorough cardiovascular, pulmonary, and musculoskeletal physical examination.

The physical examination, when conducted by an experienced examiner, takes very little time. Often, many functions can be performed at the

Table 1.3 Criteria for Determination of the Specific Activity Scale Functional Class

	Yes/ A,B, or C	No		Yes/ A,B, or C	No
1. Can you walk down a flight of steps without stopping (4.5-5.2 METs)?	Go to #2	Go to #4	(c) do recreational activities such as skiing, basketball, touch football, squash, handball (7-10 METs); or		
2. Can you carry anything up a flight of eight steps without stopping (5-5.5 METs)? Or can you	Go to #3	Class III	(d) jog/walk 5 mph (9 METs)?		
(a) have sexual intercourse without stopping (5-5.5 METs);			4. Can you shower without stopping (3.6-4.2 METs)? Or can you	Class III	Go to #5
(b) garden, rake, weed (5.6 METs);			(a) strip and make a bed (3.9-5 METs);		
(c) roller skate, fox-trot (5-6 METs); or			(b) mop floors (4.2 METs);		
(d) walk at a 4-mph rate on level ground (5-6 METs)?			(c) hang washed clothes (4.4 METs);		
3. Can you carry at least 24 lb up eight steps (10 METs)? Or can you	Class I	Class III	(d) clean windows (3.7 METs); (e) walk 2.5 mph (3-3.5 METs);		
(a) carry objects that are at least 80 lb (8 METs);			(f) bowl (3-4.4 METs); (g) play golf (walk and carry clubs) (4.5 METs); or		
(b) do outdoor work—shovel snow, spade soil (7 METs);			(h) push a power lawn mower (4 METs)?		
			5. Can you dress without stopping because of symptoms (2-2.3 METs)?	Class III	Class IV

Note. From "Comparative Reproducibility and Validity of Systems for Assessing Cardiovascular Functional Class: Advantages of a New Specific Activity Scale" by L. Goldman, B. Hashimoto, F. Cook, and A. Loscalzo, 1981, *Circulation*, **64**(6), pp. 1228, 1229. Copyright 1981 by the American Heart Association, Inc. Reprinted by permission of the American Heart Association, Inc.

same time. The physical exam can begin with a documentation of height, weight, vital signs, and body habitus. You can learn much by simply observing the patient reposition from lying to sitting and, if possible, walking. Note coordination, use of accessory muscles, unusual movement, or dyskinesis and study alignment of the arms and legs, the positioning of body parts, and posture. For the more limited patient, you can learn much of the patient's overall strength and balance by assisting her from lying to sitting or sitting to standing positions and with simple muscle strength testing. Document any problems with movement, obvious deformity of joints, or joint crepitation.

Many excellent textbooks on physical examination are currently available. These can be supplemented by training audiovisuals and by practice.

Cardiovascular Examination

During the cardiovascular exam, mentally note skin color, turgor, temperature, superficial veins, and any ulcerations and examine the lower extremities for hair loss and skin discoloration that may indicate poor circulation. Briefly assess the peripheral pulses, noting the pulse character and obvious jugular vein distension. Describe any peripheral edema and poor range of motion of the extremities that become obvious as the patient moves from position to position. Measure blood pressure in both arms; note the higher reading and use the corresponding extremity thereafter during all exercise measurements. The initial examination in the inpatient program should include an orthostatic blood pressure check as the patient moves from lying to sitting and sitting to standing. If you are experienced, you may be comfortable

Table 1.4 Index of Independence in Activities of Daily Living

A. Independent in feeding, continence, transferring, going to the toilet, dressing, and bathing

B. Independent in all but one of these functions

C. Independent in all but bathing and one additional function

D. Independent in all but bathing, dressing, and one additional function

E. Independent in all but bathing, dressing, going to the toilet, and additional function

F. Independent in all but bathing, dressing, going to the toilet, transferring, and one additional function

G. Dependent in all six functions

Other—Dependent in at least two functions, but not classifiable as C, D, E, or F

Note. This index is based on an evaluation of the functional independence or dependence of patients in bathing, dressing, going to the toilet, transferring, continence, and feeding. *Independence* means without supervision, direction, or active personal assistance. This is based on actual status and not on ability. A patient who refuses to perform a function is considered as not performing the function even if he or she is deemed able.

From "Studies of Illness in the Aged" by S. Katz et al., 1963, *Journal of the American Medical Association,* **185**(12), p. 915. Copyright 1963 by the American Medical Association. Reprinted by permission.

auscultating the heart for rate, rhythm, murmurs, S_3-S_4, and extra sounds. These parameters can change in character with exercise, especially in patients with poorly controlled congestive heart failure.

Pulmonary Examination

Next is the assessment of the pulmonary system. Examine lips and nails for cyanoses and lips for pursed lip breathing and observe the chest for obvious deformities such as kyphosis or scoliosis. Assess the patient's normal breathing pattern, noting the use of accessory muscles, the respiratory rate, and general comfort of breathing. Systematically evaluate breath sounds while the patient sits in the erect position, and note inspiratory and expiratory quality and any adventitious sounds, such as rales, rhonchi, wheezes, or friction rubs. For post–coronary artery bypass graft patients, crepitation should be assessed, because this indicates there is air in the subcutaneous tissue, which sometimes occurs from a rupture somewhere in the respiratory system.

Conclusion of Initial Consultation

Determine the patient's overall physical status by listening and examining. These skills provide valuable information you can use to anticipate the patient's responses to progressive exercise therapy. For example, be sensitive to orthostatic blood pressure responses, development of rales with exercise, an increase in the severity of rales, and changes in peripheral vascular status such as skin color and temperature. This information can be important to other consulting services and to physicians as well. The results of a thorough initial physical examination of an uncomplicated patient may be useful, but for a highly compromised, debilitated patient, these details are vital to the optimal response to therapy.

The documentation of the initial consult can be a summarized account of relevant findings of the chart review, patient interview, and physical examination. This information must then be integrated into the development of a unique plan based on these findings, a plan that includes diet modifications, activity plan, and special care or necessity for assistive devices. Also important is a brief objective for patient education, based on the patient needs, education level, and specific disease process. In order to ensure a joint effort, discuss the plan with the patient and adjust it as necessary.

Much of the initial consult will be a review of available patient data. You should emphasize the patient's prior functional capabilities and limitations based on exercise habits, activity habits, and predicted MET capacity. The cardiac rehabilitation evaluation should ultimately focus and reflect on the patient's prior, current, and anticipated future functional abilities and limitations and any potential barriers to the patient's progress.

In addition, there must be a thorough analysis of risk factors. Note patient attempts at modifying behavior and compliance with medical regimes and describe a brief risk factor intervention plan focusing on one risk.

You can develop many of the physical assessment skills based on some prior knowledge and some coaching from other professionals in the facility. Doctors, nurse specialists, physical therapists, exercise physiologists, and others possess unique abilities that are indispensable for a thorough rehabilitation examination. Most professionals are anxious to share their crafts and only need to be asked.

Risk Factor Evaluation

In the inpatient program, a realistic approach to risk factor modification becomes critically important. Overzealous goal setting can be alienating and detrimental to long-term compliance. To avoid overwhelming the patient, education efforts should focus on identification of one major risk factor that the patient is interested in modifying. These efforts must be preceded by at least a cursory evaluation of the patient's capacity to learn and interpret information. The risk factor evaluation is not only a cognitive evaluation but must also take into consideration patient learning readiness based on the patient's response to the ongoing disease process and hospitalization. With this assessment in hand, you are better able to integrate learning requirements into the patient's life.

The Therapist and Therapeutic Behavior

Your best resource, in addition to specialized exercise and education skills, is a broad-based knowledge that must include cardiology, cardiovascular surgery, pharmacology, exercise physiology, nutrition, health education, motivation techniques, psychology, nursing, physical therapy, and much more. Although you are required to be knowledgeable in all these areas, it is also vital that you are up-to-date in all the current invasive cardiology techniques, surgical practices, medical news (especially regarding cardiovascular disease), diet therapies, and any popular nonmedical remedies. Armed with this foundation of knowledge, you need to have adequate time to conduct the consultation, in order to create an environment that allows the patient to solicit the necessary information. Physicians, nurses, and other professionals are in and out of the examination rooms quickly, but you will have a distinct advantage if you spend time with your patients. This approach allows you to get to know the real patient—perhaps better than any of the other health service providers can. Time, or perhaps the lack of time urgency, can give you that window of opportunity to intercede in the patient's recovery. It also allows the patient to receive potent physical rehabilitation from someone who has a sound understanding of the disease and of the requirements for self-care and return to normal activity after discharge.

In addition to the chart review and physical exam, accurate assessments of functional status and degree of disability can be useful and unique

tools for you, as well as for other consulting services. By combining a tailored and creative progressive activity program with concise methods of documentation, risk factor modification, and learning needs assessment, you can provide a specialized service.

Exercise Therapy

Progressive exercise of the patient during hospitalization can best be accomplished by individual case management. The stepped or level inpatient rehabilitation systems used in the past cannot meet the diverse needs of patients now seen in many rehabilitation programs. Range-of-motion exercises, stretching exercises, endurance activities, and low-weight/high-repetition resistance exercises and stair climbing are important tools with which to manage the patient's individual requirements. You can best prescribe these exercises using the parameters of intensity, duration, mode, and frequency. Most patients following bypass surgery do not need range-of-motion or stretching exercises. Encourage these patients to return to hygiene, grooming, and other normal daily activities and direct endurance training using progressive ambulation and stair climbing. However, the deconditioned patient, following a long hospitalization, may require assisted range-of-motion exercises and may eventually advance to upper extremity resistance exercises, even while the patient is still maintained on a ventilator. The different therapies and exercises available to you should not be routinely applied to all patients but should be considered as tools to be selectively used when most appropriate. Creativity provides a distinct advantage for problem solving in the inpatient environment.

Frequency, Intensity, and Duration

Just as the different exercises can be applied depending upon the individual needs of the patient, so can frequency, intensity, and duration of exercise be applied. For some patients who are intolerant of exercise for reasons such as respiratory insufficiency, significant claudication, or congestive heart failure, a low-intensity/short-duration/high-frequency program may be most appropriate. For example, if the patient is able to walk independently, the prescription may be to ambulate 25 to 75 ft six to eight times per day as tolerated, at a speed less than or equivalent to 1.0 mph to avoid symptoms or distress. Or, the patient who essentially has no limitations, such as someone who has experienced an uncomplicated subendocardial myocardial infarction, may progress to exercising once a day for 20 min at the equivalent of 3.0 to 3.5 mph on a level grade to avoid symptoms or to reach a Borg Scale Rating of Perceived Exertion of 11 or 12 (see Table 1.5).

My colleagues and I have found step boxes and stair climbing to be beneficial with many patients, particularly very deconditioned patients, because stairs represent a major barrier to a patient's return to normal activities once discharged. A step box can be left in the patient's room; following education and demonstrated competency, the patient can begin to use the step box on her own. Also useful for a deconditioned patient, after the patient is screened for safety, are dynamic resistive exercises. Do not overlook upper body strength, necessary for resuming activities of daily living independently, in the inpatient setting. Introduce light resistance training early in rehabilitation. Starting with 1- to 2-lb weights and 5 to 10 repetitions, the patient can safely exercise most muscle groups of the upper body while in the sitting position. It is best for markedly deconditioned patients to work each muscle group individually and

Table 1.5 Ratings of Perceived Exertion (RPE)

Original RPE		New rating scale	
6		0	Nothing at all
7	Very, very light	0.5	Very, very weak
8		1	Very weak
9	Very light	2	Weak
10		3	Moderate
11	Fairly light	4	Somewhat strong
12		5	Strong
13	Somewhat hard	6	
14		7	Very strong
15	Hard	8	
16		9	
17	Very hard	10	Very, very strong
18			
19	Very, very hard		
20		•	Maximal

Note. The original RPE scale and the revised ratio scale may be used in exercise testing or exercise programs.

From "Psychophysical Basis of Perceived Exertion," by G.V. Borg, 1982, Medicine and Science in Sports and Exercise, 14, pp. 377-387. Copyright 1982 by American College of Sports Medicine. Reprinted by permission.

observe adequate rest periods. These exercises can be progressed and continued until the patient has a satisfactory result, or the exercises can be continued by the patient after discharge.

The duration of stay for uncomplicated bypass surgery patients and myocardial infarction patients is, for many institutions, between 6 and 8 days. This allows very little opportunity to provide all the education that was once thought important, so you will have to judge what is most important. Teaching pulse taking may unnecessarily focus the patient's attention on one skill, for example; it may be best to focus on return to activity based on symptoms rather than on heart rate parameters.

Before inpatient exercises can begin the patient must have the basic equipment. Many types of footwear, especially slippers, can affect both balance and gait, presenting a major barrier to effective progressive exercise, and may even contribute to falls. Evaluate footwear early to ensure availability of a stable, comfortable, well-fitting model with a heel counter.

Respiratory Exercises

Equally vital to many patients' rehabilitation efforts are respiratory exercises. You should have these skills and should know how to use incentive spirometry equipment used at your facility. These exercises are often initiated by the respiratory therapist, but you can conduct follow-up, observation, and skill improvement. Both professionals should teach similar technique. For patients recovering from open heart surgery, spirometry is an important part of the recovery process. In addition, you should be able to teach coughing to clear congestion, splinting of the sternum, and deep-breathing techniques. Chest auscultation becomes a valuable tool in assessing the success of chest physiotherapy or degree of respiratory insufficiency. A dyspnea grading system (Table 1.6) is a good tool for charting select patients' tolerances for rehabilitation efforts. Such a system provides another concise method of clearly documenting cardiorespiratory response and changes in response to progressive exercise. Changes in dyspnea grade can effectively alter both rehabilitation and medical therapeutics.

Getting Out of Bed

Often overlooked, but important, is the effort by the patient to move from bed to chair and assume the upright position with head up and feet down in a nonrecumbent, gravity-dependent position.

Table 1.6 Dyspnea Grades

Grade I:	Patient is normal; dyspnea occurs after unusual exertion.
Grade II:	Patient becomes breathless after going up hills or stairs.
Grade III:	Patient becomes breathless walking at normal speed on level ground.
Grade IV:	Simple activities cause breathlessness (e.g., shaving and dressing).

This activity is vital for the patient's recovery. It can delay the progressive effects of prolonged bed rest and works wonders for patient self-confidence. Chair sitting was one of the first inpatient rehabilitation therapies and has an important place today. At first, sitting in a chair for brief intervals of 10 to 30 min frequently during the day (four to five times) is recommended. Each successive day, as the patient improves, the duration is increased and frequency decreased at the patient's discretion. More is not better, so discourage long exhausting periods in the chair early in the recovery period. Chair sitting, some simple sitting exercises, and transferring from bed to chair begin to make the patient a part of the rehabilitation process.

Control of Discomfort

Encourage the patient to use prophylactic pain medications following surgery—that is, before the onset of pain, so the patient can breathe fully and deeply and move without the limiting effects of pain. You should make the patient as comfortable as possible; encourage him to use the nursing and adjunct staff to meet his personal needs. So much attention is given to progressive activity—in addition to the many tests and physician, nurse, and family visits—that the restorative therapy of rest becomes overlooked and is in short supply in the hospital. Uninterrupted sleep for several hours sometimes is the best exercise for the day. Again, more exercise is not necessarily better as the patient is healing. You and the patient must undertake the difficult task of balancing rest and activity to accomplish positive outcomes. Inquire daily if the patient is getting adequate sleep during the night, and encourage him to use sleeping medications or pain medications to accomplish a good night's rest. Furthermore, question the patient regularly as to the quality of his appetite, nutrition in the hospital, and pain relief. If the patient

is exhausted, tired, or in pain, the best therapy may be pain medication, several hours of rest, and postponement of exercise.

It is beneficial to routinely incorporate the patient in all progression of activity. The patient is a valuable member of the rehabilitation process, and optimal progression cannot be achieved without her involvement. She should know the whys and wherefores of the procedures that you apply. Every day, give the patient activity or exercise guidelines in addition to progressive ambulation.

A major challenge for you is to make the patient feel confident in her abilities to resume normal activities soon after discharge and to continue them in the future. Patients learn much from the confidence and optimism you display in reassuring them and progressing their activity. Avoid setting unnecessary limitations, making too many rules, or showing excessive concern about overactivity as the patient anticipates discharge. In general, patients do too little after discharge rather than too much. Your objective is to help the patient gain a balance between rest and activity, so she can progressively and safely increase activity and exercise at home to best promote healing and recovery as well as return to normal activities with a balanced, healthy, and optimistic attitude.

Rehabilitating Select Patient Groups

The initiation of cardiac rehabilitation in the hospital following uncomplicated myocardial infarction or coronary artery bypass surgery is routine at most centers. As the acceptance of rehabilitation has grown, the accomplishments of emergency, cardiovascular, and intensive care medicine have produced many interesting subgroups of cardiac patients. During the last 20 or 30 year period we have seen modern cardiology continue to test the limits of the human body—both its vulnerability as well as its strength and endurance. People who work with and study these patients have generated some useful information and caveats unique to their rehabilitation. The following section is a brief review of some background and recommendations for practice that you may incorporate in the care of these interesting patients.

Surgery for Left Ventricular Aneurysm

For hospitals with large open heart surgery programs, the percentage of procedures that include aneurysmectomy of the ventricle remains relatively small. However, the development of a left ventricular aneurysm is a common complication following acute myocardial infarction, with a possible incidence as high as 38% (Cosgrove et al., 1978). The long-term function of patients with symptomatic postinfarction left ventricular aneurysm can be improved by surgical treatment depending largely on preoperative left ventricular function (Buton, Stinson, Oyer, & Shumway, 1979). Surgery is accomplished with relatively low risk, and improved tolerance for activity can be expected, but the reasons for these changes are not well understood. The patient's subjective improvement is apparently not due to any substantial change in global left ventricular function. Removal of dyskinetic noncontractile scar of the left ventricle and revascularization appear to be the best combination to produce an increase of work tolerance for many of these patients. This is often associated with a corresponding improvement in New York Heart Association Functional Classification and measurable exercise capacity (Taylor et al., 1985).

A ventricular aneurysm can be defined as a noncontractile bulging of the ventricular wall. The paradoxical movement of the aneurysm during systole, called dyskinesis, becomes an important part of the changed myocardial hemodynamics. Almost all ventricular aneurysms originate in coronary artery disease and subsequent infarction. The overwhelming majority of aneurysms occur in the left ventricle's free anterior wall but are also known to occur laterally and less frequently posteriorly. Surgical repair of the postinfarction left ventricular aneurysm ideally is performed several months after injury in order to establish a healthy fibrous scar. Surgery involves excision or plication of moderate to even large areas of fibrous scar from the ventricular wall. After the scar is incised, the organized thrombus, which is found in most of the aneurysms, is carefully removed and the heart thoroughly inspected before repair and remodeling are accomplished. The left ventricular chamber size can be significantly reduced and function effectively improved, providing the remainder of the myocardium is viable.

During inpatient rehabilitation most of these patients can be progressed in a manner similar to that used for coronary artery bypass graft surgery patients. In a retrospective study of 22 patients following left ventricular aneurysm resection, we were able to show apparent differences in the type or frequency of these patients' complications when compared to other surgical cardiac rehabilitation patients (Wood, Crosby, Paternostro-Bayles, & Ab-

bott, 1986). More than 100 days of progressive activity among these patients revealed just four incidents, which occurred during an exercise session. None of these required emergency care. The average length of stay was 11 days, and the majority of the patients were discharged 8 or 9 days after surgery. Neither the surgical procedure nor the length of time after the myocardial infarction distinguished the likelihood for postsurgical, medical, or exercise problems. The only preoperative indication of complications after surgery was congestive heart failure with coexistent angina. Therefore, left ventricular aneurysm resection by itself was not a predictor of exercise complications during the early postoperative period. As with most surgical patients, concomitant medical and surgical problems differentiate the uncomplicated postoperative course and optimum functional improvement from the complicated cases with little or unpredictable improvement.

There is little reason to be concerned about disruption of the primary surgical repair, and such a concern by itself should not be a cause for limiting activities. Use the same precautions as applied to coronary artery bypass graft patients. Progress exercise by increasing the intensity and duration of walking, and use low-weight, high-repetition upper body exercises for this group. Most patients who require left ventricular aneurysm resection have in recent months sharply decreased activities secondary to their physicians' advice and symptomatic limitations. Therefore, early implementation of a total-body conditioning program appears most warranted and beneficial in this group.

Atrial Fibrillation (With a Rapid Ventricular Response)

Supraventricular tachyarrhythmias are a frequent and common complication following coronary artery bypass grafting (CABG), occurring in almost one third of the cases (Crosby, Woll, Wood, & Pifalo, 1990). Following myocardial infarction, supraventricular tachyarrhythmias and primarily atrial fibrillation usually occur in the first 72 hr, and most occur in the first 24 hr, after the initial insult (Hod et al., 1987). The recurrence of atrial fibrillation with a rapid ventricular response following its resolution is unpredictable, but the incidence is greatly reduced after pharmacological cardioversion. There are no useful predictors for the development of atrial fibrillation after myocardial infarction other than the patient's age and possibly the hemodynamics of the left atrium based on atrial dimensions and pressures.

Interestingly, unlike myocardial infarction, atrial fibrillation following CABG rarely occurs within the first 24 hr and usually occurs 48 to 72 hr later with a precipitous drop in incidence thereafter (Crosby, Woll, et al., 1990). This phenomenon may differentiate the causes of atrial fibrillation in this setting.

Risk factor profiles for the development of atrial fibrillation after surgery have been attempted without success. Again, age is the most reliable predictor. Therefore, the older the patient the more likely he is to have atrial fibrillation following coronary artery bypass surgery. The precise cause of atrial fibrillation in this setting is not known, although ischemia is thought to be contributory (Tchervenkov et al., 1983). We have shown that even in the most complicated courses following bypass surgery, the incidence of atrial fibrillation is not necessarily increased (Crosby, Pifalo, Woll, & Burkholder, 1990). Cases of symptomatic postoperative pericarditis, reexploration, and perioperative myocardial infarction did not increase the incidence of these dysrhythmias. Also, it is now well established that total aortic cross-clamp time, the number of bypasses, creatine kinase levels, anemia, and beta blocker withdrawal do not contribute to atrial fibrillation after surgery (Crosby, Pifalo, et al., 1990).

The predominant form of a resting heart rate greater than 120 bpm found in the inpatient program at Allegheny General Hospital is atrial fibrillation with a rapid ventricular response. Rapid atrial fibrillation in patients without previous histories of the rhythm is frequently self-terminating or is pharmacologically cardioverted, or the ventricular rate is controlled. Electrical D/C cardioversion, especially following open heart surgery, is usually unnecessary.

In a prospective study of 249 patients following elective coronary artery bypass graft surgery, we were not able to demonstrate a relationship between any activity, either by the patient or attending medical personnel, and the onset of supraventricular tachyarrhythmias (Crosby, Woll, et al., 1990). Numerous activities were evaluated, including coughing, transfer, chest physiotherapy, walking, exercise therapy, and back rest position at the time of onset. Any association between these arrhythmias and patient or staff activities appears to be coincidental. Apparently the efforts of the nurse or rehabilitation personnel do not cause or even contribute to the onset of these dysrhythmias.

In many hospitals, D/C cardioversion is used only after several days of unsuccessful drug trials or if the rhythm is poorly tolerated by the patient. Other than the sensation of palpitations, most patients with well-preserved left ventricular function will not demonstrate any symptomatic intolerance with these rhythms. Heart rates for inpatient exercise are usually limited to below 120 bpm. However, in this group allowances can be made if the patient is asymptomatic and has a stable blood pressure. The heart rate may be elevated, but stroke work and stroke volume should remain low, and cardiac output and $\dot{V}O_2$max are at near-normal resting values. With this in mind, you may allow heart rates to fluctuate to 130 bpm without limiting the patient's progress. After the ventricular rate is controlled the patient should resume normal activities, and progressive exercise may safely begin 24 hr later. There appears to be no reason to withhold activity or exercise after these rhythms are under control and the patient is without symptoms.

Postoperative Anemia

Routine coronary artery bypass surgery imposes tremendous physiological trauma, from which most patients take several months to fully recover. In addition to repairing bone and tissue, the body must replace a considerable amount of red blood cells. The average hemoglobin of patients on Day 3 after open heart surgery at Allegheny General Hospital is less than 10 gm/dl. Blood transfusion is not routine and is performed only when the patient's symptoms appear related to postoperative anemia. Many patients are discharged without problems, though their hemoglobin levels are as low as 7.5 gm/dl.

Following surgery, anemia is usually isovolemic, with a reduction of more than one third of the circulating red blood cells. This type of anemia causes a decrease in blood viscosity and peripheral resistance. In addition, there is an increased need for oxygen delivery to the tissues to compensate for the lowered oxygen-carrying capacity of the blood. This results in a metabolically induced dilation, which further lowers peripheral vascular resistance (Grossman & Braunwald, 1984). All the mechanisms for the total reduction in cardiovascular pressures with anemia have not yet been explained. Acutely induced anemias reduce the coronary vascular resistance whereas chronic anemias may enhance the growth of coronary collateral circulation (Grossman & Braunwald, 1984).

Symptoms may not develop in otherwise normal patients with mild or moderate anemia during usual hospital activity. Measurements of resting cardiac output do not often significantly change until the hemoglobin reaches 7 to 9 gm/dl. However, studies do show that hemoglobin is an important factor affecting oxygen delivery and exercise capacity, particularly at peak exercise (Woodson, 1984).

The primary symptoms of fatigue and exertional dyspnea will depend on the severity of the anemia and the presence of an underlying cardiovascular disease. In the presence of cardiovascular disease, anemia can lower the threshold of angina. Other factors that may affect the patient's symptomatic response to acute anemia are how fast the anemia developed and the patient's prior physical condition.

If anemia develops gradually and is longstanding, patients can tolerate levels as low as 7 gm/dl and compensate enough to meet most daily physical requirements. Although uncommon, congestive heart failure with pulmonary edema in the absence of heart disease can occur with extremely severe anemia (Rosenthal, Handin, & Braunwald, 1984).

There is the possibility that anemia may inhibit tissue healing, although this has been difficult to validate experimentally. Prolonged, low-tissue oxygen tension does impair healing significantly (Collins, 1986). However, adequate tissue perfusion does seem more important than the oxygen-carrying capacity of blood for normal healing. Hemorrhage or anemia alone may not alter tissue oxygen tension, but elevated blood viscosity can have profound effects on local oxygen tension (Collins, 1986).

The effects of mild to moderate anemia on exercise tolerance and hemodynamics have been clearly demonstrated in nonanemic subjects who are made anemic (Woodson, 1984). In this study, hemoglobin was reduced while isovolemia was maintained. Results showed that with an acute reduction in hemoglobin from 14.8 to 10.4 gm/dl, maximal oxygen consumption does fall, despite an increase in cardiac output at maximal exercise. In this study the increase in maximal cardiac output was due to an increase in stroke volume; heart rate remained essentially unchanged. The study shows that reduction in $\dot{V}O_2$max with acute anemia causes a drop of blood oxygen-carrying capacity, which is partially compensated by the increase in cardiac output. When hemoglobin is reduced, there is a roughly proportional reduction in $\dot{V}O_2$max and exercise capacity. Typically, people compensate for anemia during submaximal exercises with relative increases in cardiac output, heart rate, and ventilation rate. At low intensities, moderate increases in work load are well tolerated as shown by increased cardiac output (Woodson, 1984). All signs and symptoms usually disappear when the hemoglobin concentration is restored to normal.

Isovolemic patients with low hemoglobin/hematocrit levels should be progressed symptomatically. Anemia can be well tolerated without a disruption in the patient's course, especially postcoronary artery bypass grafting. The inpatient's activity levels are relatively light, ranging from 1.5 to 3.5 METs, and in most cases when hemoglobin is 10 gm/dl or more, the patient is asymptomatic. Patients are seen with hemoglobin from 5 to 7 gm/dl due to religious practices; such patients are often pale, dusky, and tachycardic at rest. They can have relatively uncomplicated postoperative courses and resume normal activities, although at slower than usual rates. The major concerns for the clinician are the assessment and maintenance of isovolemia and the patient's symptomatic response to progressive activity. Orthostatic blood pressure evaluations are important in these patients, as are observations for heart rate response, skin color and temperature, and significant peripheral vasoconstriction during activity.

Right Ventricular Infarction

Right ventricular infarction is a frequent and significant complication of acute inferior and posterior myocardial infarction of the left ventricle. The hemodynamic consequences of acute myocardial infarction largely depend on the extent of left ventricular involvement. In as many as one-third of acute inferior myocardial infarctions there is a significant right ventricular involvement that may affect the patient's clinical course and treatment during the initial hospitalization (Isner & Roberts, 1978). This pathologic phenomenon has generated interest in establishing diagnostic criteria using invasive, noninvasive, and bedside techniques for early recognition of significant right ventricular injury.

Initial complications associated with right ventricular infarction include high incidences of atrioventricular blocks, hypertension, complex ventricular dysrhythmias, and cardiogenic shock. In spite of these problems, short-term prognosis may not differ from prognosis for left ventricular involvement alone (Cohn, Guiha, Broder, & Limas, 1974). Right ventricular ejection fractions that are acutely depressed can return to near normal as early as 3 weeks later.

Relationships have been demonstrated between acute inferior myocardial infarction complicated by a hemodynamically evident right ventricular involvement and a propensity to develop clinically important ventricular dysrhythmias experienced in late outpatient cardiac rehabilitation (Crosby, Paternostro-Bayles, Cottington, & Pifalo, 1989). These complications may result in more frequent referrals to physicians, more hospital admissions, and ultimately an increase in the use of medications, specifically nitrates, antiarrhythmics, and digitalis. These complications, however, and their outcomes do not appear to affect the right ventricular infarction patient's ability to safely make equivalent improvements in her overall functional capacity during treatment.

Patients with significant right ventricular involvement in acute myocardial infarction may have more complications, and you should take this into consideration during rehabilitation. However, most patients can be expected to return to a near normal functional capacity, even in the environment of hugely depressed right ventricular hemodynamics. Long term prognosis and activity restrictions should no doubt reflect the amount of left ventricular destruction and remaining myocardium at risk.

Cardiac Transplantation

The effects of exercise following orthotopic cardiac transplantation in the late postoperative period patient have been well described in the literature. In brief, the heart rate response to exercise is delayed in part because of the lack of cardiac innervation. The peak heart rate achieved in response to maximal effort is reduced, and this heart rate response remains essentially unchanged even years after transplantation. Resting heart rates are higher after transplantation than those of nontransplant subjects because of the higher intrinsic rate of the denervated sinoatrial node. Higher resting heart rates are seen in younger patients, and the resting heart rates appear to decrease as the patients age. There is a normal demand for peripheral blood flow at rest. The normal cardiac output is maintained with a resting tachycardia and a smaller stroke volume. During light exercise the Frank Starling mechanism can produce an increase in cardiac output substantial enough to meet peripheral requirements. However, during more vigorous activity, any further increase in cardiac output depends on circulating catecholamine-induced chronotropic and inotropic central responses.

A number of mechanisms interact to varying degrees to bring about the training effect in transplant patients. But, strengthening of peripheral muscles plays an important role in return to optimal function. You can achieve this by providing the healthy transplant recipient with a well-balanced rehabilitation program with strong emphasis on large-muscle training beginning early in her recovery.

Because of the relatively low work loads used in inpatient programs, the prolonged warm-up and cool-down periods recommended for the outpatient program are not necessary. A significantly increased heart rate cannot be anticipated at 2 to 3.5 METs. The transplanted heart can compensate by increasing the stroke volume with no increase in heart rate at no detriment to the patient. You can exercise these patients at light levels without seeing the predictable slow increase of heart rates and slow recovery response. Cardiac output will increase considerably with work load at all levels of exercise. Higher-than-normal filling pressures in nontransplant patients may produce symptoms of dyspnea, but interestingly, this is not necessarily the case in transplant patients (Hosenpud et al., 1989). Some studies report that reduced functional capacity may be more related to abnormal filling pressures than to restriction of exercise cardiac output. Inpatients should not reach these exercise-induced limitations.

An important consideration is donor/recipient heart and body size matching. A patient who receives a relatively small heart in proportion to her body size requires a higher resting heart rate and higher resting filling pressure to maintain the required cardiac output. Evidence supports the concept that patients who receive smaller hearts are excessively filled at rest and therefore have no cardiac reserve available in exercise (Hosenpud et al., 1989). The opposite may also be true: Patients who receive larger hearts may have additional cardiac reserve at rest. However, the size of the transplanted heart is not available to you, so you must progress exercise based on patient symptoms. The transplanted heart may remodel over time but does not appear to achieve a normal relation between ventricular volume and body size of the recipient. It is unclear whether persistently elevated resting heart rates play a role in altering heart size. Despite near-normal resting hemodynamics, most transplant patients will have a marked degree of exercise intolerance. This exercise intolerance is due to several factors that initially are related to postsurgical status and prolonged functional disability.

A long history of congestive heart failure with associated chronic elevation of blood norepinephrine concentrations at rest pretransplant will be a factor that contributes to the immediate posttransplant recovery. This state may alter the effect of circulating catecholamine function as a result of receptor desensitization or down regulation due to chronic hyperstimulation. A decreased clearance of circulatory catecholamines may further alter hemodynamics in the early postoperative period (Ganguly, 1989). Physical and psychological stressors for prolonged periods are associated with high levels of circulating catecholamine and chronic heart disease. In addition, the absence of contribution from the denervated heart can alter norepinephrine and epinephrine release. In summary, most of these patients will probably have modified responses to circulating catecholamines during exercise due to several factors. This in combination with a prolonged deconditioning will play an important role in the responses you observe immediately after transplantation.

Rest and exercise hemodynamics will be abnormal both early and late after transplantation in healthy heart transplant recipients. The etiology of these findings is uncertain and most likely multifactorial. Nevertheless, such patients have considerable cardiac reserve to allow for most inpatient activities and activities of daily living. Patients should resume activity as completely as possible and progress activity as quickly as tolerated, with prompt addition of low-weight, high-repetition resistance exercises early in their programs. High doses of prednisone may significantly alter wound healing by contributing to untoward sternal dehiscence, although this has not been described in the literature. Therefore, you should prohibit pushing, pulling, or heavy lifting during the first 3 to 6 months after surgery. Overemphasis on warm-up or cool-down early in the program causes the patient unnecessary concern and frustration regarding normal activities (warm-up and cool-down are important for heavy exercise, but most of these patients will not tolerate strenuous activity). Stair climbing should be incorporated into the program and is an important part of the home program, because managing stairs is a major barrier to many even in the late recovery period. During the early postoperative hospitalization, many transplant patients do surprisingly well and do not suffer the severe side effects of chronic steroid therapy. They enjoy the uplifting experience of markedly improved heart function and therefore feel vigorous and optimistic in the first several weeks.

Education

The role of patient education in the hospital environment remains vital. In fact, in many facilities education is the primary function of the cardiac rehabilitation staff. However, learning is a complicated and variable conundrum even in a controlled environment. In the uncontrolled setting of an acute care hospital, following a life-threatening event with a largely heterogeneous patient population, adult learning is a side effect rather than a viable pursuit. Nevertheless, education remains the major objective of many professionals in this field in spite of the lack of evidence that significant learning occurs here. I am concerned that adult education in the hospital is sometimes conducted to meet the teaching needs of the educator, as opposed to the immediate learning needs of the patient. I don't mean to imply that patient knowledge deficits aren't important or to question the intentions of professional staff, but I believe we must refocus inpatient education efforts.

The environment for education has changed as dramatically as the requirements for exercise therapy. The length of stay for most uncomplicated patients following myocardial infarction or coronary artery bypass surgery is as little as 5 to 8 days. For several of these days, the patient usually has little opportunity for contact with cardiac rehabilitation staff. The remaining days are punctuated with tests and physician and family visits, and are heavily weighted by a growing uncertainty of the future—both near and distant.

A thorough evaluation during the initial consult, as described earlier, can create a unique professional relationship as you examine the patient and inquire about his concerns. Exercise therapy further enhances the therapeutic relationship and provides you opportunities to meet some educational objectives. Most of the dialogue between you and the patient can remain general in nature and should focus on the patient's immediate well-being. You must decide on which specific educational goals you will focus and should make them brief. Direct risk-factor education and modification at one influential risk factor, or at the most two. Emphasizing several risk factors may be overwhelming even for a healthy individual and therefore counterproductive for the patient.

These limited efforts can be worthwhile if you are selective, concise, and, when necessary, definitive in what you say to the patient. This most certainly must be supplemented with high-quality printed information. Numerous high-quality patient education pamphlets and books are available that will meet many of the patient's individual needs. You can further enhance learning with adjunctive information, such as slides and videos, which are pertinent to your patient groups and the physician's personal recommendations. If you have one learning goal for the patient, it should be that the patient reads the written education material (once, if not twice) after she is discharged and calls with any questions or concerns.

We should be selective in our information sharing and cognizant of our overdependence on the many "dos and don'ts." Individualize your advice by making sure it applies. For example, why tell a patient to limit stair climbing to one flight per day, when the patient may never routinely encounter steps or may have to use steps three times per day? Be accommodating, specific, and above all patient.

Conclusion

Like most viable professions, cardiac rehabilitation has been in constant evolution since its inception. This change is due not just to new patient populations but also to the growing knowledge and skills of the practitioners. Time and experience have resulted in a greater respect for the services we provide, and concomitantly we are being entrusted with increasingly more challenging patient groups. This process is evident in inpatient and outpatient programs alike.

We must continue to ask questions, fine tune and expand our skills, and exchange ideas and methods. The practice of cardiac rehabilitation must become more uniform in its application by a skilled professional staff. As well as being educators, we must be the experts on the use of therapeutic exercise in an expanding number of chronic deconditioning diseases. This is no more evident than in the inpatient programs, where the list of absolute contraindications to exercise becomes shorter and shorter.

Further Reading

American Association of Cardiovascular and Pulmonary Rehabilitation. (1991). *Guidelines for cardiac rehabilitation programs*. Champaign, IL: Human Kinetics.

American College of Sports Medicine. (1988). *Resource manual for guidelines for exercise testing and prescription*. Philadelphia: Lea & Febiger.

American College of Sports Medicine. (1990). *Guidelines for exercise testing and prescription* (4th ed.). Philadelphia: Lea & Febiger.

Wenger, N.K. (1989). Rehabilitation of the patient with coronary heart disease. New information for improved care. *Postgraduate Medicine, 85*, 369-380.

References

Borg, G.V. (1982). Psychophysical basis of perceived exertion. *Medicine and Science in Sports and Exercise, 14*, 377-387.

Buton, N.A., Stinson, E.B., Oyer, P.E., & Shumway, N.E. (1979). Left ventricular aneurysm, preoperative risk factors and long-term postoperative results. *Journal of Thoracic and Cardiovascular Surgery, 77*(1), 65-73.

Cohn, J.N., Guiha, N.H., Broder, M.I., & Limas, C.J. (1974). Right ventricular infarction. *American Journal of Cardiology, 33*, 209-214.

Collins, J.A. (1986). Blood transfusions and disorders of surgical bleeding. In D.A. Sabiston (Ed.), *Textbook of surgery* (pp. 99-115). Philadelphia: Saunders.

Cosgrove, D.M., Loop, F.D., Irragawal, M.J., Groves, L.K., Taylor, P.C., & Golding, L.A. (1978). Determinants of long-term survival after ventricular aneurysmectomy. *Annals of Thoracic Surgery, 26*(4), 357-362.

Crosby, L.H., Paternostro-Bayles, M., Cottington, E., & Pifalo, W.B. (1989). Outpatient rehabilitation after right ventricular infarction. *Journal of Cardiopulmonary Rehabilitation, 7*, 286-291.

Crosby, L.H., Pifalo, W.B., Woll, K.R., & Burkholder, J.A. (1990). Risk factors for atrial fibrillation after coronary artery bypass surgery. *The American Journal of Cardiology, 66*, 1520-1522.

Crosby, L.H., Woll, K.R., Wood, K.L., & Pifalo, W.B. (1990). Effect of activity on supraventricular tachyarrhythmias after coronary artery bypass surgery. *Heart & Lung, 19*(6), 666-670.

Ganguly, P.K. (1989). Catecholamines and cardiovascular disorders: pathophysiologic considerations. *American Heart Journal, 118*(4), 868-872.

Goldman, L., Hashimoto, B., Cook, E., & Loscalzo, A. (1981). Comparative reproducibility and validity of systems for assessing cardiovascular functional class: Advantages of a new specific activity scale. *Circulation, 64*(6), 1227-1235.

Grossman, W., & Braunwald, E. (1984). High

cardiac output rates. In E. Braunwald (Ed.), *Heart disease—A textbook of cardiovascular medicine* (pp. 807-822). Philadelphia: Saunders.

Hod, H., Lew, A.S., Keltai, M., Cercek, B., Geft, I.L., Shah, P.K., & Ganz, W. (1987). Early atrial fibrillation during evolving myocardial infarction: A consequence of impaired left atrial perfusion. *Circulation, 75,* 146-150.

Hosenpud, J.D., Morton, M.J., Wilson, R.A., Pantely, G.A., Norman, D.J., Cobanogliu, M.A., & Starr, A. (1989). Abnormal exercise hemodynamics in cardiac allograft recipients one year after cardiac transplantation. *Circulation, 80,* 525-532.

Isner, J.M., & Roberts, W.C. (1978). Right ventricular infarction complicating left ventricular infarction secondary to coronary heart disease. *American Journal of Cardiology, 42,* 885-894.

Katch, F., & McArdle, W. (1988). *Nutrition, weight control, and exercise* (3rd ed.). Philadelphia: Lea & Febiger.

Katz, S., Ford, A.B., Moskowitz, R.W., Jackson, B.A., & Jaffe, M.W. (1963). Studies of illness in aged, the index of ADL: A standardized measure of biological and psychosocial function. *Journal of the American Medical Association, 185*(12), 914-919.

Rosenthal, D.S., Handin, R.I., & Braunwald, E. (1984). Hematologic-oncologic disorders and heart disease. In E. Braunwald (Ed.), *Heart disease: A textbook of cardiovascular medicine* (pp. 1676-1703). Philadelphia: Saunders.

Taylor, N.C., Barber, R., Crossland, P., Wraight, E.P., English, A.H., & Petch, M.C. (1985). Does left ventricular aneurysmectomy improve ventricular function in patients undergoing coronary bypass surgery? *British Heart Journal, 54,* 145-152.

Tchervenkov, C.I., Wynands, J.E., Symes, J.F., Malcolm, I.D., Dobell, A.R., & Morin, J.E. (1983). Persistent atrial activity during cardioplegic arrest: A possible factor in the etiology of post-operative supraventricular tachyarrhythmias. *Annals of Thoracic Surgery, 36,* 437-443.

Wood, K.L., Crosby, L.H., Paternostro-Bayles, M., & Abbott, R.A. (1986). Inpatient medical and exercise complications in left ventricular aneurysm resection patients. *Journal of Cardiopulmonary Rehabilitation, 6,* 433.

Woodson, R.D. (1984). Hemoglobin concentration and exercise capacity. *American Review of Respiratory Disease, 129*(Suppl. 2), 72-75.

Chapter 2

Early Outpatient Rehabilitation

Martha D. Livingston, RN, MS, MBA, FAACVPR

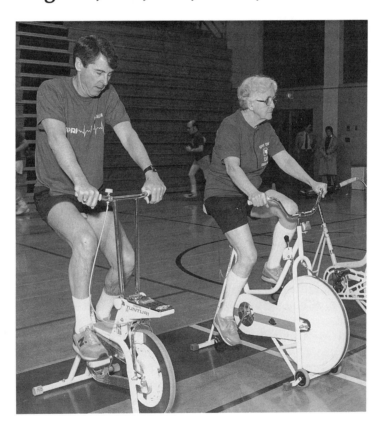

Much has been written about what cardiac rehabilitation can accomplish (Consolvo, 1990; Kallio, Hamalainen, Hakkila, & Luurila, 1979; O'Connor et al., 1989). However, to date, much of the education and behavior change efforts in Phase II cardiac rehabilitation programs have been applied as adjuncts during the exercise portion of the therapeutic regime.

This chapter explores current theory of behavior change, beginning with assessment of behaviors, measurement of behavior change through goal setting, and outcome data collection. This chapter parallels the AACVPR (1991) guidelines and establishes a plan for meeting these guidelines for education and behavior change.

Learning Objectives

1. To understand methods for evaluating health risk behaviors

2. To understand the components of a behavior change plan

3. To understand the mechanisms involved in maintaining new behaviors and managing lapse and relapse

4. To meet the objectives of the Joint Commission on Accreditation of Healthcare Organizations by measuring final outcomes and achievements in health risk behavior change

---

The clinical management of patients following acute coronary events has evolved significantly, from 4 to 8 weeks of bed rest and sedation to early ambulation, structured aerobic exercise, and resumption of normal activities. Traditionally, exercise therapy has been the core component of the early outpatient cardiac rehabilitation program. Typically, patients received 12 weeks of telemetry-monitored exercise therapy and educational information to modify cardiac risk factors.

Consolvo (1990) noted that comprehensive programming can produce substantial reductions in coronary heart disease. Earlier, Kallio et al. (1979) reported on a multifactorial intervention program among patients following myocardial infarction. The authors noted a reduction in deaths from coronary heart disease, although the rate of nonfatal myocardial infarctions rose. A reduction in body weight, blood lipid levels, and blood pressure values persisted for 3 years. O'Connor et al. (1989) found the odds ratios for cardiovascular-related deaths to be substantially lower in "exercise plus other interventions" trials than in "exercise only" trials.

Unfortunately, little effort has been made to accommodate individual needs based on the severity of illness, other coexisting medical problems, lifestyle preferences, and desired outcomes (Wenger, 1989). As a result of programs failing to address the individual, Wenger has advocated developing a delivery system for health care needs that embodies a patient care model—viewing the patient as an individual customer. Programs must be able to quickly incorporate new information that becomes available regarding how to slow or reverse the atherosclerotic process. Moreover, em-

phasis needs to be placed on helping participants integrate this information into lasting behavioral change (Wenger, 1989). Eliot (1988) noted that compliance is markedly improved when the plan of therapy is tailored to the patient's lifestyle.

This chapter is aimed at helping transform the traditional components of education and exercise into a well-targeted, individualized plan of care, the central aim of which is to achieve favorable long-term behavioral change.

The model used in this chapter (see Figure 2.1) has evolved from and complements a model recently put forth by the American Association of Cardiovascular and Pulmonary Rehabilitation (1991). The patient's objectives drive the entire model, dictating the type and level of education, counseling, and exercise therapy you will provide. The length of therapy in any one area is predicated on the outcomes achieved. You and the patient set goals and objectives after thoroughly analyzing the patient's risk factors. Education and behavior change counseling help enhance the patient's success in attaining the desired outcomes. Risk stratification is used to delineate appropriate surveillance parameters for exercise therapy.

Risk Assessment

Multiple factors impact the development and progression of coronary heart disease (American Heart Association [AHA], 1973; Truett, Cornfield, & Kannel, 1967). Thus, the objective assessment of risk factors can provide information that you need to plan an effective, well-targeted intervention program aimed at disease reduction. The as-

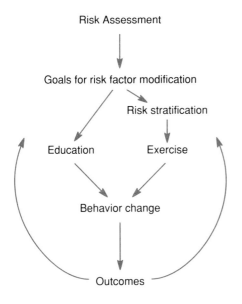

Figure 2.1 Model for early outpatient cardiac rehabilitation.
Note. Data from *Guidelines for Cardiac Rehabilitation Programs* by the American Association of Cardiovascular and Pulmonary Rehabilitation, 1991, Champaign, IL: Human Kinetics.

sessment should include controllable as well as uncontrollable risk factors. You should compare each data point to well-established parameters which, where appropriate, are age and sex specific. For example, total cholesterol as measured fasting equals 277 mg/dl compared to the National Cholesterol Education Program's normal risk level of 200 mg/dl. In addition to displaying the value, the data point should be weighted according to its role in promoting disease. Because several factors may be related to each other (Gotto, 1986), you may need to consider the values in these areas when you are assigning a risk ranking. Such a system can help the patient prioritize areas for change.

Dietary Patterns

Dietary patterns affect various risk factors—hypertension, hypercholesterolemia, obesity, hypertriglyceridemia, and diabetes (Grundy, 1990). As a result, you should evaluate the patient's total caloric intake; the percent of calories derived from fat, saturated fat, protein, and carbohydrates; and the amount of dietary cholesterol, sodium, and fiber consumed. Desirable values are outlined in The Expert Panel report (1988). You must interface data from other risk factors with certain dietary values when you are determining desirable values:

triglycerides with carbohydrates, ideal body weight with total caloric intake, low-density lipoprotein (LDL) and total cholesterol with percent of calories derived from total and saturated fat.

NUTRITION ANALYSIS SOFTWARE

Methods for evaluating dietary patterns range from a simple analysis of dietary preferences to more thorough, computer-scored 3- and 7-day dietary recalls. Generally, the computer analysis will yield more specific information. Analyze both typical and atypical eating patterns (e.g., weekdays vs. weekends). The most marked differences between software packages lie in the report format. Systems that support excellent graphics can serve as very important educational tools. (See Figure 2.2.)

Nutritional analysis programs are designed to analyze the nutrients in an individual's diet. The expense and complexity of these programs vary enormously. Some are inexpensive ($50) and can be used by lay people; others are quite costly ($2,500) but sophisticated enough to be used in the research setting. You should evaluate several aspects of the program:

1. How are foods entered? Must you look up codes in a manual, or can the food name be typed directly into the computer?
2. How big is the data base, and how many nutrients per item are analyzed? Some data bases carry only 500 foods; others several thousand. Many packages analyze a few basic nutrients (such as calories and protein), whereas others evaluate up to 30 separate nutrients.
3. How flexible is the software? Can you modify the data base to suit the program's needs? Is it easy to select food amounts? Can frequently eaten foods be added to the data base?
4. Is the documentation adequate? What graphics will the program produce?

Several nutritional analysis programs:

1. Diet and Exercise Analysis, EXERTEC Company, 3813 Griffin Lane, Harrisburg, PA 17110. $495
2. Michael Jacobson's Nutrition Wizard, CSPI, 1875 Connecticut Avenue NW, Suite 300, Washington, DC 20009. $99.95

3. Nutrition and Exercise Evaluation System, Institute for Aerobics Research, 12330 Preston Road, Dallas, TX 75230. $995
4. Nutritionist III, N-Squared Computing, 3040 Commercial Street SE, Suite 240, Salem, OR 97302. $1391

ate total cholesterol, HDL and LDL cholesterol, and triglyceride levels. For maximum accuracy, blood lipid levels should be drawn after a 12-hr fast, 8 to 10 weeks after the event, and not immediately following an exercise session. Newly established guidelines define low, intermediate, and high risk levels (Castelli, Abbott, & McNamara, 1983; Rifkind & Segal, 1983).

Blood Lipids

Elevated serum cholesterol has been firmly established as a major risk factor for coronary artery disease (Grundy, 1990; National Institute of Health, 1985; Reardon, Nestel, Craig, & Harper, 1985; Truett, Cornfield, & Kannel, 1967). Furthermore, low-density lipoprotein (LDL) and high-density lipoprotein (HDL) cholesterol each function independently in promoting disease progression; LDL is directly and HDL inversely related (Kannel, Castelli, & Gordon, 1979). You need to evalu-

Diabetes

The Framingham data (Kannel & McGee, 1979) identified the independent contribution of diabetes or an elevated fasting blood sugar to the development of coronary artery disease. In addition, glucose intolerance is linked to obesity and is associated with elevated triglyceride levels, hypertension, and elevated LDL and low HDL cholesterol values (Caspersen & Heath, 1988). You can screen for diabetes through the measurement of the fasting blood sugar.

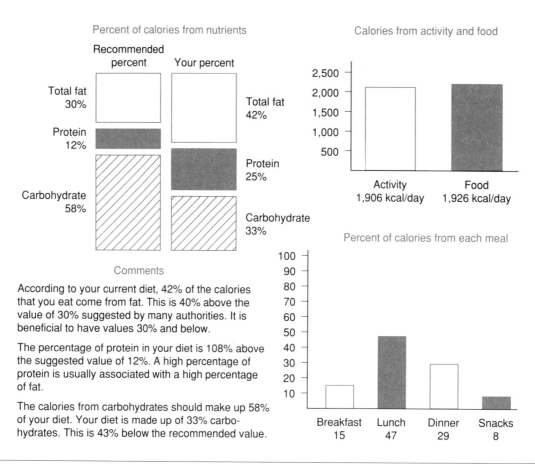

Figure 2.2 Sample graphics from a nutrition analysis software package.
Note. From The Exertec Company, 3813 Griffin Lane, Harrisburg, PA, 17110. Reprinted by permission.

Stress

Type A personality traits impact one's overall risk for the development of coronary artery disease (Haynes, Feinleib, & Kannel, 1980; Matthews & Haynes, 1986). Recently, research has analyzed several components of the Type A personality and has singled out hostility and anger as the emotions most strongly related to the development of disease (MacDowall, Dembroski, Dimsdale, & Hackett, 1985). Structured interviews tend to provide the most valid and reliable data for patient assessment. However, when such an interview is not practical, the Cook-Medley Hostility Scale (Cook & Medley, 1954) may be a useful screening tool for identifying individuals who may benefit from additional counseling.

Body Fat

Obesity refers to a body composition that has a disproportionate amount of fat. Generally, obesity results from a person's consuming more food calories than he expends through physical activity and exercise. Obesity has been linked to adult-onset diabetes, hypertension, and hypercholesterolemia. Hubert, Feinleib, McNamara, and Castelli (1983) reported obesity to be an independent risk factor for coronary artery disease.

Body composition can be determined through a variety of techniques. Although hydrostatic weighing is a more accurate method of assessment, the analysis of skin-fold measurements may be more practical and safer for a cardiac population. Jackson and Pollock (1978) and Jackson, Pollock, and Ward (1980) provided equations for estimating body density, body fat, and ideal body weight. In addition, it may be useful to calculate the body mass index (BMI) to determine the risk associated with the degree of excess weight. You can calculate the BMI by applying height and weight data to a formula or to a nomogram (Bray, 1983).

Smoking

The impact of cigarette smoking on cardiovascular and lung disease is irrefutable (Holbrook, Grundy, Hennekens, Kannel, & Strong, 1984). Moreover, the impact is dose dependent; the risk of disease increases as the number of cigarettes smoked per day rises. A similar dose relationship exists after the habit is terminated; the more cigarettes the person smoked before quitting, the more dramatic the

reduction of risk after the person quits. The benefit of smoking cessation is most pronounced 2 years after cessation when the risk for heart disease incurred by having been a smoker (twice that of non-smokers) returns to normal risk enjoyed by non-smokers (Rosenberg, Kaufman, Helmrich, & Shapiro, 1985). Thus, when predicting the impact of cigarette smoking, gather data regarding how much and for how long the patient smoked and the date of cessation.

Hypertension

The incidence of cardiovascular disease (coronary heart disease as well as stroke) increases incrementally as blood pressure rises. Moreover, the longer blood pressure remains elevated, the greater the risk (Joint National Committee on the Detection, Evaluation, and Treatment of High Blood Pressure, 1984). Kannel et al. (1979) found that individuals who remain hypertensive after a myocardial infarction are at increased risk over their normotensive counterparts for a repeat event or death. Elevated blood pressure is often found in conjunction with obesity, diabetes, smoking, inactivity, and unhealthy dietary habits. The Joint National Committee on the Detection, Evaluation, and Treatment of High Blood Pressure (1984) provides important guidelines for assessing blood pressure levels.

Inactivity

A sedentary lifestyle has been categorized as a major independent risk factor for the development of coronary artery disease (AHA, 1990). Studies report lower rates of heart attack and death among those who engage in vigorous leisure activities (Morris, Everitt, Pollard, Chave, & Semmence, 1980), occupational activities (Paffenbarger & Hale, 1975), and total daily activities (Kannel, Gordon, Sorlie, & McNamara, 1971). Although there appears to be an independent effect, physical activity may promote favorable change in the levels of other risk factors as well. In addition, physical activity reduces the incidence of coronary heart disease and may improve the likelihood of a patient's survival following a myocardial infarction (Morris, 1953; Paffenbarger, Wing, & Hyde, 1978; Peters, Cody, Fischoff, Bernstein, & Pike, 1983; Powell, Thompson, Caspersen, & Kendrick, 1987). Several sources provide cardiorespiratory fitness classification tables from which you can determine fitness levels (AHA, 1972; Cooper, 1977). Evidence also suggests that exceeding a 9 and 10 metabolic equivalent (MET) level for women and men, respectively, may not significantly impact mortality (Blair et al., 1989).

Personal History

Evidence of known cardiovascular disease must be documented. Clearly, the patient's medical history as well as her resting and exercise electrocardiograms (ECG) can help you establish overall risk (Cooper, 1977). The prognostic value of the exercise ECG has been studied by many investigators (Froelicher, 1987; Giagnoni et al., 1983; Uhl & Froelicher, 1983).

Family History

A family history of coronary heart disease, particularly disease affecting family members under the age of 60, has long been thought to increase one's risk for the disease (Snowden et al., 1982). However, Khaw and Barrett-Connor (1986) suggested that a family history of heart disease does not itself increase the risk of myocardial infarction. Rather, the history of other risk factors such as hypercholesterolemia, hypertension, and diabetes among first-degree relatives increases the patient's risk.

Goals

Evidence suggests that changing undesirable risk factors after a coronary event may favorably impact morbidity and mortality as well as disease progression (Brown et al., 1990; Canner et al., 1986; Kannel, Sorlie, Castelli, & McGee, 1980; Leon et al., 1990; Sparrow, Dawber, & Cotton, 1978). The degree of success of behavioral interventions in modifying cardiac risk factors varies. Generally, approaches have revolved around an educational format (Godin, 1989). However, in order to effectively achieve long-term change, the patient must acquire new cognitive or behavioral skills (Russell, 1986). Godin (1989) reported that interventions with targeted, goal-directed outcomes that incorporate individual counseling have met with the most success. Perri and Richards (1977) found that individuals who maintained long-term behavior change employed more strategies over a longer period of time.

After you have compiled data from the risk assessment, you should schedule a patient conference to discuss the results. Ideally, this should occur within the first 2 weeks of program participation. A concise, graphic display of the data (see Figure 2.3) may help the patient identify important areas to target for change. You, the patient, and the physician must reach a consensus as to the ideal risk profile for which the patient should aim and must prioritize the areas for change. It may be helpful to outline how the modification of one risk area may favorably impact others. Write clear, specific, short-term objectives for the areas of highest priority, assign areas of responsibility, and provide the patient with the necessary tools to achieve the targeted outcome. Lastly, make a date to evaluate the progress and fine tune the program. The first follow-up conference should be 1 week after initiation of the plan to ensure that any problems are quickly addressed before the patient perceives them as insurmountable. Revise or add additional objectives as appropriate and continue to hold follow-up sessions at intervals appropriate to allow the patient to achieve small incremental objectives. These follow-up sessions may be informal checks during an exercise session or scheduled appointments lasting 20 min to 1 hr.

Education

People who experience difficulty in changing behavior fall principally into two categories. The first category involves individuals who have insufficient knowledge of the disease or its treatment to facilitate the change, reject the medical diagnosis, or reject the medical prescription (Russell, 1986). For this group, the principal intervention is patient education.

Knowledge obtained through education represents a critical element necessary to affect behavior change. "Knowledge is the gathering of cognitive information in order to understand an event, process or phenomenon" (AACVPR, 1991, p. 21). The patient must be able to understand the process as well as the cause and effects of various actions in order to implement behavior change.

Patients must have opportunities to learn what is necessary to implement behavior change. Traditionally, educational material has encompassed anatomy, physiology, pathophysiology, treatment regimens, modification of all cardiovascular risk factors, resumption of sexual activity, and psychosocial and work-related issues. Educational content must be firmly grounded in state-of-the-art practice and must follow nationally recognized standards and guidelines (AACVPR, 1991).

Provide the patient with a spectrum of educational options from which to choose in each area.

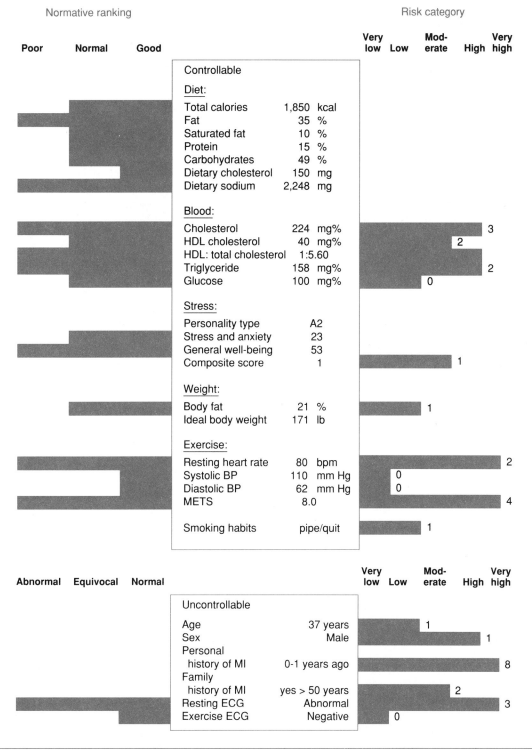

Figure 2.3 Risk assessment profile report. ECG = electrocardiogram; HDL = high-density lipoprotein; MI = myocardial infarction.

Note. From Patient Management System. Central DuPage Hospital, Danada Wellness Center, Winfield, IL. Reprinted by permission.

For example, for nutrition education, offer resources from a lending library, one-on-one counseling with a dietitian, and nutrition/cooking classes. A patient's beliefs about what will or will not best meet his needs play an important role in how successfully the patient is able to integrate the information. From a management perspective, it is not fiscally prudent to house the entire spectrum of services internally; rather, gather a pool of referral sources to be used by patients and physicians alike. Consider including programs of varying depth and cost.

Although there does not appear to be a consensus, several studies suggest one patient education methodology may be preferable over another (Karvetti, 1981; Morley, Ribisl, & Miller, 1984). Because individuals rely most frequently on one of three ways of processing information (Robbins, 1986), you should provide opportunities for individuals to hear, see, and do that which you are teaching. If you tell a patient something, follow up the statement with written material. Irrespective of the methodology used, make sure that the educational content is at the appropriate reading comprehension level (Boyd & Citro, 1983) and considers the ethnic, socioeconomic, and age characteristics of the patient.

Behavior Change Counseling

The second category of individuals who have difficulty changing behavior include those who lack the self-management skills to establish a new health behavior as a habit or intermittently self-debate due to a conflict with other priorities (Russell, 1986). For this category, behavior counseling may be appropriate.

The purpose of behavior counseling is to help the patient understand her current behavioral pattern and guide the patient to develop and use specific skills that produce and maintain the desired changes. The patient is central to the process, an objective coinvestigator (Marlatt & Gordon, 1985). The patient defines the problem and through her response to questions determines and integrates the solutions, assuming full responsibility for the behavior and its redirection. You function as the facilitator (Robbins, 1989).

The process incorporates these essential stages: preparation, change, and maintenance (see Table 2.1). Behavior change counseling strives to separate the behavior from the person (Foreyt, Goodrick, & Gotto, 1981; Marlatt & Gordon, 1985; Russell, 1986; Watson & Tharp, 1989); takes an educational approach (Marlatt & Gordon, 1985; Watson & Tharp, 1989); and incorporates behavioral skills (Brownell & Rodin, 1990; Marlatt & Gordon, 1985; Russell, 1986; Watson & Tharp, 1989), cognitive restructuring (Foreyt, Goodrick, & Gotto, 1981; Marlatt & Gordon, 1985; Robbins,

Table 2.1 Behavior Change Checklist

Rapport

Art of asking questions

The Preparation
1. Outcome clarity—the behavior change desired
2. Data collection—the behavior record
3. Identification of high-risk situations and self-efficacy ratings
4. The internal operating system
   Beliefs—current self-image, new self-image
   Values—hierarchy, evidence procedure
   Goals—add balance
5. Rules—motivation threshold . . . **must change now**
6. Tools for success—new resources
   Skills
   a. Record keeping
   b. Shaping
   c. Stimulus control—cue elimination
   d. Substitution
   e. Assertion
   f. Anger management, communication skills, time management
   Cognitive restructuring
   a. Reframe the situation
   b. Imagery, modeling, future pacing
   c. Rehearsal
   Social support
   Rebalancing lifestyle

The Change

Maintenance . . . relapse prevention
1. Understanding urges and cravings
2. Steps to take when lapse occurs—individualized lapse cards
3. Lapse analysis

1989; Watson & Tharp, 1989), lifestyle rebalancing (Marlatt & Gordon, 1985), and relapse prevention (Foreyt, Goodrick, & Gotto, 1981; Marlatt & Gordon, 1985; Watson & Tharp, 1989).

The success of this process rests on the premise that you are able to develop and maintain rapport with the patient at all times and are skilled in the art of asking questions. Rapport is the first tool in the process of behavior change.

Rapport is the ability to enter someone else's world, to make that person believe that you understand him, that you have a strong bond. Most of us establish rapport easily and without effort. We establish rapport by creating things in common—common interests or associations—and through our communication, the words we choose, our tonality, and our body language (Robbins, 1986). Rapport between you and the patient is necessary for gaining compliance (Eliot, 1988).

The second tool is the use of questions. Questions help the patient weed through all of the extraneous material and get to the heart of the matter. Be gently persistent with your questioning. Ask empowering questions, such as, What are your choices? What would happen if . . . ? How can you make this even better now? What can you learn from this? Ask questions in a way that elicits a specific response. Avoid *why* questions because they will cause the patient to focus only on the problem (Robbins, 1986; Robbins, 1989).

It is important for the patient to understand the behavior change process. Marlatt and Gordon (1985) likened this to knowing the wiring diagram (i.e., self-efficacy, beliefs, references, expectancies, causal links) of a black box (i.e., the brain). By knowing the wiring diagram and how different processes influence one another and one's behavior, the patient can better control the operations of the black box. Furthermore, ask the patient to function as a cotherapist, to develop a scientific attitude toward deciphering the wiring diagram. Such a relationship helps the patient develop a detached, objective attitude instead of a guilty, defensive one. This empowers the patient to become a change agent rather than a victim.

The Preparation

The preparation phase encompasses many critical elements: establishing outcome clarity; collecting data; identifying and analyzing high-risk situations; understanding the internal operating system (beliefs, values, goals, and rules); and teaching tools to sustain the change (skills, cognitive restructuring, social support and lifestyle rebalance).

Outcome Clarity

What is the patient's desired outcome or goal? What does the patient believe about the behavior change process? In helping to clarify the patient's outcome, keep the following points in mind:

1. The outcome must be initiated and maintained by the patient (Russell, 1986). In other words, the patient must be able to take personal control of the outcome and cannot depend upon others (Marlatt & Gordon, 1985).

For example, a patient who uses a health club as her sole means of exercise and depends on someone else for transportation to the health club is not in total control of the exercise regimen.

2. The outcome must be appropriately contextualized (Robbins, 1986; Robbins, 1989; Russell, 1986). Be certain that the patient's reasons for wishing to make a change are appropriate. A patient may state, ''I wish to be thin so I will have a more active social life.'' For this person, long-term maintenance of desired body weight may be difficult, because the patient's social life may not solely depend upon his weight.

3. Short-term, small, immediate goals produce better results than long-term, large, distant goals (Bandura & Simon, 1977; Russell, 1986).

4. If the patient states goals in a very general manner, seek to add clarity by asking for specifics (Robbins, 1986). Does ''stop smoking'' mean to refrain from the use of cigarettes alone or all tobacco products? Often it is better to specify performance rather than outcome (Russell, 1986). For example, it may be more appropriate for a patient to aim for consuming a certain percentage of fat rather than lowering cholesterol by $X\%$, because certain biochemical interactions may be beyond the person's control.

5. Goals framed in terms of moderation as opposed to total abstinence may cause less guilt and self-blame when a lapse occurs. This, however, is not appropriate for certain behaviors such as smoking, alcohol, or drug abuse (Marlatt & Gordon, 1985).

Data Collection

Data collection is a critically important step, because it provides you with an accurate description of the behavior that the patient wishes to change and helps to identify the interrelationships between the patient and other associated behaviors (Brownell & Rodin, 1990; Marlatt & Gordon, 1985; Russell, 1986; Watson & Tharp, 1989).

One's behavior, thoughts, and feelings are embedded in contexts; the events that precede them are antecedents and those that follow are consequences (Watson & Tharp, 1989) (See Table 2.2).

To solve a problem, the patient must pay attention to details, identifying those that appear to be

Table 2.2 ABCs of Changing Behavior

Antecedents (A)	Behaviors (B)	Consequences (C)
When did it happen? Whom were you with? What were you doing? Where were you? What were you saying to yourself?	Actions, thoughts, feelings	What happened as a result? Was it pleasant or unpleasant?
You can change the triggering events for a behavior by building in antecedents that lead to wanted behavior and by removing antecedents that lead to unwanted behavior.	You can change actions, thoughts, feelings, or behaviors themselves by practicing desirable acts or substituting desirable alternatives for unwanted acts.	You can change the events that follow your behavior by reinforcing desired actions and not reinforcing unwanted behavior.

Note. Adapted from Watson & Tharp (1989, pp. 13 & 90).

critical to the problem. Listing details will help the patient focus clearly on what the targeted goal should be.

Research in problem solving suggests that individuals who complete detailed analyses improve their problem-solving abilities more than those who do not (D'Zurilla & Goldfried, 1971; Nezu & D'Zurilla, 1981). The patient's ability to comply with the data collection process will predict her ability to put the program into action (Russell, 1986). Often, this exercise alone may be enough to elicit sufficient change in behavior, because it helps the patient gain insight into the factors that stimulate the behavior's occurrence and support its recurrence, and because the exercise increases awareness of choices and alternative approaches. As Marlatt and Gordon (1985) wrote, this exercise helps the patient get a lay of the land; it provides the patient with his location on the map and the nature of the surrounding territory. In analyzing the data, consider how informed the patient is relative to the area targeted for change. Additional education may be the only catalyst required.

Instruct the patient to keep a written record of the behavior for a 2-week period. This is generally sufficient time to encompass the patient's regular and irregular schedules (e.g., work and travel schedules, or differences in weekdays vs. the weekend) and all potential stressors. To ensure the accuracy and detail of the record, the patient must record the behavior at the time of the event (Marlatt & Gordon, 1985). To facilitate this, provide a diary that can easily be carried in a shirt pocket or purse. Construct the behavior record (see Table 2.3) so that each entry will include the following items: time of day, place, with whom, cues, emotional state (mood), thoughts, degree of the urge (0-5), simultaneous activity (antecedents), consumption or results (behavior), and resulting emotional state and other anchors (consequences) (Russell, 1986).

Encourage the patient to specify not only situations in which the targeted behavior occurs but also incidents in which the behavior is successfully controlled. In addition, examine infrequent desirable behaviors that the patient may wish to enhance as substitute behaviors (Russell, 1986), for example, exercise.

Last, determine what programs have or have not worked for the patient in the past. Identifying programs that were not successful can tell you a lot about the patient. Seek to determine what specifically did not work in each incidence. The patient may have labeled an entire program a failure when in fact only a single aspect was ineffective (Marlatt & Gordon, 1985; Robbins, 1989).

Identification and Analysis of High-Risk Situations

The behavior record will help to identify potential high-risk situations. A high-risk situation is "any situation that poses a threat to the individual's sense of control (self-efficacy) and increases the risk of potential relapse" (Marlatt & Gordon, 1985, p. 37).

Table 2.3   Behavior Record

| Time | Antecedent | | | | | Behavior | Consequences | | |
	Place	With whom	Mood	Thoughts	Simultaneous activity	Degree of urge (0-5)		Mood	Thoughts	Activities

Three categories of high-risk situations are responsible for 75% of all lapses (Cummings, Gordon, & Marlatt, 1980):

1. Negative emotional states/moods/feelings such as anger, frustration, anxiety, and boredom
2. Interpersonal conflict such as an ongoing or relatively recent argument or confrontation with a spouse, family member, friend, or employer/employee
3. Social pressure, whether it be direct or indirect

Create a list of potential high-risk situations and assess the patient's self-efficacy by mutually ranking her coping capacity for each situation. What degree of temptation is the patient likely to experience and what coping responses will she employ in each situation? Begin to identify strengths and weaknesses. The degree of self-efficacy will vary depending upon the patient's past performance, observation of others' performances, influence of social pressure, level of emotional arousal, and expectations from the treatment program (Bandura, 1977; Edell, Edington, Herd, O'Brien, & Witkin, 1987). The patient's own past success in dealing with the high-risk situation exerts the most important influence (Bandura, 1977b). When self-efficacy is reduced, the patient will tend to give up sooner in a difficult situation.

A number of investigators have developed self-efficacy scales (Annis, 1982; Condiotte & Lichtenstein, 1981; Glynn & Ruderman, 1986). Most tools ask the patient to rate the likelihood that he will have difficulty in controlling the target behavior in a particular situation. However, Annis (1982) posed a different question: Using a four-point scale (*never*, *rarely*, *frequently*, *almost always*), the patient identifies the occurrence of the target behavior in certain situations over the past year. The logic is that if the behavior occurred in the past, it will probably occur in the future as a response to a high-risk situation. Using Table 2.4, create your own self-efficacy scales by adding and/or subtracting items on the list as you tailor it to the specific behavior pattern.

The Operating System

The Chinese character for change is composed of the symbols for danger and opportunity. Change represents positive and negative consequences. Each time our world or something inside us

Table 2.4 Situational Self-Efficacy Checklist

How difficult is it for you to control your behavior . . .

| | Level of difficulty | | | | |
| | None | Moderate | | | Most |
	1	2	3	4	5
1. After work.....................					
2. When bored					
3. When depressed					
4. When angry					
5. When alone					
6. When with friends					
7. When traveling...............					
8. When irritable					
9. At the end of the day......					
10. At a bar........................					
11. At a restaurant					
12. When confronted with the item (cigarettes, alcohol, food)					
13. With family members					
14. Before a meal					
15. After eating...................					
16. When you feel stressed....					
17. When you feel tired					
18. After an argument					
19. When hungry.................					
20. When nervous................					
21. When there is peer pressure					
22. When you want to increase your enjoyment.....					
23. When you are up against a deadline......................					
24. When you see a visual reminder or hear something.......................					
25. When you want to test your willpower...............					
26. When you want to celebrate					
27. As self-punishment					
28. When impatient..............					
29. When thinking about the item......................					

changes, we have to rethink who we are, where we are going, how we will do things, and what we want to do. Each person brings a web of expectations, judgments, and attitudes to life (Jaffe & Scott, 1988); these are one's beliefs, values, and rules (Robbins, 1986). Knowing one's core beliefs and values is essential to navigating through change successfully without losing sight of one's core roots.

Beliefs

Beliefs are underlying assumptions, feelings of certainty about what something means. They are generalizations, a means by which to judge and evaluate a situation. Beliefs drive our actions and reactions to a situation. They are statements like "the world is . . . ," "I am . . . ," "people are . . ." (Robbins, 1986). One way to explore one's own beliefs in operation is to listen closely to the words one uses when thinking (self-talking) about a topic (Jaffe & Scott, 1988). For example, a person may believe that diets can lead to weight loss or that diets never work. Beliefs reveal much about our internal dialogue or self-talk and our attitudes. Our prior experiences shape our beliefs and expectations; beliefs and expectations shape behavior.

We have beliefs about ourselves, our capabilities, and the type of people we are, and we have beliefs about the world, organizations, jobs, and other people. Beliefs can be positive or negative, expansive or limiting, accurate or inaccurate (Jaffe & Scott, 1988; Robbins, 1986; Watson & Tharp, 1989).

Beliefs about oneself can be off base in three ways (Jaffe & Scott, 1988):

1. One can think too little of oneself, being excessively critical or demanding.
2. One can be too easily satisfied with oneself, stopping short of what one is capable of becoming.
3. One can have unrealistic or misplaced beliefs.

In addition, there are two maladaptive beliefs that individuals often hold (Goldfried, 1979):

1. The belief that constant love and approval are necessary from everyone all the time
2. The belief that all important undertakings must be performed to perfection

A negative belief is a conviction that something is not possible. People often deny the possibility that the future can be decisively different and instead project that the past will continue indefinitely into the future (Jaffe & Scott, 1988). The past does not equal the future (Robbins, 1986); however, negative beliefs can be very powerful. If a person does not believe he can do something, often the

person behaves in a way that upholds that belief (Watson & Tharp, 1989).

There are several questions you can ask to break down a patient's disempowering beliefs. "Do you really believe that?" "Is it logical?" "Must everyone *smoke* constantly?" "Does this belief help promote your goals?" "What is a better, more empowering belief?"

Another way to change limiting or negative beliefs is through imagination (Robbins, 1986; Robbins, 1989; Watson & Tharp, 1989). We cannot do anything that we cannot first imagine ourselves doing (Jaffe & Scott, 1988). Instruct the patient to visualize herself accomplishing the task. The clearer, more detailed, and precise the image is, the more fully the patient will be on the road to achieving the goal. As the patient visualizes this goal, make sure he associates feelings that are pleasurable, positive, and energizing.

As the patient transforms a limiting or negative belief into a positive, empowering one, ensure that it becomes more concrete and specific (Jaffe & Scott, 1988). Consider the difference: "I can't make all the changes my doctor wants me to make" and "I will find a way to reduce my triglyceride levels through modifying my diet and achieving my ideal body weight." One reason that negative beliefs defeat us is because they are so overpoweringly global (Watson & Tharp, 1989). By accepting a more reasonable belief, the patient can change the controlling antecedent and begin focusing behavior in a new direction. Table 2.5 is a sample work sheet for eliciting one's beliefs.

It is critical that the patient have a clear picture of her future self-image—one of an active, coping, independent individual who has successfully achieved her goal. Often, people have great difficulty seeing themselves as nonsmokers, former drinkers, or thin people, because their self-images are tied up with the old behavior patterns. If this is the case, have the patient write a brief statement describing her present self-image. Next ask the patient to write another statement reflecting how she will view herself after successfully changing the target behavior. Compare the two accounts, noting areas that may identify potential conflict (Marlatt & Gordon, 1985).

Values

Values are emotional states or feelings in which we invest time, energy, and even money to satisfy. They are private, personal, internal beliefs about what is most important to us, what is right

Table 2.5 Beliefs

Definition: Beliefs are underlying assumptions, feelings of certainty about what something means. They are generalizations that drive our actions and reactions to a situation.

Global beliefs: Life is, I am, people are . . .	Does the belief limit you?	New empowering belief

Rules: I must, he should, they can, we will . . .
What rules do you have about the behavior you wish to change?

and wrong, what we should and should not do. Values come from a variety of sources—family, peers, friends, self-made heroes, religious figures, co-workers, and teachers. We have values for our lives, careers, and relationships. Most people are not sure what their values are; as a result, they are unhappy because they are not making progress toward what they believe to be the most important. They become bogged down with the immediate, reacting to events rather than spending time on what really matters to them (Robbins, 1986).

You can elicit a patient's values by asking, "What is important to you in your life?" or "What do you need in a relationship or a job?" You are attempting to elicit the emotional states (*ends values*) the patient wishes to achieve (Robbins, 1986). Examples of ends values include love, happiness, honesty, success, respect, freedom, creativity, and passion. *Means values* move us toward our ends values (Robbins, 1986). For example, one may value family; family is a means value (not an emotional state) that gives us a valued emotional state such as love, belonging, or security.

All values have a hierarchy of importance (Robbins, 1986), and we will always strive to satisfy that which is most important. To determine the hierarchical order, for example, of the values *love, success, honesty,* and *creativity,* ask the patient which is more important, love or success. If the answer is *love,* move to the next value and compare *love* and *honesty.* If the patient chooses *love* again, move on to the next value until the list is complete and the most important value has been elicited. Repeat the process until you obtain a complete rank order.

Last, specify an evidence procedure for each value (Robbins, 1986). In other words, how will the patient know when he is loved or successful? Make sure the evidence procedure is appropriate. Notice the difference between the two evidence procedures for the value *success:* an annual income of $750,000, or a person's knowing that each day he has done his best to give back to the world a little more than he took.

Values, which can be identified with the help of Table 2.6, can provide you with important insight into how a patient's behavior change program can be constructed. Consider a patient who wants to lose weight. When asked what is most important to him in life, he responds, "success, money, and happiness." Money is a means value. To find out what the ends value is, ask, "What is important to you about money?" His response might be "the freedom and security that having money affords me." Next the patient may rank the values from ascending to descending order in the following way: *happiness, success, freedom,* and *security.* You may then obtain his evidence procedures by asking, "How do you know when you are happy?" ("I feel good and am more active and outgoing") and "How do you know when you are successful?" ("I feel it inside, others tell me, and I accomplish tasks").

You now have several important pieces of information that you can use to structure a program to complement the patient's internal operating system. First, you can use happiness as a motivator. Second, you should build in an external reinforcement system and make the program task oriented. However, because *freedom* is the third highest value, the program needs to be flexible as well.

Goals

Goals are things a person wants to do (Robbins, 1989). If a person specifies a behavior he should state it in the present tense as if he has already accomplished the goal. This will cause the individual to want what he has already done or achieved (Jaffe & Scott, 1988).

Goals add an element of balance to life. Often we become so absorbed in one aspect of life that we may cut ourselves off from other meaningful activities or relationships (Jaffe & Scott, 1988). Goals help the patient rebalance his lifestyle (Marlatt & Gordon, 1985), and they suggest sources of pleasurable, substitute activities (Watson & Tharp, 1989). Clear, precise goals can direct and motivate the patient to fulfill her highest values. As the patient writes down goals (see Table 2.7), encourage her to be playful, to let her mind race, to write goals that will provide more balance to her life. For each goal, the patient identifies a time frame for accomplishment (e.g., 1 month, 6 months, or 1 year). She selects the top three 1-year goals and, for each, writes a compelling statement as to why she absolutely must achieve this goal. Next, for each goal she writes two action steps that she will take the next 2 weeks to begin achieving each goal (Robbins, 1986). The therapist guides in these activities to make sure the goals are reasonable.

Rules

A person's rules often keep her from getting what she wants. Rules fall into several categories: "Must" or threshold rules are the most powerful, followed by "should" or personal standard rules and "can" rules or rules of possibility (Robbins, 1989). A person's rules may not be congruent with the targeted behavior. His "should" or "can" rules may not be strong enough to motivate him to make a change. Most addictive behaviors involve a conflict of motives. The desire for immediate gratification is often in direct conflict with the desire for abstinence (Marlatt & Gordon, 1985; Russell, 1986; Watson & Tharp, 1989). In addition, people will do more to avoid pain than they will to gain pleasure (Robbins, 1989). Until the patient perceives more pain associated with indulging in the behavior than pleasure associated with the immediate gratification, the behavior will continue. The level of motivation and commitment to change the target behavior closely correlates with the degree of success achieved (Marlatt & Gordon, 1985). Marlatt and Gordon (1985) described this as the "threshold of motivation," which must be strong enough to effect the actual change. Many factors can increase motivation: increased risk of damage to physical or psychological well-being associated with the behavior; guilt or dissatisfaction with dependence on the substance or activity; social disapproval from spouse, family, friends, or

Table 2.6 Values

Definition: Values are emotional states or feelings in which we invest time, energy, and even money to satisfy. They are individual beliefs about what is important to us.

Ends value: A state you wish to achieve
Means value: Moves you to an ends value

What is important to you in life?	Is it a means value?	If yes, what does the means value give you?	Hierarchical order	How do you know when you achieve this value?

Table 2.7 Goals

Goals specify a behavior; they are things you want to do. Consider things that may add more balance to your life.

Goals	Time frame	Priority

Compelling statement

Explain why you absolutely **must** achieve these goals within the next year.

Goal 1:	Action steps
	1.
	2.
	3.

peers; and economic costs. People who want to institute behavior change believe they should change. It is not until their shoulds become musts that they will be successful (Robbins, 1989).

The easiest way to increase a patient's motivation threshold is to ask questions that push the person to a point where change becomes an absolute must (Robbins, 1989). The following are examples of such questions.

- How much has (*the behavior*) cost you in your life?
- What have you lost as a result of (*the behavior*)?
- How bad does this make you feel?

- In how many ways have you cheated yourself by (*the behavior*)?
- In what ways has (*the behavior*) affected your relationships, career, and health? (Use items that are important to the patient.)
- By continuing (*the behavior*), what kind of role model are you for your children?
- Five years from now, how much more will (*the behavior*) have cost you? How will you look, feel, and act? How much more will you have missed out on?

When you have made the patient fully aware of the negative consequences of the behavior, break the pattern by drastically changing the subject (Robbins, 1989). You can do this by asking a totally unrelated question. The point is not to devastate the patient but to bring her to the point where her "can" and "should" rules become "must" rules.

Tools for Success

You must provide the patient with general problem-solving skills and specific coping techniques. Teach the patient to be on the lookout for high-risk situations and to take preventive action as early as possible. Instruct the patient to look at the coming week, determine likely high-risk situations, and create a plan. Advanced planning increases a person's sense of personal responsibility and fosters self-efficacy (Marlatt & Gordon, 1985). However, not all high-risk situations can be foreseen. For these, one must rely on coping skills.

Skills

In developing the patient's repertoire of skills and techniques, ask her what she thinks will work best in the situation (Russell, 1986; Marlatt & Gordon, 1985). It is important to provide the patient with solid techniques, but the skills should be flexible enough to meet the demands of the particular situation; avoid reliance on rote memorization (Marlatt & Gordon, 1985). Last, the patient must possess enough knowledge to effectively use the tool.

Self-Monitoring Record Keeping
Foreyt, Goodrick, and Gotto (1981) stated that the most important skill is the ability to accurately monitor the behavior through record keeping. A detailed written record of the behavior can be used to refute cognitive distortions such as rationalization and denial (Marlatt & Gordon, 1985). In addition, a record provides immediate feedback on progress and compliance with the regimen and will highlight new high-risk situations (Martin & Dubbert, 1984).

Shaping
Initially it is important to keep the treatment plan simple and easy to follow (Russell, 1986). In addition, it is critical that the patient experience success implementing the regimen. Early success will have a significant impact on increasing self-efficacy (Edell et al., 1987). *Shaping* is a method of succes-

sive approximation; it means acquiring skill one step at a time. Once the patient masters the first step, another is added. To ensure early success, start with steps the patient feels confident he can successfully implement and maintain (Watson & Tharp, 1989). Martin and Dubbert (1984) called shaping the most vital tool for effecting a new persistent behavior pattern. Dieters who hold excessively stringent standards for compliance often violate them by binge eating. Hawkins and Clement (1980) found that dieters who set steps to gradually reduce their caloric intake realize success and are more likely to develop self-control.

Stimulus Control—Cue Elimination
Most behavior is preceded by a stimulus called an antecedent. An antecedent becomes a cue to a behavior when the behavior is reinforced in the presence of the stimulus and not reinforced in its absence. Over time, the stimulus will control the performance of the behavior; when the individual perceives the stimulus, the behavior is automatically performed (Watson & Tharp, 1989). Stimulus control is often found with such behaviors as smoking, reactions to stress, and overeating. It follows that if the stimulus is eliminated, the resulting behavior will be controlled (Watson & Tharp, 1989), that is, out of sight, out of mind. Thus, it is important that the patient eliminate all possible cues from the environment before and after changing the targeted behavior to reduce temptation and prevent backsliding. Doing so signals the patient's commitment to therapy. As reinforcement of the cue diminishes, so will its control over the behavior until eventually this control is completely eliminated (Marlatt & Gordon, 1985).

Substitution
Substituting a desired behavior for an undesired one is preferable to merely suppressing the bad habit. Selecting an incompatible behavior is a good tactic, particularly if the incompatible behavior itself is desirable (e.g., exercise as a substitute for smoking) (Russell, 1986). The patient must not substitute one addictive behavior for another; it is unwise to use alcohol as a substitute for smoking (Marlatt & Gordon, 1985). Instruct the patient to create a list of substitute activities. It is important that the patient view many of these activities as positive substitutes; this will reduce the sense of deprivation during the first few days after the behavior change is instituted (Marlatt & Gordon, 1985; Watson & Tharp, 1989).

Assertion

An assertive individual is able to express thoughts and feelings in an appropriate, straightforward, honest manner while taking into account the feelings of others (Watson & Tharp, 1989). Goldfried (1979) found that timid people often are willing to give up their beliefs the moment they come under scrutiny. As a result, these people may have difficulty standing up for themselves and may easily bow to social pressure. Assertiveness training helps these individuals positively affirm their decisions, improving behavioral compliance.

Anger Management, Communication Skills, and Time Management

These are additional skills that may help the patient achieve and maintain the desired behavior changes (Marlatt & Gordon, 1985; Russell, 1986; Watson & Tharp, 1989).

Cognitive Restructuring

Behavior is a product of one's focus, emotional state, and physiology. In order to change behavior, a person needs to acquire the tools to change focus and emotional state (cognitive restructuring), which in turn will impact physiology and thus behavior (Robbins, 1989).

Cognitive restructuring means changing a person's beliefs about her social skill deficits (Marlatt & Gordon, 1985). A person's life is her focus. People who fail in life do so because they major in minor things (Robbins, 1986), that is, they concentrate on things that are not important or that are negative. Thus, if a person continually focuses on negative things, the minutiae of life, or all the things that can go wrong (possible problems), that person is putting herself in a state that supports negative behavior and results in failure (Robbins, 1989).

Reframe the Situation

Reframing a situation merely changes the way a person views a situation. The patient does this either by altering the pictures she makes in her mind or changing what she says to herself (self-talk) (Robbins, 1986).

To change the pictures, the patient should de-emphasize them—make them dull, black and white, smaller, blurry, or a still frame. The patient can add humor, making the participants talk like Donald Duck or adding big feet or huge red noses. Or the patient can view the situation from a dis-

tance, step outside the picture; this is called dis-association (Robbins, 1986; Robbins, 1989). By disassociating herself from the event, the patient becomes less emotionally involved and can observe the situation more objectively (Marlatt & Gordon, 1985; Watson & Tharp, 1989). Conversely, the patient should make an OK or good situation even better, enlarging the picture, making it panoramic and more colorful, adding sound, actively stepping into the situation, and fully enjoying the experience (Robbins, 1989).

The patient can use reframing to lessen the strength of paired associations (Marlatt & Gordon, 1985). For example, the patient may enjoy the creamy rich taste of cheesecake, using it as frequent positive reinforcement. Consider the strength of this association if every time the patient sees a cheesecake he also pictures a large St. Bernard dog shaking its head, drool from the corners of its mouth covering the piece of cheesecake.

One can reframe a situation by the words selected to describe it. A person should aim to soften the intensity for negative events. Notice how differently a person feels if she changes "I'm so angry" to "I'm a little peeved." Conversely, she can add intensity and emotion to the positive. Instead of saying "I'm OK," she can say "I'm terrific." Robbins (1989) called this *transformational vocabulary*.

Self-talk has a powerful effect on emotional state (Watson & Tharp, 1989). The patient should eliminate *failure* from her vocabulary. There are no failures, just outcomes and results (Robbins, 1986). This is critical when a person is faced with a lapse. Instead of letting a patient torture himself over a slip, coach him to view it as a single, isolated event from which he can gain new insight (Marlatt & Gordon, 1985; Watson & Tharp, 1989). Hall, Bass, and Monroe (1978) found negative emotional states and depression to be inversely correlated with weight loss. Wortman and Dintzer (1978) wrote that an individual may philosophically construct reasons for an event's occurrence that give the event special meaning, in contrast to focusing on the "mechanical causality" of the incident itself.

Imagery, Modeling, and Future Pacing

Some people have difficulty imagining themselves doing things that they are unable to perform in real life. In fact, until a person can imagine herself doing something, she will be unable to perform it. Because a patient may have no reference for such a behavior, it is often easier for her to imagine someone else (a model) performing the act (Robbins, 1989). The patient should choose a model similar to himself or herself in age and sex. The patient imagines the model facing the same difficulties that the patient faces, successfully coping with the problem, and being positively reinforced for it. Now, using these same resources, the patient should actually step into the situation, replacing the model, and successfully handle the problem just as the model did (Watson & Tharp, 1989). This combines the techniques of imagined modeling (Watson & Tharp, 1989) and covert modeling (Kazdin, 1976).

In addition, the patient can find and imitate individuals who in real life embody the desired behavior traits. If observation doesn't reveal a crucial part of a model's performance, the patient should ask the individual to explain that which is not observable (Robbins, 1989). Through the imitation of competent models, the patient can receive a large boost in self-efficacy expectations (''if she can do it, so can I'') (Bandura, 1977a; Robbins, 1989).

You can help a patient rehearse behavior in his imagination. This is called imagined rehearsal (Watson & Tharp, 1989) or future pacing (Robbins, 1989). Coach the patient to picture himself in a high-risk situation—a restaurant, bar, or party—and rehearse in his mind his coping responses to that situation. To establish a framework within which the patient can develop additional choices, you may find the following lead-in phrases (Robbins, 1989) helpful:

- Let's suppose you have already quit smoking. What will you do to keep your hands busy?
- If you lost 10 pounds, how would your daily activities change?
- Pretend that you have successfully confronted your boss. How will you deal with the situation the next time it arises?

Jaffe and Scott (1988) have developed the Jaffe Scott Personal Power Grid that depicts four quadrants divided into areas that can and cannot be controlled. Certainly a person should put the bulk of her energy into aspects of life that can be controlled. By controlling aspects of her life, a patient feels rewarded, in that the energy she has invested makes a difference; she has a feeling of success, accomplishment, and increased self-efficacy. Instruct the patient to make a list of all those things she can and cannot control in a high-risk situation. Now have her break down the uncontrollable items into parts that can be controlled. For some

items, there is a gray area between what one can or cannot control. It is important that the patient test the limits of her abilities by pushing into this risk zone. Often the patient is amazed by the number of things that can be controlled in a difficult situation.

Coach the patient through an imagined relapse. Make certain that guilt and self-blame are rechanneled into positive self-talk and constructive behaviors (Marlatt & Gordon, 1985).

All new traits and skills must be rehearsed in the real world. Models and imagined rehearsals are excellent preparation for real life; however, it is not until one has rehearsed these new responses in real life that they become integrated, viable resources (Thase & Moss, 1976).

Much of the target behavior's lure is the anticipated positive outcome that has become associated with the behavior. Marlatt (1985) attempted to decouple this relationship by coaching the individual through a planned lapse. Before allowing the patient to engage in the behavior, ask him to vividly imagine all of the wonderfully positive consequences that he expects to experience—the sights, sounds, feelings, tastes, and smells. Then have the patient engage in the behavior. This exercise helps him realize the actual act does not produce the imagined results.

Social Support

Before initiating the actual behavior change, the patient must have a solid and deep social support system. Foreyt, Goodrick, and Gotto (1981) wrote that this can be a very powerful motivator, and its effect has been well documented with regard to exercise adherence (Daltroy & Godin, 1989; Oldridge, 1984). Support systems provide encouragement, moral support, and social reinforcement. Enlist the help of the spouse and other family members, as well as people with whom the patient has frequent contact, such as co-workers. Instruct the patient to ask for help in specific ways. Ask the patient to consider participating in a group of like individuals, or pair two clients together as buddies. In such groups, patients can share experiences and solutions and can offer, as well as receive, support (Marlatt & Gordon, 1985). It is important for the patient to have contact with someone in the support network on a daily basis for the first several weeks.

Be aware of patients who want to make this change alone (Marlatt & Gordon, 1985). Often they do not want anyone to know about their efforts, because they fear failure. Instruct such a patient to revisit her list of beliefs, rewriting disempowering ones. Making a public commitment and enlisting social support increases the chances of success (Levy, 1977).

Rebalancing Lifestyle

A comprehensive behavior change program should strive to improve the patient's overall lifestyle. With a balanced lifestyle, the patient will find it easier to cope with high-risk situations. Often a person becomes weighted down with activities perceived as external demands or threats (''shoulds'') and lacks time for pleasurable, self-fulfilling activities (''wants''). A person who feels she is faced with too many shoulds often has a sense of self-deprivation and a corresponding desire for indulgence and gratification. The indulgence is often rationalized with ''I deserve a break!'' To temper the need for negative indulgences, the patient must achieve a healthy lifestyle balance. Individuals attempting to refrain from addictive behaviors are more likely to experience relapses if their lifestyles are unbalanced (Marlatt & Gordon, 1985).

Waitley (1983) suggested that to gain a broad perspective of lifestyle balance, the patient should complete a ''wheel of fortune'' that depicts family and community support as well as physical, spiritual, social, mental, professional, and financial aspects. Jaffe and Scott (1988) emphasized the importance of the way energy is distributed between one's work and personal life, and between giving to and receiving from others.

Marlatt and Gordon (1985) devised an exercise that is more immediate and specific. Because it is important to take time each day to engage in worthwhile, positive indulgences in an attempt to balance shoulds and wants, he suggested that the patient keep a daily want-should tally sheet. This can help the person understand her overall pattern of daily activities and the corresponding rating of each (1 = a want, 7 = a should, 4 = an equal mix). When you and the patient review the tally sheet, some questions will arise. Are the shoulds all clumped together? Are shoulds postponed until the very last minute? Can the patient insert some wants into the schedule to minimize the development of a high-risk situation?

Examples of wants include habitual aerobic exercise, meditation, relaxation exercise, a massage or hot bath, a good book, coffee with a friend, sexual activity, religious activities, and community service work. Use the individual's list of goals as a springboard for ideas.

The Change

Select a date to institute the program and be sure the date does not coincide with a high-risk situation. The actual date should be a celebration, for it marks the beginning of a journey to improved health, increased sense of accomplishment, and new freedom. Marlatt and Gordon (1985) recommended that the patient sign a statement of commitment, listing her reasons for undertaking the process, incorporating higher beliefs and values, and describing the final outcome. It is important for you and the patient to realize that in many ways quitting is the easiest step. The maintenance of the new behavior is where the work lies.

Maintenance—Relapse Prevention

The maintenance phase begins as soon as the behavior change is initiated. The incidence of lapse, a single slip, and subsequent relapse is greatest during the 1st 3 months, with the highest frequency occurring in the 1st month (Brownell & Rodin, 1990; Marlatt & Gordon, 1985). As the patient learns from each lapse, the rate of relapse stabilizes beginning with the 4th month (Hunt, Barnett, & Branch, 1971).

It is important for the patient to understand that urges and cravings are conditioned responses. Most urges are triggered by external factors. They have specific life expectancies; they arise, peak, and then subside and pass away. It is a myth that a craving or urge will continue to intensify and will only be relieved through indulgence in the behavior. Conversely, giving in to the urge strengthens it and increases its probability of recurrence. Instruct the patient to recognize and label an urge for what it is. She should view an urge with detachment, watch it rise, crest, and then subside like a wave. By detaching herself, she will tend to identify less with the craving and not be overwhelmed by it. Once the patient has identified the urge, she should stop and ''take five.'' This time will allow her to detach herself, look around, and recognize her choices. Marlatt and Gordon (1985) suggested that individuals carry cards that provide ''emergency procedures'' for the situations (see Table 2.8). Concrete instruction is essential, because the patient is at greatest danger for continuing to engage in the behavior immediately following the lapse.

When a lapse does occur, it is critical that the patient view the slip as a single, isolated event, an error from which he can learn valuable information. He must not equate the slip with an irreversible failure. Moreover, a slip does not signal a treatment failure. How the person internalizes the event is a pivotal determinant to whether the lapse will progress to a full-blown relapse. Immediately help the patient analyze why the lapse occurred. Review the variables on the behavior record, concentrating on external factors that are specific and controllable. It is important to praise the patient for controlling the depth of the slip. Help him look for things he can do differently the next time; add new resources and reinforce existing resources as appropriate. Do not allow the patient to discuss past slips at this time. Reinforce the need to continue keeping detailed records, including both controlled and uncontrolled incidents. These records will identify persistent as well as new high-risk situations. Be alert for individuals who use rationalization and denial as means of coping with the incident (Marlatt & Gordon, 1985; Watson & Tharp, 1989).

Exercise Therapy and Risk Stratification

Risk stratification will help you determine a patient's prognosis for future cardiac events and survival. The literature is replete with variables describing the risk categories. DeBusk, Kraemer, and Nash (1983) studied 100 survivors of a documented myocardial infarction; their study provides general guidance for a three-tiered risk-stratification model. This model relates risk of future cardiac events to the extent of myocardial ischemia and left ventricular dysfunction. The high-risk category reflects myocardial dysfunction. The intermediate category includes parameters suggestive of resting or exercise-induced residual myocardial ischemia. The low-risk category is for those who have neither myocardial ischemia nor left ventricular dysfunction.

Recently, the American College of Physicians (1988) and the AACVPR (1991) published risk stratification classification tables. In addition, the American College of Sports Medicine (ACSM) (1991) has outlined patient characteristics associated with an increased risk for cardiac events during exercise.

Table 2.8 Lapse Attack Card

1. Stop, remain calm, and read this card. Act now!
2. Step out of the situation. Urges and cravings are like waves; they rise, crest, and fade away.
3. Renew your commitment to changing your behavior (write an empowering statement why you must change now).

Remember, **the past does not equal the future.**

This is a single isolated event from which I will learn.

Focus now on all your successes.

4. Review what led up to this point.
5. Make an immediate plan to improve the situation.

_____

_____
(List key resources to access now.)

_____

You always have a choice!

6. Wait; before continuing to _____ , call _____ .

Believe and you can!

You are in control. There is always a way!

Note: Adapted from Robbins (1986); Marlatt & Gordon (1985).

Following is a compilation of these data and resources:

Low Risk

† Uncomplicated clinical course in hospital (De-Busk et al., 1983)
† No evidence of myocardial ischemia (Beller & Gibson, 1986; DeBusk et al., 1983; DeBusk et al., 1986; McNeer et al., 1978; Weiner et al., 1987)
† Functional capacity ≥7 METs (DeBusk et al., 1983)
† Normal left ventricular function (ejection fraction [EF] ≥50%) (Beller & Gibson, 1986; DeBusk et al., 1983; DeBusk et al., 1986)
† Absence of significant ventricular ectopy (Bigger, Fleiss, Kleiger, Miller, & Rolnitzkey, 1984)
† Intermediate risk group ≥3 months S/P event

Intermediate Risk

† ST segment depression ≥2 mm flat or down sloping (Beller & Gibson, 1986; DeBusk et al., 1983; DeBusk et al., 1986; McNeer et al., 1978; Waters et al., 1985)
† Reversible thallium defects (Beller & Gibson, 1986; Hung, Goris, Nash, Kraemer, & DeBusk, 1984)
† Moderate left ventricular function (EF 35 to 49%) (DeBusk et al., 1986)
† Changing pattern or new development of angina pectoris (AACVPR, 1991; ACSM, 1991; Cole & Ellestad, 1978; Mark et al., 1987)
† Failure to comply with exercise prescription (ACSM, 1991; American College of Physicians, 1988)
† Inability to monitor heart rate (American College of Physicians, 1988)
† High-risk group ≥6 months S/P event
† Prior or multivessel percutaneous transluminal coronary angioplasty (PTCA) (Wenger et al., 1990)

High Risk*

† Prior myocardial infarction or infarct involving ≥35% of left ventricle (Beller & Gibson, 1986; DeBusk et al., 1986; Madsen et al., 1984; Waters et al., 1985; Weiner et al., 1987)

† EF ≤35% at rest (DeBusk et al., 1983)
† Fall in exercise systolic blood pressure, or failure of systolic blood pressure to rise more than 10 mm Hg on exercise tolerance test (DeBusk et al., 1983; Hammermeister, DeRouen, & Dodge, 1979; Krone, Gillespie, Weld, Miller, & Moss, 1985; Van Camp & Peterson, 1989; Waters et al., 1985)
† Persistent or recurrent ischemic pain 24 hr or more after hospital admission (DeBusk et al., 1983; Waters et al., 1985)
† Congestive heart failure syndrome in hospital (Beller & Gibson, 1986; DeBusk et al., 1983; DeBusk et al., 1986; Van Camp & Peterson, 1989)
† Cardiomegaly (Bruce & DeRouen, 1978; Hammermeister et al., 1979)
† High-grade ventricular ectopy (Bigger et al., 1984; Hammermeister et al., 1979; Van Camp & Peterson, 1989)
† Functional capacity ≤5 METs on symptom-limited test (Bruce & DeRouen, 1978; Hung et al., 1984; McNeer et al., 1978; Weiner et al., 1987) with abnormal systolic blood pressure response (Froelicher, Perdue, Pewen, & Risch, 1987) or peak heart rate ≤135 bpm (McNeer et al., 1978; Van Camp & Peterson, 1989)
† ≥2 mm ST segment depression at peak heart rate ≤135 bpm (DeBusk et al., 1983; DeBusk et al., 1986)
† Survivor of cardiac arrest (ACSM, 1991; Van Camp & Peterson, 1989)
† Non–Q wave infarct (Wenger, 1989) in patients ≥70 years (Nicod et al., 1989)
† Failed PTCA (Wenger et al., 1990)

*Selected patients who undergo cardiac valve surgery may fall into this category if they have additional medical problems such as pulmonary hypertension, moderate to severe left ventricular dysfunction, ventricular dysrhythmias, renal or hepatic dysfunction, or low functional capacity (Wenger et al., 1990).

Low-risk patients have a mortality of less than 2% the 1st year following acute myocardial infarction or coronary artery bypass surgery. Intermediate-risk patients have a 10 to 25% mortality rate, and high-risk patients have greater than a 25% mortality rate. Studies report that 30 to 50% of patients who have experienced acute myocardial infarction and 75% who have undergone coronary artery bypass surgery fall into the low-risk category (DeBusk, 1989; DeBusk et al., 1986). An analysis of 100 consecutive patients who entered a Phase II cardiac rehabilitation program at the Danada

Wellness Center of Central DuPage Hospital in Wheaton, Illinois showed that 12% were stratified as low risk, 38% intermediate risk, and 50% high risk (see Table 2.9).

Table 2.9 Distribution of Phase II Cardiac Rehabilitation Patients Across Risk Categories and Corresponding ECG Notations During Exercise

| | Stratification categories | | |
	Low	Intermediate	High
Demographics:			
N	12	38	50
Men (%)	90	88	75
Age (years)	44	46.7	50.3
Telemetry abnormalities:			
PVCs > 10/min	3	11	16
ST > 1-1/2 mm	1	5	4
Actions taken:			
Physician intervention	1	8	15
Medication change	0	7	9

Note. PVC = premature ventricular contraction; ST = segment depression on an ECG.

Prior to initiating exercise therapy, you should determine a patient's risk stratification category. You can determine the appropriate category by reviewing selected clinical variables during the hospitalization, results of cardiac catheterization, exercise tolerance test, echocardiography, or 24-hr holter monitor. ACSM (1991) has compiled a list of clinical contraindications for participation in exercise. When a patient indicates such clinical parameters, exercise should be delayed or discontinued until appropriate clinical intervention has been taken to correct the problem. New data from Jugdutt, Michbrowski, and Kappagoda (1988) suggest that some individuals with large anterior myocardial infarctions demonstrate worsening wall motion with exercise. Hess and colleagues (1988) demonstrated in a small group of patients with exercise-induced myocardial ischemia the development of structural alterations in the affected areas. Although the last two studies were based on a relatively small sample size, these subsets deserve special attention.

Exercise Mechanisms

Regardless of the patient's risk stratification category, you should write the exercise prescription from the exercise tolerance test, using ACSM guidelines (1991) and taking into account the patient's age, sex, habitual physical activity, musculoskeletal integrity, and any other related medical problems (Franklin, Hellerstein, Gordon, & Timmis, 1989). The mechanisms of the exercise class have been reported elsewhere (Franklin et al., 1989; Giese, 1988). Individuals in the lower risk stratification categories generally tolerate an early resumption of prior activity levels (DeBusk et al., 1986).

The length of the patient's participation in the program should be driven by the risk stratification category and the goals and desired outcomes that were established at the time of the risk assessment. Prepare early to augment the patient's exercise regimen with a home program. A good policy is that members in the lower risk stratification categories exercise without incident in the upper end of their exercise prescriptions before discharge to a home setting.

Use of Continuous ECG Monitoring

The necessity of continuous ECG monitoring for all patients during exercise therapy has been questioned. After reviewing data from 167 centers and 2,351,916 patient exercise hours, Van Camp and Peterson (1989) found no difference in the frequency of cardiovascular complications between centers that used continuous ECG monitoring and those that used intermittent monitoring. Earlier, Haskell (1978) postulated that the lower incidence of sudden death that he reported among continuously ECG-monitored patients may be due to closer medical supervision and lower exercise intensities. Moreover, no data have been reported indicating that cardiovascular complications associated with exercise occur more frequently during the early outpatient recovery period (Haskell, 1978; Hossack & Hartwig, 1982). The data to date are still equivocal relative to monitoring. One indisputable benefit in certain patients is the alteration of their medical regimen as a result of monitoring.

The American College of Cardiology (1986) has listed criteria for the ECG monitoring of patients. This list parallels very closely the criteria for the high-risk stratification category. Recently, the AHA (1990) defined four classes of individuals (one class without CAD and three classes with CAD) and enumerated activity, supervision, ECG, and blood pressure monitoring guidelines for each class. Based upon the AHA citing, it is our practice at Danada Wellness Center that all high-risk patients receive continuous ECG monitoring during exercise. After patients show stable ECG responses to exercise, intermittent monitoring is instituted for patients in the low- and intermediate-risk categories. Due to our experience with the incidence of ECG findings and the resultant medical intervention (see Table 2.9), patients in the intermediate-risk category are monitored somewhat longer than patients in the low-risk group. All patients are monitored when the intensity of the exercise prescription is substantially increased. Erb, Fletcher, and Sheffield (1979) suggested ECG monitoring of one in three sessions; this monitoring decreases over time. Mitchell, Franklin, Johnson, and Rubenfire (1984) maintained that a 4-week program of continuous monitoring during exercise therapy is sufficient for patients who undergo careful preliminary screening. Before instituting intermittent ECG monitoring, verify the accuracy of the patient's pulse-taking technique. In addition, the staff must be able to immediately ascertain a rhythm via quick look paddles off of the defibrillator before a policy of intermittent monitoring is instituted.

Outcome Measures

With this model, outcome measures are based upon the attainment of the objectives established at the outset of the program. You can make a series of comparisons from four data points for each objective. The data collection points are the starting value(s), ideal goal(s), intermediate goal(s), and actual ending value(s). It may be most useful to compare starting, actual, and ideal values and create an average score between the intermediate targets and each corresponding actual ending value. Moreover, make comparisons in each goal area. This analysis can serve as a motivational tool for the patient as she summarizes her progress. The analysis highlights areas in which the patient has done well and depicts areas where additional change is needed to bring her closer to the target.

As the patient continues to achieve intermediate objectives in an area, you need to incorporate the next level of change into the treatment plan and help the patient apply the appropriate resources to facilitate its achievement. In those areas where the patient has met all objectives, place the participant in a maintenance mode with the appropriate adjustment of program component use. When the outcomes are poor, review the objectives: Are they appropriate? Is additional behavior change counseling or education needed? Sometimes an objective is no longer appropriate

and should be dropped. As a result, there will be times, for example, when an individual no longer participates in the structured exercise setting but continues to see you for behavior change counseling. Moreover, it may be appropriate for a patient to reenter the model if there is a deterioration in his clinical status (Leon et al., 1990) or if you note backsliding in a risk factor area.

You can expand the analysis to collectively evaluate the outcomes of all participants in the program. It may be helpful to analyze the outcomes according to risk stratification category. For each category, evaluate the amount of resources consumed (number of monitored and unmonitored exercise sessions, units of counseling), complications during program participation, and long-term morbidity and mortality data. In addition to fulfilling JCAHO (1990) requirements, these data can be used to evaluate your effectiveness and provide important information to referral sources and insurance vendors.

Further Reading

Caspersen, C.J., & Heath, G.W. (1988). The risk factor concept of coronary heart disease. In American College of Sports Medicine (Ed.), *Resource manual for guidelines for exercise testing and prescription* (pp. 111-125). Philadelphia: Lea & Febiger.

Eliot, R.S. (1988). Achieving compliance. In R.S. Eliot (Ed.), *Stress and the heart: Mechanisms, measurements, and management.* Mt. Kisco, NY: Future.

Marlatt, G.A., & Gordon, J.R. (Eds.) (1985). *Relapse prevention: Maintenance strategies in the treatment of addictive behaviors* (pp. 213-220). New York: The Guilford Press.

References

American Association of Cardiovascular and Pulmonary Rehabilitation (1991). *Guidelines for cardiac rehabilitation programs.* Champaign, IL: Human Kinetics.

American College of Cardiology. (1986). Position report on cardiac rehabilitation. *Journal of American College of Cardiology,* **7,** 451-453.

American College of Physicians. (1988). Cardiac rehabilitation services. *Annals of Internal Medicine,* **15,** 671-673.

American College of Sports Medicine. (1991). *Guidelines for exercise testing and prescription* (4th ed.). Philadelphia: Lea & Febiger.

American Heart Association. (1972). *Exercise testing and training in apparently healthy individuals*. Dallas: Author.

American Heart Association. (1973). *Coronary risk handbook*, **73**, 80-285, Dallas: Author.

American Heart Association. (1990). AHA medical scientific statement: Exercise standards. *Circulation*, **82**, 2286-2322.

Annis, H.M. (1982). *Inventory of drinking situations*. Toronto: Addictions Research Foundation.

Bandura, A. (1977a). Self efficacy: Toward a unifying theory of behavioral change. *Psychological Review*, **84**, 191-215.

Bandura, A. (1977b). *Social learning theory*. Englewood Cliffs, NJ: Prentice Hall.

Bandura, A., & Simon, K.M. (1977). The role of proximal self-intentions in self regulation of refractory behavior. *Cognitive Therapy and Research*, **1**, 177-193.

Beller, G.A., & Gibson, R.S. (1986). Risk stratification after myocardial infarction. *Modern Concepts of Cardiovascular Disease*, **55**, 5-10.

Bigger, J.T., Fleiss, J.L., Kleiger, R., Miller, J.P., & Rolnitzkey, L.M. (1984). The relationships among ventricular arrhythmia, left ventricular dysfunction and mortality in the first two years after myocardial infarction. *Circulation*, **69**, 250-258.

Blair, S.N., Kohl, H.W., Paffenbarger, R.S., Clark, D.G., Cooper, K.H., & Gibbons, L.W. (1989). Physical fitness and all-cause mortality: A prospective study of healthy men and women. *New England Journal of Medicine, 262*, 2395-2401.

Boyd, M.D., & Citro, K. (1983). Cardiac patient education literature: Can patients read what we give them? *Journal of Cardiac Rehabilitation*, **3**, 513-516.

Bray, G.A. (1983). Diet and exercise as treatment for obesity. In H.L. Conn, E.A. DeFelice, & P.T. Kuo (Eds.), *Health & obesity* (pp. 79-104). New York: Raven Press.

Brown, G., Albers, J.J., Fisher, L.D., Schaefer, S.M., Lin, J.T., Kaplan, C., Zhao, Z.Q., Bisson, B.D., Fitzpatrick, V.F., & Dodge, H.T. (1990). Regression of coronary artery disease as a result of intensive lipid-lowering therapy in men with high levels of apolipoprotein B. *New England Journal of Medicine, 323*, 1289-1298.

Brownell, K.D., & Rodin, J. (1990). *The weight maintenance survival guide*. Dallas: Brownell & Hager.

Bruce, R.A., & DeRouen, T.A. (1978). Exercise testing as a predictor of heart disease and sudden death. *Hospital Practitioner*, **13**, 69-75.

Canner, P.L., Berge, K.G., Wenger, N.K., Stamler, J., Friedman, L., Prineas, R.J., & Friedewald, W. (1986). Fifteen years mortality in Coronary Drug Project patients; Long-term benefit with niacin. *Journal of American College of Cardiology*, **8**, 1245-1255.

Caspersen, C.J., & Heath, G.W. (1988). The risk factor concept of coronary heart disease. In American College of Sports Medicine (Ed.), *Resource manual for guidelines for exercise testing and prescription* (pp. 111-125). Philadelphia: Lea & Febiger.

Castelli, W.P., Abbott, R.D., & McNamara, P.M. (1983). Summary estimates of cholesterol used to predict coronary heart disease. *Circulation*, **67**, 730-734.

Cole, J.P., & Ellestad, M.H. (1978). Significance of chest pain during treadmill exercise: Correlation with coronary events. *American Journal of Cardiology*, **41**, 227-232.

Condiotte, M.M. & Lichtenstein, E. (1981). Self-efficacy and relapse in smoking cessation program. *Journal of Consulting Clinical Psychology*, **49**, 648-658.

Consolvo, D.A. (1990). Efficacy and administration of cardiac rehabilitation: A review. *Journal of Cardiopulmonary Rehabilitation*, **10**(6), 246-254.

Cook, W.W., & Medley, D.M. (1954). Proposed hostility and pharisaic virtue scales for the MMPI. *Journal of Applied Psychology*, **38**, 414-418.

Cooper, K.H. (1977). *The aerobics way*. New York: Bantam Books.

Cummings, C., Gordon, J.R., & Marlatt, G.A. (1980). Relapse: Strategies of prevention and prediction. In W.R. Miller (Ed.), *The addictive behaviors: Treatment of alcoholism, drug abuse, smoking and obesity* (pp. 291-322). Oxford, UK: Pergamon Press.

Daltroy, L.H., & Godin, G. (1989). The influence of spouse approval and patient perception of spouse approval on cardiac patient participation in exercise program. *Journal of Cardiopulmonary Rehabilitation*, **9**, 363-367.

DeBusk, R.F. (1989). American College of Physicians position paper: Evaluation of patients after recent acute myocardial infarction. *Annals of Internal Medicine*, **110**, 485-488.

DeBusk, R.F., Blomqvist, C.G., Kouchoukos, N.T., Luepken, R.V., Miller, H.S., Moss, A.J., Pollock, M.D., Reeves, T.J., Selvester, R.H., Strason, W.B., Wagner, G.S., & Willman, V.L. (1986). Identification and treatment of low-risk patients after acute myocardial infarction and coronary artery bypass graft surgery. *New England Journal of Medicine*, **314**, 161-166.

DeBusk, R.F., Kraemer, H.C., & Nash, E. (1983). Stepwise risk stratification soon after myocardial infarction. *American Journal of Cardiology*, **52**, 1161-1166.

D'Zurilla, T.J., & Goldfried, M.R. (1971). Problem solving and behavior modification. *Journal of Abnormal Psychology*, **78**, 107-126.

Edell, B.H., Edington, S., Herd, B., O'Brien, R.M., & Witkin, G. (1987). Self-efficacy and self-motivation as predictors of weight loss. *Addictive Behaviors*, **12**, 63-66.

Eliot, R.S. (1988). Achieving compliance. In R.S. Eliot (Ed.), *Stress and the heart: Mechanisms, measurements and management* (pp. 213-220). Mt. Kisco, NY: Future.

Erb, B.D., Fletcher, G.F., & Sheffield, T.L. (1979). Standards for cardiovascular exercise treatment program. American Heart Association subcommittee on rehabilitation target activity group. *Circulation*, **59**, 1084A-1090A.

The Expert Panel. (1988). Report of the National Cholesterol Education expert panel on detection, evaluation, and treatment of high blood cholesterol in adults. *Archives of Internal Medicine*, **148**, 36-69.

Fletcher, G.F., Froelicher, V.F., Hartley, L.H., Haskell, W.L., & Pollock, M.L. (1990). Exercise standards: A statement for health professionals from the American Heart Association, *Circulation*, **82**, 2286-2322.

Foreyt, J.P., Goodrick, G.K., & Gotto, A.M. (1981). Limitations of behavioral treatment of obesity: Review and analysis. *Journal of Behavioral Medicine*, **4**, 159-174.

Franklin, B.A., Hellerstein, H.K., Gordon, S., & Timmis, G.C. (1989). Cardiac patients. In B.A. Franklin, S. Gordon, & G.C. Timmis (Eds.), *Exercise in modern medicine* (pp. 44-80). Baltimore: Williams & Wilkins.

Froelicher, V.F. (1987). *Exercise and the heart: Clinical concepts*. Chicago: Year Book Medical.

Froelicher, V.F., Perdue, S., Pewen, W., & Risch, M. (1987). Application of meta-analysis using an electronic spreadsheet to exercise testing in patients after myocardial infarction. *American Journal of Medicine*, **83**, 1045-1051.

Giagnoni, E., Secchi, M.B., Wu, S.C., Morabito, A., Oltrona, L., Mancarella, S., Volpin, N., Fossa, L., Bettazzi, L., Arangio, G., Sachera, A., & Folli, G. (1983). Prognostic value of exercise EKG testing in asymptomatic normoten-sive subjects. *New England Journal of Medicine*, **309**, 1085-1089.

Giese, M.D. (1988). Organization of an exercise session. In American College of Sports Medicine (Ed.), *Resource manual for guidelines for exercise testing and prescription* (pp. 244-247). Philadelphia: Lea & Febiger.

Glynn, S.M. & Ruderman, A.J. (1986). The development and validation of an eating self-efficacy scale. *Cognitive Therapy and Research*, **10**, 402-420.

Godin, G. (1989). The effectiveness of interventions in modifying behavioral risk factors of individuals with coronary heart disease. *Journal of Cardiopulmonary Rehabilitation*, **9**, 223-236.

Goldfried, M.R. (1979). Anxiety reduction through cognitive behavioral intervention. In P.C. Kendall & S.D. Hollon (Eds.), *Cognitive-behavioral interventions: Theory, research and procedures* (pp. 117-149). New York: Academic Press.

Gotto, A. (1986). Interactions of the major risk factors for coronary heart disease. *American Journal of Medicine*, (Suppl.), 48-55.

Grundy, S.M. (1990). *Cholesterol and atherosclerosis: Diagnosis and treatment*. Philadelphia: Lippincott.

Hall, S.M., Bass, A., & Monroe, J. (1978). Continued contact and monitoring as follow-up strategies: A long-term study of obesity treatment. *Addictive Behaviors*, **3**, 139-147.

Hammermeister, K.E., DeRouen, T.A., & Dodge, H.T. (1979). Variables predictive of survival in patients with coronary disease: Selection of univariate and multivariate analyses from clinical, electrocardiographic, exercise, angiographic and quantitative angiographic evaluation. *Circulation*, **59**, 421-430.

Haskell, W.L. (1978). Cardiovascular complications during exercise training of cardiac patients. *Circulation*, **57**, 920-924.

Hawkins, R.C., & Clement, P. (1980). Development and construct validation of a self-report measure of binge eating tendencies. *Addictive Behaviors*, **5**, 219-226.

Haynes, S.G., Feinleib, M., & Kannel, W.B. (1980). The relationship of psycho-social factors to coronary heart disease in the Framingham study. *American Journal of Epidemiology*, **11**, 37-58.

Hess, O.M., Schneider, J., Nongi, H., Carroll, J.D., Schneider, K., Turina, M., & Krayen-buehl, H.P. (1988). Myocardial structure in patients with exercise-induced ischemia. *Circulation*, **77**, 967-977.

Holbrook, J.H., Grundy, S.M., Hennekens, C.H., Kannel, J.W.B., & Strong, J.P. (1984). Cigarette smoking and cardiovascular diseases. *Circulation*, **70**, 1114A-1117A.

Hossack, K.F., & Hartwig, R. (1982). Cardiac arrest associated with supervised cardiac rehabilitation. *Journal of Cardiac Rehabilitation*, **2**, 402-408.

Hubert, H.B., Feinleib, M., McNamara, P.M., & Castelli, W.P. (1983). Obesity as an independent risk factor for cardiovascular disease: A 26 year follow-up of participants in the Framingham Heart Study. *Circulation*, **67**, 968-976.

Hung, J., Goris, M.L., Nash, E., Kraemer, H.C., & DeBusk, R.F. (1984). Comparative value of maximal treadmill testing, exercise thallium myocardial perfusion scintigraphy, and exercise radionuclide ventriculography for distinguishing high and low risk patients soon after myocardial infarction. *American Journal of Cardiology*, **53**, 1221-1227.

Hunt, W.A., Barnett, L.W., & Branch, L.G. (1971). Relapse rates in addiction programs. *Journal of Clinical Psychology*, **27**, 455-456.

Jackson, A.S., & Pollock, M.L. (1978). Generalized equations for predicting body density of men. *British Journal of Nutrition*, **40**, 497-504.

Jackson, A.S., Pollock, M.L., & Ward, A. (1980). Generalized equations for predicting body density of women. *Medicine and Science in Sports and Exercise*, **12**, 175-182.

Jaffe, D.T., & Scott, C.D. (1988). *Take this job and love it*. New York: Simon & Schuster.

Joint Commission on Accreditation of Healthcare Organizations. (1990). *Accreditation manual for hospitals*. Chicago: Author.

Joint National Committee on the Detection, Evaluation, and Treatment of High Blood Pressure. (1984). The 1984 report of the Joint National Committee on the Detection, Evaluation, and Treatment of High Blood Pressure. *Archives of Internal Medicine*, **144**, 1045-1056.

Jugdutt, B.I., Michbrowski, B.L., & Kappagoda, C.T. (1988). Exercise training after anterior Q wave infarction: Importance of regional left ventricular function and topography. *Journal of American College of Cardiology*, **12**, 362-372.

Kallio, V., Hamalainen, H., Hakkila, J., & Luurila, O.J. (1979). Reduction in sudden deaths by a multifactorial intervention programme after acute myocardial infarction. *Lancet*, **2**, 1091-1094.

Kannel, W.B., Castelli, W.P., & Gordon, T. (1979). Cholesterol in the prediction of atherosclerotic disease. New perspectives based on the Framingham study. *Journal of Internal Medicine*, **90**, 85-91.

Kannel, W.B., Gordon, T., Sorlie, P., & McNamara, P.M. (1971). Physical activity and coronary vulnerability: The Framingham study. *Cardiology Digest*, **6**, 28-32.

Kannel, W.B., & McGee, D.L. (1979). Diabetes and cardiovascular disease: The Framingham study. *Journal of the American Medical Association*, **241**, 2035-2038.

Kannel, W.B., Sorlie, P., Castelli, W.P., & McGee, D. (1980). Blood pressure and survival after myocardial infarction: The Framingham study. *American Journal of Cardiology*, **45**, 326-330.

Karvetti, R.L. (1981). Effects of nutrition education: Changes in the diet of myocardial infarction patients. *Journal of the American Dietetic Association*, **79**, 660-668.

Kazdin, A.E. (1976). Effects of covert modeling, multiple models, and model reinforcement on assertive behaviors. *Behavior Therapy*, **7**, 211-222.

Khaw, K.T., & Barrett-Connor, E. (1986). Family history of heart attack: A modifiable risk factor? *Circulation*, **74**, 239-244.

Krone, R.J., Gillespie, J.A., Weld, F.M., Miller, J.P., & Moss, A. (1985). Low level exercise testing after myocardial infarction: Usefulness in enhancing clinical risk stratification. *Circulation*, **57**, 64-70.

Leon, A.S., Certo, C., Comoss, P., Franklin, B.A., Froelicher, V.F., Haskell, W.L., Hellerstein, H.K., Marley, W.P., Pollock, M.L., Ries, A., Sivarajan Froelicher, E., & Smith, L.K. (1990). Scientific evidence of the value of cardiac rehabilitation services with emphasis on patients following myocardial infarction: Section 1. Exercise conditioning component. *Journal of Cardiopulmonary Rehabilitation*, **10**, 79-87.

Levy, R.L. (1977). Relationship of an overt commitment to task compliance in behavior therapy. *Journal of Behavior Therapy and Experimental Psychiatry*, **8**, 25-29.

MacDowall, J.M., Dembroski, T.M., Dimsdale, J.E., & Hackett, T.P. (1985). Components of Type A, hostility and anger. Further relationships to angiographic findings. *Health Psychology*, **4**(23), 137-152.

Madsen, E.B., Gilpin, E., Henning, H., Ahnve, S., LeWinter, M., Ceruto, W., Joswig, W., Collins, D., Pitt, W., & Ross, J. (1984). Prediction of late mortality after myocardial infarction from variables measured at different times during hospitalization. *American Journal of Cardiology*, **53**, 47-54.

Mark, D.F., Hlatky, M.A., Harrell, F.E., Lee, K.L., Califf, R.M., & Pryor, D.F. (1987). Exercise treadmill score for predicting prognosis in coronary artery disease. *Annals of Internal Medicine*, **106**, 793-800.

Marlatt, G.A., & Gordon, J.R. (Eds.) (1985). *Relapse prevention: Maintenance strategies in the treatment of addictive behaviors*. New York: Guilford Press.

Martin, J.E., & Dubbert, P.M. (1984). Behavioral management strategies for improving health and fitness. *Journal of Cardiac Rehabilitation*, **4**, 200-208.

Matthews, K.A., & Haynes, S.G. (1986). Type A behavior pattern and coronary disease risk: Update and critical evaluation. *American Journal of Epidemiology*, **123**, 923-960.

McNeer, J.F., Margolis, J.R., Lee, K.L., Kisslo, J.A., Peter, R.H., Kong, Y., Behar, V.S., Wallace, A.G., McCants, C.B., & Rusati, R.A. (1978). Role of the exercise test in evaluating patients for ischemic heart disease. *Circulation*, **57**, 64-70.

Mitchell, M., Franklin, B., Johnson, S., & Rubenfire, M. (1984). Cardiac exercise programs: Role of continuous electrocardiographic monitoring. *Archives of Physical Medicine and Rehabilitation*, **65**, 463-466.

Morley, D., Ribisl, P.M., & Miller, H.S. (1984). A comparison of patient education methodologies in outpatient cardiac rehabilitation. *Journal of Cardiac Rehabilitation*, **4**, 434-439.

Morris, J.N. (1953). Coronary heart disease and physical activity of work. *Lancet*, **2**, 1053.

Morris, J.N., Everitt, M.G., Pollard, R., Chave, S., & Semmence, A. (1980). Vigorous exercise in leisure time: Protection against coronary heart disease. *Lancet*, **2**, 1207-1210.

National Institute of Health. (1985). Lowering blood cholesterol to prevent heart disease. National Institute of Health consensus development conference statement. *Journal of the American Medical Association*, **253**, 2080-2086.

Nezu, A.M., & D'Zurilla, T.J. (1981). Effects of problem definition and formulation on the generation of alternatives in the social problem-solving process. *Cognitive Therapy and Research*, **5**, 265-271.

Nicod, P., Gilpin, E., Dittrich, H., Polikar, R., Itjalmarson, A., Blacky, A.R., Henning, H., & Ross, J. (1989). Short and long-term clinical outcome after Q wave and non–Q wave myocardial infarction in a large patient population. *Circulation*, **79**, 528-536.

O'Connor, G.T., Buring, J.E., Yusuf, S., Goldhaber, S.Z., Olmstead, E.M., Paffenbarger, R.S., & Hennekens, C.H. (1989). An overview of randomized trials of rehabilitation with exercise after myocardial infarction. *Circulation*, **80**, 234-244.

Oldridge, N.B. (1984). Compliance and dropout in cardiac exercise rehabilitation. *Journal of Cardiac Rehabilitation*, **4**, 166-177.

Paffenbarger, R.S., & Hale, W.E. (1975). Work activity and coronary heart mortality. *New England Journal of Medicine*, **292**, 545-550.

Paffenbarger, R.S., Wing, A.L., & Hyde, R.T. (1978). Physical activity as an index of heart attack risk in college alumni. *American Journal of Epidemiology*, **108**, 161-175.

Perri, M.G., & Richards, C.S. (1977). An investigation of naturally occurring episodes of self-controlled behaviors. *Journal of Counseling Psychology*, **24**, 178-183.

Peters, R.K., Cody, L.D., Fischoff, D.P., Bernstein, L., & Pike, M.C. (1983). Physical fitness and subsequent myocardial infarction in healthy workers. *Journal of the American Medical Association*, **249**, 3052-3056.

Powell, K.E., Thompson, P.D., Caspersen, C.J., & Kendrick, J.S. (1987). Physical activity and the incidence of coronary heart disease. *Annual Review of Public Health*, **8**, 253-287.

Reardon, M.F., Nestel, P.J., Craig, I.H., & Harper, R.W. (1985). Lipoprotein predictors of the severity of coronary artery disease in men and women. *Circulation*, **71**, 881-888.

Rifkind, B.M., & Segal, P. (1983). Lipid research clinics program reference values for hyperlipidemia and hypolipidemia. *Journal of American Medical Association*, **250**, 1869-1872.

Robbins, A. (1986). *Unlimited power: The new science of personal achievement*. New York: Simon & Schuster.

Robbins, A. (1989). *Certification training: Power of choice*. Unpublished seminar material, Robbins Research Institute, San Diego.

Rosenberg, L., Kaufman, D.W., Helmrich, S.P., & Shapiro, S. (1985). The risk of myocardial infarction after quitting smoking in men under 55 years of age. *New England Journal of Medicine*, **312**, 1511-1514.

Russell, M.L. (1986). *Behavioral counseling in medicine: Strategies for modifying at-risk behavior*. New York: Oxford University Press.

Snowden, C.B., McNamara, P.M., Garrison, R.J., Feinleib, M., Kannel, W.B., & Epstein, F.H. (1982). Predicting coronary disease in siblings— A multivariate assessment. *American Journal of Epidemiology*, **11**, 217-222.

Sparrow, D., Dawber, T.R., & Cotton, T. (1978). The influence of cigarette smoking on prognosis after myocardial infarction. *Journal of Chronic Disease, 31,* 425-432.

Thase, M.E., & Moss, M.K. (1976). The relative efficacy of covert modeling procedures and guided participant modeling on the reduction of avoidance behavior. *Journal of Behavior Therapy and Experimental Psychiatry, 7,* 7-12.

Truett, J., Cornfield, J., & Kannel, W. (1967). A multivariate analysis of the risk of coronary heart diseases in Framingham. *Journal of Chronic Diseases, 20,* 511-524.

Uhl, G.S., & Froelicher, V.F. (1983). Screening for asymptomatic coronary artery disease. *Journal of American College of Cardiology, 1,* 946-955.

Van Camp, S.P., & Peterson, R.A. (1989). Identification of the high risk cardiac rehabilitation patient. *Journal of Cardiopulmonary Rehabilitation, 9,* 103-109.

Waitley, D. (1983). *Seeds of greatness: The ten best kept secrets of total success.* Old Tappan, NJ: Revell.

Waters, D.D., Bosch, X., Bouchard, A., Morse, A., Roy, D., Pelletier, G., & Theroux, P. (1985). Comparison of clinical variables and variables derived from a limited predischarge exercise test as predictors of early and late mortality after myocardial infarction. *Journal of the American College of Cardiology, 5*(1), 1-8.

Watson, D.L., & Tharp, R.G. (1989). *Self-directed behavior: Self-modification for personal adjustment.* Pacific Grove, CA: Brooks/Cole.

Weiner, D.A., Ryan, T.J., McCabe, C.H., Luk, S., Chaitman, B.R., Sheffield, L.T., Fisher, L.D., & Tristani, F. (1987). Value of exercise test in determining the risk classification in the response to coronary artery bypass grafting in three vessel coronary artery disease: A report from the CASS registry. *American Journal of Cardiology, 60*(4), 262-266.

Wenger, N.K. (1989). Rehabilitation of the patient with coronary heart disease. New information for improved care. *Postgraduate Medicine, 85,* 369-380.

Wenger, N.K., Balady, G.J., Cohn, L.H., Hartley, H., King, S.B., Miller, H.S., & Weiner, D.A. (1990). *Cardiac rehabilitation services following PTCA and valvular surgery: Guidelines for use.* Position statement to the National Center for Health Services Research. American College of Cardiology.

Wortman, C.B., & Dintzer, L. (1978). Is an attributional analysis of the learned helplessness phenomenon variable? A critique of the Abramson-Seligman-Teasdale reformulation. *Journal of Abnormal Psychology, 87,* 75-90.

Chapter 3

Phases I and II: Practical Application

Linda K. Hall, PhD

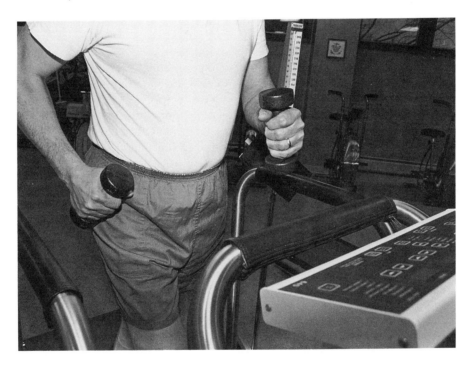

In chapters 1 and 2 you were introduced to the types of patients referred to a cardiac rehabilitation program, methods of evaluating these patients, and designs for beginning cardiac rehabilitation and changing behavior. This chapter deals with the methodology of creating Phase I and Phase II programs, obtaining referrals from physicians, and moving the patient through the therapeutic plan.

Learning Objectives
1. To recognize the mechanisms of patient referral
2. To establish an orderly plan for applying case management techniques to patients in Phases I and II

3. To develop general guidelines for progressing patients from/to Phases I, II, III, and IV

4. To identify some examples of educational materials for patients and families in Phases I and II

Cardiac rehabilitation has evolved over the last 30 years into a model that has generally been traditional in its application of a fairly rigid therapy to all patients. This therapy was formulated based on patient populations that are now classified as "low risk" or those who went through the hospital with an unremarkable clinical course or experienced no medical, physiological, or anatomical complications. But with the accumulation of experience and research, cardiac rehab is moving toward an application model that focuses on the intermediate- and high-risk populations who need rehabilitation and our time, attention, and resources. For example, as few as 3 years ago exercise would not have been prescribed for a patient who had an ejection fraction below 30%. Now a large number of patients have that clinical parameter and are being prescribed exercise.

The focus on intermediate- and high-risk patients has brought a transition from a very structured, itemized program for each patient, with exercise regimented and strictly controlled, to a case-managed program that can be adjusted as the disease, patient, progress, or signs and symptoms indicate. We can use our skill and experience in conjunction with the many modalities available to better accomplish patient-specific goals.

You should be beginning to see the changes occurring in the management of patients. In chapters 1 and 2, neither author talked about a specific prescription or a way in which to "step" a patient through a specific phase because practicing case management cardiac rehabilitation precludes this. I suggest you work back and forth between chapters 1 and 2 and this one as I show you methods of implementing the programs needed for the models that have been outlined. I will be describing not only the program but also a philosophy of cardiac rehabilitation that will guide the program. The inpatient mechanics I discuss are for the most part the structure of the program at Allegheny General Hospital, Pittsburgh, Pennsylvania, and the outpatient mechanics are in place at both Allegheny General and The Christ Hospital, Cincinnati, Ohio. I use these programs because I have directed both and have worked with their staffs to evolve case management rehabilitation programs that reflect current standards (AACVPR, 1991; ACSM, 1991; AHA, 1990)

Inpatient Cardiac Rehabilitation

To apply cardiac rehabilitation, you need patients. Rehab cannot start without a physician's referral because applying an exercise therapy to a patient is considered practicing medicine. Once you have established your policies and procedures and have applied rehabilitation on a case-by-case referral basis, physicians will begin to trust your program and increase their referrals (see Table 3.1). Standing orders from cardiovascular surgeons make sense because surgery patients are more likely to be a homogenous group. Referral orders from cardiologists, internists, and family practice physicians should be made case by case. Because case management means risk stratification and individualized therapy, not every patient is a candidate for cardiac rehabilitation.

Exercising the Patient

Exercise medium- to high-risk or markedly debilitated patients daily, or twice daily, as the case dictates. In some cases it helps for both physical therapy and cardiac rehabilitation staff members to visit the same patient, providing, for example, both gait training and endurance training.

Prescribing exercise in the inpatient setting requires a judgment call based on what the patient is experiencing at the moment. If the patient's condition is stable, start her on a program that increases in duration and intensity each day. If she is having rhythm problems such as ventricular tachycardia or blood pressure problems such as hypotension or hypertension, or if she is very tired and weak, adjust exercise accordingly (e.g., cancel exercise or have her exercise at the bedside).

Table 3.1 Procedures for Enhancing Physician Referrals

1. Establish a focus group of physicians who will provide you with information about what to include in your department policies and procedures. Ask them what they require in a program in order to refer to it.
2. Use current guidelines (AACVPR, 1991; ACSM, 1991; AHA, 1990) to set up your policies and procedures, and make the guidelines available to all physicians who would refer to your program.
3. Have your medical director conduct a yearly grand rounds to update physicians about new procedures or services.
4. Conduct in-service seminars on all cardiac floors within the hospital to keep all care givers informed about cardiac rehabilitation. Remember, these people communicate with physicians.
5. Practice state-of-the-art cardiac rehabilitation and accept only referrals that are appropriate for your service.
6. Communicate with and ask for advice from the referring physician regarding patient medical problems.
7. Understand each physician's practice model and also her own lifestyle habits; approach the physician from that perspective.

Nurse and physician notes will tell you a lot about the patient's medical condition. Also, you should talk with the patient and look for signs and symptoms. Is her skin pink? When you press the skin does it go white and then turn pink? Is the patient breathless, panting, or puffing? Is there a hint of pain in her eyes? Is she flinching and wincing beyond what is normal? Is her pulse rapid? How is her blood pressure? Can she move from lying to sitting to standing slowly? Is she nauseous? If you conducted an in-depth initial consult as was described in chapter 1, you will have a baseline from which to start each day. The patient should feel better and should have more energy and fewer problems each day.

Progress the patient each day, increasing her exercise capacity and getting her ready to face the physical environment that going home will present. Use the hospital stairs between floors for stair-climbing practice, and indicate when the patient may practice alone. Bicycle ergometers are useful for patients who have difficulty walking.

Prior to a patient's discharge, the inpatient exercise specialist meets with the patient to discuss a plan for activity and for resuming usual activities of daily living when he gets home. The specialist gives him written instructions, activity

SAMPLE PROCEDURE

Anytime a patient is registered at Allegheny General Hospital for cardiothoracic surgery, information about the patient becomes available over the computer system that is connected throughout the hospital. The Cardiac Rehabilitation Department gets a daily surgery schedule and has standing orders to see anyone scheduled for cardiothoracic surgery. The consulting physician may order cardiology consults which are typed into the computer by the ward manager. The cardiac rehabilitation clinical coordinator assigns the patient to a specific staff member in the department. Staff members carry 7 to 10 cases on their daily work sheets. Seven to eight of the patients are active and are seen daily, and the rest are inactive cases, for example, patients who are staying in surgical or medical intensive care for prolonged periods and are not being actively rehabilitated on the floor. Once a patient is assigned to a staff member, the patient stays with that same staff member throughout his stay in the

hospital. The initial consult is the first meeting, when the thorough examination discussed in chapter 1 is completed. Particular attention is paid to what the patient wants to know and accomplish. Also the staff member becomes a resource for the family of the patient.

Each day the staff member reviews the chart for any updates on laboratory and test results, medication changes, or changes in patient status that may have arisen since the previous visit. The staff member starts each visit with a check to see how the patient is feeling emotionally, mentally, and physically. At that time the staff member applies therapy according to changes in the patient's clinical, mental, and emotional status. Often a patient who qualifies as low risk (DeBusk et al., 1986) is exercised with a staff member for 2 or 3 days and then assigned to exercise on her own. Staff members check on the patient on a regular basis, education continues, and family questions and problems are addressed.

guidelines, a 6-week at-home walking program, and an introduction to the American Heart Association diet (see Appendix A).

Education and Risk Intervention

Inpatient cardiac rehabilitation programs traditionally have set incredibly high goals for patient education and risk factor intervention. When patients are tested to see what they remember, quite often they score lower than 60%. Make a list of all of the areas of information you are able to teach and provide materials for (see Table 3.2), and ask patients to rank the areas according to what they believe they need to know before being discharged. Use these rankings as guidelines for patient education. Patients will attend to what they want to know and will not pay any attention to information that doesn't interest them.

It is essential to instruct patients about what to do when they get home. Each patient should set a daily schedule, such as the following: get up, bathe, dress (this is important, because getting

Table 3.2 Patient Education Preference List

_____ What exactly happened to my heart, and what will I feel if it happens again?

_____ What should I do if I experience the heart pain and problems that I had the first time?

_____ What will I be able to do when I go home from the hospital?

_____ When will I be able to resume sexual activity?

_____ Will I be able to play golf, garden, mow the grass, and be active again?

_____ When can I go back to work?

_____ How can I quit smoking?

_____ How can I reduce my cholesterol levels?

_____ How can I lose weight?

_____ How can I reduce my salt intake?

_____ What is stress, and how can I moderate it?

_____ How should I start exercising?

_____ How can I manage my blood pressure better?

_____ Why am I sad, depressed, or angry? How do I deal with it?

_____ How do these testing procedures work: catheterization, treadmills, thallium, cardiac ECG pacing?

_____ How do pacemakers and Cardiac Care Unit machines work?

dressed means the patient is well, and staying in pajamas means that she isn't), rest, eat breakfast, rest, do light housework, rest, exercise, rest, eat lunch, rest, exercise, rest, and so forth.

Outpatient Cardiac Rehabilitation

When should patients start Phase II? When and if the physician orders it. Patients are able to start exercise with no increased morbidity or mortality the day after they are discharged. For patients at Mount Sinai in Milwaukee, Wisconsin, and the Mayo Clinic in Rochester, Minnesota, the last inpatient visit is a scheduled session in the outpatient clinic, and Phase II begins 1 or 2 days after patients have gone home. The AACVPR (1991) guidelines recommend that Phase II begin within 2 weeks of the patient's discharge. A low-risk patient who is home for 6 weeks before he starts rehabilitation may return to unhealthy habits, such as smoking, not exercising, overeating, and eating high-fat foods. However, a patient who does exercise and is in adequate condition to return to work may not require physical rehabilitation. It's possible that after you interview the patient, assess his intervention into his own risk factors, and determine the activity level he has achieved and the level he wants to achieve, you may decide that cardiac rehabilitation is not necessary. If this is the decision, refer the patient back to the physician and leave your phone number with the patient in case he has questions about exercise. This is an ethically responsible practice and may have positive long-term consequences for your program, because the physician will appreciate your nonintervention.

Phase II is a prescribed exercise and educational intervention for which the patient must have a physician referral. Phase II services are billed with current physician terminology (CPT) codes that are described as physician services (see chapter 12). Because of the CPT code regulations, the medical director or medical advisory board must play an integral part in the rehabilitation program. Exercise tests require the interpretation of a physician, exercise prescriptions are noted and signed by a physician, and any change in the patient's program that indicates a change in therapy is reported to and initialed by a physician. A physician must be available in the area for any emergency.

The AACVPR (1991) and the AHA (1990) guidelines recommend that all patients be risk stratified (see pages 44-46, chapter 2) and exercise therapy be applied accordingly. Risk stratification requires the Phase II program to operate on a case management basis rather than the old concept of 36 sessions for all patients. The AACVPR guidelines include a list of clinical criteria for monitoring/nonmonitoring (essentially, those who are in the high-risk category are monitored). The AHA establishes that a low-risk patient does not need monitoring, and a moderate- or high-risk patient may be monitored for 6 to 12 sessions or until the patient has a stable response.

Following is a recommended process for case management in Phase II.

1. The patient is referred to rehabilitation with a physician's written referral note. A recent (within 1 month) graded exercise test (GXT) accompanies the patient, or one is ordered.

2. A case manager or therapist is assigned to the patient and interviews the patient for salient data not already included in the patient's chart: risk factor history, exercise and recreational history, work history, information about what the patient likes to do and wants to do, physical limitations, cognitive limitations, and emotional stability. (Cognitive and emotional limitations are usually uncovered through observation of nonverbal cues.)

3. The case manager prescribes exercise that will condition and strengthen the patient so she can return to the activities of her choosing. The patient chooses risk factors to be addressed, and the case manager develops an education program using the behavior change strategies outlined in chapter 2. The case manager must strictly adhere to the AACVPR (1991), ACSM (1991), and AHA (1990) guidelines when determining risk stratification and when monitoring patients.

A number of companies have designed very sophisticated monitoring systems that allow hospitals to monitor patients while they exercise at home. According to the AHA (1990), "Such programs have the disadvantage of lacking immediately available emergency medical care, but the advantage of no required clinic visit. The equipment is not generally available, but these programs would be particularly useful in following up high-risk cases in which clinics are not readily available" (p. 2316). Patients can be monitored in a similar and much less expensive way with transtelephone ECG monitoring that uses finger telemeters. A hospital that purchases an expensive monitoring machine can make a great deal of money by monitoring all of the potential Phase II patients who live too far away from the hospital to attend clinic programs. However, all of the current guidelines recommend monitoring only high-risk patients (AACVPR, 1991; AHA, 1990).

The lengths of the exercise and education programs are determined by the patient's progress. If the patient has been a lifelong exerciser, the exercise program may last as few as two or three visits, perhaps with the patient returning once every 4 weeks for a progress check or if the patient has questions or feels the need for a visit. The same patient may be in an educational program for stress management that runs once or twice a week for 6 weeks. But a patient who is terribly debilitated, has a low ejection fraction, and has no history of exercise may attend a Phase II class for 6 to 10 weeks. Or, she could be monitored until all parameters are stable in response, and stay in the Phase II class until she reaches a conditioning plateau. At that point the patient may progress to Phase III and on to Phase IV; this transition is individualized to meet the patient's needs and desires.

Additionally, the patient may vary exercise modes for enjoyment and may vary the method of using the exercise mode (e.g., using different walking speeds and grades, pedaling speeds and resistance, or rowing speeds and distance) to meet the same MET levels. Interval and fartlek training techniques can be used for most patients to provide an interesting workout. For example, walking 3 to 3.5 mph at zero grade is around 3 to 3.5 METs; the patient can achieve the same MET level by walking 1.7 to 2.5 mph at 2.5% grade or 1.7 to 2.0 mph at 5% grade. Be sure to train patients to run their own equipment. Check the speeds, grades, and work loads as you move around the room and talk with the patients. Monitor a patient's first two to three visits closely to make sure that the patient understands getting on and off, starting and selecting speeds, and work loads. Give patients "stop exercise" guidelines relative to heart rate, breathing, and general feelings of their bodies. Is the patient sweating, panting, or out of breath? Does she feel pain in arm and leg muscles? Is there chest pain? Educate the patient when to stop based not only on heart rate but also on a general total body feeling and a perception of the effort of exertion.

Case Management Tip

If you are going to case manage the patient, how can you be with the patient during exercise, watch the monitor, and take rhythm strips? Turn the monitor around, get out from behind the monitor and on the exercise floor, and take strips and blood pressures only once during each mode of exercise or when symptoms warrant. When my staff members were instructed to do this they became concerned that they might miss V-tach or some other untoward rhythm. I suggested that they would be better able to handle a patient who was compromised by the rhythm if they were standing next to the patient rather than sitting behind the ECG monitor. Monitors have alarms and will print ECG strips when the rhythm indicates it needs to print. Being beside the patient talking to him results in better education and more rapid progress and also allows you to intercede faster when trouble does arise. See Figure 3.1 for the new method we use at Allegheny General Hospital for charting exercise progress for patients in Phase II. Yes, we do take ECG strips, date and code them, staple them together, and enter them into the patient's chart. One ECG strip is taken per mode and at entry and exit, or to document a rhythm disturbance.

The Exercise Prescription

What type of exercise should you prescribe, and how should you monitor it? Chapter 5 describes exercise prescription for all phases of cardiac rehabilitation. You must understand exercise physiology and a healthy person's physiological responses to exercise. It is also important to understand the pathology of heart disease and the effects of that pathology on physiological function. Through exercise, attempt to move the patient from the pathology end of the continuum toward the healthy response end. Refer to chapter 5 for specifics of exercise prescription.

Transitions From Phase to Phase

With the publication of the AACVPR (1991) guidelines and the separation of exercise and education, case management has become one of the new ways of implementing the mandates of the guidelines. A major question that practitioners face is, How will I know when the patient needs to move from Phase II to Phase III and from III to IV? All patients are different and therefore will progress at different speeds, both in physical reconditioning and

lifestyle changes. Following are questions to ask when you transition patients from phase to phase or discharge them to their own programs to be done at home or at an exercise facility of their choice.

1. Has the patient reached a plateau in his exercise conditioning? Is he able to increase the intensity of his exercise?
2. Has the patient reached a level of exercise intensity that allows her to return to work, reenter recreational activities as she wishes, and feel good about energy levels and her control of daily exercise/activity programs?
3. Has the patient achieved the goals that he set at the beginning of Phase II for exercise, activity, and conditioning?
4. What does the patient want to do next: stay in an organized program, go to a community fitness facility, or be responsible for her own program?
5. What is the patient's status regarding his risk factors? Is he compliant, in control, in need of help, seeing dietitians or smoking counselors, or working in stress management programs?

Patients will know when they are ready to transition, and you will too. The important thing is to not keep them too long; get them back to controlling their own lives.

At Allegheny General we administer all four phases and have set limits on the length of time patients may stay in Phase III. We found that some patients developed umbilical-cord relationships with our department and eventually "owned" exercise slots in our program. When we wanted to move these patients or put Phase II patients in their slots, we had some very angry "regulars." Because of that we have now separated all of our phases, holding classes for each phase on different days of the week. Patients may remain in Phase III for 6 months and then must transition to some other program, exercise on their own, or move to Phase IV.

Conclusion

Due to the introduction of risk stratification, cardiac rehabilitation is now conducted from a case management perspective which is relative to actual application of therapy. It is no longer "36 monitored sessions whether the patient likes it or not." Each person is a special case with an individualized program. The program is developed

Exercise Summary—Phase II and III Programs

Name: _____ Age: _____ THR: _____ FC: _____ Lipid date: _____ MD: _____

History: _____

_____

Risk factors: _____   Medication(s): _____

Education sessions: 1 2 3 4 5 6 7 8 9 10

Goal: _____

Plan: _____

Evaluation: _____

Goal: _____

Plan: _____

Evaluation: _____

Goal: _____

Plan: _____

Evaluation: _____

Note: _____

Date/ weight	Entry						Exercise I						Exercise II						Exercise III					Exit	
	HR	BP		Mode	HR	BP	RPE	Min	Mode	HR	BP	RPE	Min	Mode	HR	BP	RPE	Min	Mode	HR	BP	RPE	Min	HR	BP
1)																									
Comments:																						Signature:			

Date/ weight	Entry						Exercise I						Exercise II						Exercise III					Exit	
	HR	BP		Mode	HR	BP	RPE	Min	Mode	HR	BP	RPE	Min	Mode	HR	BP	RPE	Min	Mode	HR	BP	RPE	Min	HR	BP
2)																									
Comments:																						Signature:			

Figure 3.1 Exercise summary form. (THR = target training heart rate; FC = functional capacity; HR = heart rate; BP = blood pressure; and RPE = rate of perceived exertion). *Note.* Repeat through 10 sessions.

From Allegheny General Hospital. Reprinted by permission.

by the patient, the physician, and the exercise leader with special attention paid to the patient's wishes regarding return to work and recreational activities and his or her interest in particular risk factor reduction. Clear and concise descriptions of methods to reduce risk factors are contained in chapter 2. Risk factor reduction is perhaps the most critical area on which the therapist must focus. Behavior change is a process, not an event. Thus, risk factor reduction takes hard work, time, and individualized effort.

References

American Association of Cardiovascular and Pulmonary Rehabilitation. (1991). *Guidelines for cardiac rehabilitation*. Champaign, IL: Human Kinetics.

American College of Sports Medicine. (1991). *Guidelines for exercise testing and prescription* (4th ed.). Philadelphia: Lea & Febiger.

American College of Sports Medicine. (1988). *Resource manual for guidelines for exercise testing and prescription*. Philadelphia: Lea & Febiger.

DeBusk, R.F., Blomqvist, C.G., Kouchoukos, N.T., Luepker, R.V., Miller, H.S., Moss, A.J., Pollock, M.L., Reeves, T.J., Selvester, R.H., Stason, W.B., Wagner, G.S., & Willman, V.L. (1986). Identification and treatment of low-risk patients after acute myocardial infarction and coronary-artery bypass graft surgery. *New England Journal of Medicine*, **314**, 161-166.

Fletcher, G.F., Froelicher, V.F., Hartley, L.H., Haskell, W.L., & Pollock, M.L. (1990). Exercise standards: A statement for health professionals from the American Heart Association. *Circulation*, **82**, 2286-2322.

Chapter 4

Outpatient Maintenance

Ruth E. Townsend, MS
Linda K. Hall, PhD

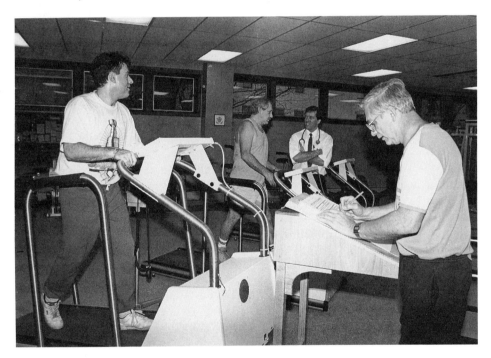

This chapter shows how you can help the patient comply by providing a program that maintains what the patient has accomplished in Phase II and allows a little more latitude in the way the patient accomplishes goals. After providing some historical background, the chapter describes program options you may consider as you develop the Phase III and Phase IV programs. Additionally, this chapter poses some questions that practitioners in the field should ask and some possible answers to those questions.

Learning Objectives

1. To recognize the traditional model of Phase III/Phase IV cardiac rehabilitation programs

2. To question the structure of current Phase III/Phase IV programs

3. To suggest some alternative solutions to methods and structure that are already in place

We'd like to thank Kathy Berra for her input and editing assistance on this chapter.

According to Wenger (1984), one should look at rehabilitation efforts in relation to the patient's phase of illness, because the patient's need for care varies considerably from phase to phase. Phases III and IV of the cardiac rehabilitation continuum may be thought of as maintenance of an exercise and lifestyle habits program. Ideally, regular activity/exercise and healthy lifestyle habits such as eating a low-fat diet, reducing stress, and not smoking begin in the Phase I (chapter 1) and Phase II (chapter 2) programs. The maintenance phases continue the efforts begun in Phases I and II and play an important role in the reinforcement of healthy lifestyles as well as the prevention of lapse and relapse behaviors.

Historical Perspective

With the advent of risk stratification, there may be significant changes in the structure and function of Phases III and IV, which may mean that rather than the description of Phases II, II, and IV, the delineation may need to become inpatient and outpatient. Formalized programs of cardiac rehabilitation began in the 1960s. At that time the key objective of most programs was preparing the individual for return to work, and quite often a number of these programs were funded by research grants and government sources. For example, the Cardiopulmonary Research Institute (CAPRI) in the state of Washington was partially funded by the Washington/Alaska Regional Medical Program to develop answers to some basic organizational problems. Eventually these programs moved from research and study to health care delivery, because grant support was reduced and they had to become self-supporting (Pyfer & Doane, 1973). Most patients who went through these programs were able to return to sedentary jobs at 6 to 10 weeks post-MI and to more physical or stressful positions at 10 to 14 weeks post-MI (Naughton, 1973). In the 1970s and early 1980s the patients were typically referred to the program at 12 to 24 weeks post-MI. At this time graded exercise testing was becoming more prevalent, and the tests were used as en-

try criteria for outpatient cardiac rehab programs at all levels (Wilson, Fardy, & Froelicher, 1981).

In the late 1960s and early 1970s, patients were typically referred by their physicians and were encouraged to participate for 3 to 6 months. Historically, dropout or noncompliance was a problem; however, a fair number of patients remained in the maintenance phase indefinitely, as they do now. After reviewing studies from 1976 through 1986, the National Center for Health Services Research and Health Care Technology Assessment (1987) concluded that the average compliance to a program for a lifetime is about 33%. Here we ask the first question in reviewing or restructuring thinking related to Phases III and IV. Is not 33% an excellent number? Does it perhaps reflect the number of clients who may select an ongoing organized program? Maybe an additional 33% are exercising at home without need for an organized program, which means that 66% of patients may be compliant. We may need to review what we are asking of our patients. Not everyone will need or want an organized program; not everyone will be able to get to an organized program. Maybe we need to work with patients to give them every avenue to select exercise/activity programs that will work for them, whether programs involve organized groups or individual at-home programs.

The major difference seen in the long-term outpatient programs of the 1980s and 1990s compared to earlier years may lie in the speed with which some patients transition into those programs. The new guidelines from the AACVPR (1991) and the AHA (1990) indicate that the need for monitoring and surveillance differs with risk stratification, and some low-risk patients will arrive in Phase III programs much sooner (see chapter 2).

Current Programs

Phase III/Phase IV cardiac rehabilitation programs are ideally extensions of the Phase II program but in many cases are the beginning of the rehabilitation process for cardiac patients. Therefore, before maintenance can take place, participants need to achieve optimal functional capacity. Additionally, they may need to attain an educational foundation and an understanding of behavior change practices. For a number of patients these new behaviors include the following:

- Compliance with medication regimens
- Compliance with a number of behavioral changes such as
  - a low-fat, low-salt, low-cholesterol diet,
  - smoking cessation,
  - increases in daily exercise and activity,
  - managing stress, and
  - weight loss
- Taking responsibility for their own health care

These goals and objectives appear to cover a broad spectrum of activities and education and to require well-trained and educated staff. However, these goals are within the capabilities of community programs. Quite often community programs serve a large number of patients who may have limited funds or insurance coverage, or patients for whom hospital facilities are geographically inaccessible. Additionally, these programs may occur in facilities with multiple programs that may include other family members.

Program Design

The first things we should look at are the goals and objectives of the organization undertaking the development of the program. In developing a program you must address several questions, and a later section of this text will help you know which questions to ask and why (see Introduction to Part II). The questions should be broadly stated to include total community perspectives, for example, Is this type of service needed in the community? Will the medical community support this type of program? Is my facility respected for its ability to provide adult health education and lifestyle programs? Will I be able to draw on the medical community for support in the form of referrals as well as administrative support?

If your program is a community program in a building separate from a hospital and in a facility that has other programs, you will need to consider questions such as space availability, parking and commuter access, showers, locker rooms, safety, equipment, and the breadth of activities as well as services you will be able to offer. What opportunities are available for exercise outside the cardiac rehabilitation program? Participants may be

referred to the following: the local YMCA/YWCA, Jewish Community Center, health and fitness spa, fitness facility located at work, community recreation center, or other exercise facility available in the community. There is no research proving that a maintenance program has to be established by a medical facility. DeBusk et al. (1986) consistently challenge the field of cardiac rehabilitation with this question: Many people do not go into outpatient programs, so where do they go? They exercise at home, at health clubs, or at exercise facilities with no formal cardiac program. The AHA (1990) states that activity guidelines should be provided to patients who do not participate in supervised programs.

A number of patients who leave Phase II programs and who have fitness facilities at work, belong to YMCAs, or have their own treadmills and bicycles at home still attend Phase III and Phase IV programs. Why? Because they feel they need the contact with health care professionals and other recovering cardiac patients. We present these questions to force you to think about where, why, and when you need to structure a Phase III/Phase IV program.

The Medical Advisory Board

Once you have decided to start a Phase III/Phase IV program and you have the facility and potential services outlined, it is important to then create a medical advisory board. Who is on the board is important from medical, safety, and political points of view. Each hospital that will potentially provide referrals to the program should be represented by a physician, and each large medical group in the city should be represented. The facility director and legal counsel should be part of this board also. The board provides guidance on the following issues:

1. Policies and procedures, especially
   - medical emergency procedures,
   - risk stratification for patient medical status,
   - exercise prescription,
   - exercise testing, and
   - surveillance and personnel training requirements

2. Financial and budgetary matters

3. Goals and objectives of the program, including
   - quality assurance objectives,

- lifestyle change and education objectives, and
- outcome objectives

4. Research and record keeping

Most importantly this board provides a major marketing tool for referrals. For this reason it is important that no major potential medical referring group is slighted when you set up the board. At the same time you should keep the board small enough to be effective in its ability to advise and consent.

Staffing the Program

Exercise physiologists, recreation specialists, RNs, physicians, and physical therapists who have training and knowledge necessary for rehabilitation (AACVPR, 1991) are all able to manage or work in outpatient programs. The University of Wisconsin–La Crosse's Phase III/Phase IV program is directed by a professor in the master's degree program for cardiac rehabilitation and adult fitness, and the exercise leaders are graduate teaching assistants. In a number of YMCAs, the community Phase III/Phase IV programs are directed by medical personnel and staffed by YMCA-trained advanced exercise leaders.

Other support staff should include dietitians, physical therapists, psychologists, and occupational therapists. These staff may be employed by the program or may be volunteers. In addition there may be advisory or consulting staff.

For general concepts concerning staffing a Phase III/Phase IV program, refer to chapter 7. The major questions that need to be answered about the staffing mix and patient-to-staff ratios are these: What will be the policies and procedures with regard to emergency procedures? What are national recommendations and state mandates relative to supervision? The AACVPR (1991) recommends that supervision be within a 10:1 to 15:1 ratio range. The AACVPR Guidelines provide a chart on page 40 of their document which describes utilization of personnel in supervision of exercise therapy. The supervision is stratified much the same as for patients that are risk stratified. This should be applied accordingly to your facility (see Table 4.1). The levels of certification, licensure, and training for staff are directly related to the level of supervision mandated by the medical advisory board and by national, state, and local guidelines.

The most effective team to run the Phase III/Phase IV program is an exercise specialist/physiologist and a cardiac rehabilitation–trained nurse. Both have the expertise required to provide the services that are needed day to day. The nurse requirement is decided by the way in which emergency procedures and policies are established. If the policies and procedures require that an emergency cart, defibrillator and standing orders for Advanced Cardiac Life Support (ACLS) shall be in the emergency plan, then a nurse, para-

Table 4.1 Utilization of Program Personnel in Supervision of Exercise Therapy

Personnel category	Patient risk for exercise-related cardiovascular complications		
	High (hospitalized)	High/Interm. (ambulatory)	Low (maintenance)
Supervising physician	IA	IA/IS	IS
Program director/coordinator	IA	IA	IS
Registered nurse	IA	IA*	NA
Exercise specialist/leader	IA	IA	IA

Note. IA = immediately available in the facility if requested by personnel authorized to visually supervise the exercising patient; IS = indirect supervision, that is, individual provides substantial influence for policy and procedure development affecting exercise services delivered to patients; also, substantially involved in planning, review of progress, and discharge assessments for each individual patient's exercise intervention; * = should be in the exercise room; NA = not applicable.

From *Guidelines for Cardiac Rehabilitation Programs* (p. 40) by American Association of Cardiovascular and Pulmonary Rehabilitation, 1991, Champaign, IL: Human Kinetics. Copyright 1991 by A.A.C.V.P.R. Reprinted by permission.

medic, or physician must be present during exercise as they are the only medical people licensed to carry out ACLS directives and standing orders.

The critical questions that the medical advisory board must ask as it sets the policies that will determine the staffing requirements are as follows:

1. The level of emergency provision must equal the level of provision at any other facility where people with similar conditions are exercising and being active. That is, what is provided at a YMCA, a Jewish Community Center, a university club, or other areas?
2. Will the policy and procedures require an emergency cart to include drugs, defibrillator, intravenous (IV) equipment, and intubation apparatus? If so, then appropriate personnel with standing orders and license to operate this cart should be present.

In essence, the question is, What level of emergency service does Phase III/Phase IV require? That is answered by your board, the area emergency service deliverers, and your legal counsel. If you are to have emergency carts, defibrillators, intubation, and IV equipment on hand, then you must have an employee who is licensed to put standing orders and the equipment into action. Further, that employee must be on the premises, visually in contact with the participants.

Budget and Finance

Budgetary considerations for running a Phase III/Phase IV program are difficult to pinpoint. The reasons for this are many and include the following:

1. Quite often the facility is shared with other programs, such as universities, colleges, community centers, or YMCAs/YWCAs. As a result, there may be a charge for the use, no charge, or a nominal fee for utilities only.
2. In a number of programs the staff members' salaries come from a larger facility or organization, or the management staff may be volunteer, as is the case in the La Crosse Exercise Program at the University of Wisconsin–La Crosse. (Also, the daily exercise staff of that program received stipends as graduate teaching assistants; this did not add to the budget of operating the Phase III/Phase IV program.) Medical supervisory people, if there are any, may be voluntary. Creative staffing is critical, because salaries

may be as much as 75 to 80% of the budget. That means the difference between operating in the red and breaking even. Here are some ideas on how to get free or minimal-cost supervising staff. (a) Offer a free membership to the facility and its programs to physicians, nurses, and paramedics. (b) Invite potential staff members to exercise at the same time they supervise, thereby taking care of their own needs as well as your needs. (c) Advertise free aerobic and other classes to medical personnel who are willing to be supervisors. (d) Give free weight room certificates or swimming pool passes to students in graduate programs in exercise physiology. (e) Affiliate with the local university as a field study site for experience in exercise leadership. Remember that students who work in programs must be trained to understand the requirements of the work and also must be appropriately supervised.
3. The program may be a shared expense of many hospitals operating in a community facility.
4. The program may operate on grants or funding from business and industry to facilitate employees' return to work and reduce health care costs for the businesses.

Refer to the chapters on staffing (7) and budget and finance (13) for the basics of operating a program. An example of a budget and operating expenditures appears in Table 4.2.

A major factor involved in starting a program is determining sources of funding. Third party reimbursement, with the exception of a few "gold star" policies (which pay 100% reimbursement for medical expenses, and for prevention and extended rehabilitation), does not reimburse for Phase III/Phase IV cardiac rehabilitation. Because of this the program must be affordable for patients. A program that costs $6 per session will total about $900 a year. For most people, especially those over age 65 on fixed incomes, that is a considerable amount of money. The average cost per participant for Phase III and IV is around $300 to $500 per year. To meet the expenses outlined in Table 4.1, a program would require 75 to 85 participants.

It is important to seek funding from various resources in the community: hospitals, YMCAs, businesses and industry, the AHA, universities and colleges, and other private and research companies. Fiscal responsibility is especially important to organizations such as these. It is wise to ask

Table 4.2 Initial Expenditures for a Phase III Program

Budget

Initial expenditure:

Planning

Marketing and fund raising	1,098

Equipment

Oxygen tank, cart, regulator, air, nasal canula	351
Silicone resuscitator	141
Suction pump and tubing	259
Drug box and supplies	162
Blood pressure unit (2)	100
Stethoscope (2)	22
Blanket	32
Emergency cart with storage	2,000
Schwinn Air-Dyne Bicycle (2)	1,406
Bodyguard 955 Bicycle (2)	798
Avita 950 Rowing Machine	270
Detecto Scale	300
Bulletin board	43
File boxes (2)	40
ECG supplies—paper, electrodes	20
Office supplies—pencils, file folders, forms, program manual, copies	300
Educational brochures	50
Folding chairs (20)	324
Open house	200
	$6,818

Operating expenses (May 1988-December 1988)

Salaries*	9,180
Benefits*	285
Payroll taxes*	726
Supplies (other than initial expenditures)	200
Telephone—lease, installation	380
Postage	125
Rent	2,811
Defibrillator maintenance contract	300
Printing	150
Travel	96
Liability insurance (professional, property, general)	2,500
Miscellaneous	300
	$17,053
Total	$24,969

Note. This is a 6-month start-up budget for 15 patients, 6 hours/week to increase to 30 patients in the second year. ECG = electrocardiogram; * = part-time nurse (6 hours/week), part-time exercise physiologist (15 hours/week).

other program managers how they are doing and how they manage financially.

Patient Services

According to the AACVPR (1991), ''patients are moved into the exercise maintenance stage when stabilized cardiovascular and physiological responses to exercise have been obtained and the desired outcome from exercise therapy has been achieved or no additional progress is evident'' (p. 4). The maintenance program is available for those who wish to continue group exercise and who desire continued education, surveillance, and attention to help them maintain compliance with lifestyle and behavior change. Essentially, any patient who has been a Phase I and Phase II participant may become a Phase III or maintenance candidate. Other maintenance program candidates are people who have not manifested the disease but have strong family histories of heart disease and lifestyle and risk factor profiles that call for a guided exercise and lifestyle program.

Data suggest that the risk for untoward events in maintenance and exercise programs is very small (Haskell, 1978; Van Camp & Peterson, 1986). Several major considerations ensure that the risk is minimal and lay the foundations for patient safety. These factors include referral and entry criteria, intake evaluations by the Phase III staff, exercise prescription, and self-monitoring by participants.

Referral and Entry Procedure

This is a policy and procedural mechanism established by the advisory board of the Phase III/Phase IV program. All participants should be referred into the program by their physicians. This may be the primary care physician, such as a family practice physician, internal medicine specialist, or a general practitioner. In other cases a cardiologist, physiatrist, or cardiovascular surgeon may be the referring physician. Accompanying the referral should be a general health history including the recent clinical course of treatment in the hospital, postdischarge information, and Phase II information. Along with this data should be a resting ECG and a current maximal sign or symptom treadmill/ergometer exercise test. Guidelines for entrance into and exit from a Phase III program are found in Table 4.3.

At this point in the referral process you can initiate the beginnings of an excellent communication

Table 4.3 Example of Entry and Exit Guidelines for a Phase III Program (3-6 Months)

Entry Guidelines

- Patient has been out of the hospital 4-6 weeks and completes a graded exercise test within 3 months of entry into the program
- Patient has satisfied Phase II exit guidelines
- Patient has a minimum functional capacity of 5 METs (a patient with a lower functional capacity should enter a Phase II program)
- Patient does not have to have participated in Phase I and Phase II programs
- Patient is at high risk for coronary heart disease
- Patient needs exercise guidelines (as opposed to medical surveillance or restrictions)

Exit Guidelines

- Patient has participated at least 3-6 months
- Patient has a functional capacity of 6 METs or more
- Patient has performed satisfactorily in Phase III in the judgment of staff
- Patient has normal hemodynamic responses to level of home exercise (see Phase II guidelines)
- Patient is free from angina with moderate exercise
- Patient can self-monitor
- Patient understands what constitutes a healthy lifestyle

network between the program, the referring physician, and the participant. As a part of the referral process, the referring physician should play an integral role in communicating the expected outcomes that she has for the participant. The program representative communicates the plan that has been developed for the participant and apprises the referring physician regularly (once every 6 months, or sooner if questions arise) of the patient's progress. The communication relationship developed between the program and the physician serves as a marketing tool for continued referral. At no time should the physician see the program as a threat to the relationship she has established with the patient.

Intake Evaluation

Once the information has been gathered from the referral process, it should be organized into the following categories: past history, current history, clinical course of most recent episode, test results, exercise test, and general information. You, or a

Phase III/Phase IV staff member should review this information and note what is missing and request any additional tests that may be required. It is essential that the information needed to set up a safe program is available. It is also essential that you do not require the participant to provide information he has given what may seem like a thousand times before and that may be found in the inpatient record. At this time ask the participant to review any new feelings, physical symptoms, and changes that he has noticed since last seeing his referring physician.

This information is collected, an exercise prescription is determined (chapter 5), expected outcomes for lifestyle change and behavior modification are established, and a plan for working toward those outcomes is written (chapter 2). The plan is written as a joint venture with the participant and the staff member. The patient sets the measurable levels. All of this is presented to the medical director of the program, who reviews and signs the program.

What degree of telemetry monitoring is done in a Phase III/Phase IV setting? The answer is that as a general rule, none. If a participant reports an abnormal heart rate, rhythm, or new symptoms suggestive of angina, then blood pressure and resting 12 lead ECG may be performed. Quick scans may be done with the paddles from the defibrillator. This is a method regularly used at William Beaumont Hospital in Royal Oak, Michigan, where over a period of 12 months, 14% of the patients demonstrated 25 incidences that required further medical attention (Grais, Franklin, Bonzheim, & Gordon, 1991). Another reason you may do a quick scan is to see if the participant is reaching the heart rate that is prescribed and is monitoring it accurately. People who require continuous telemetry monitoring are in a high-risk category and need to be in Phase II.

Exercise Prescription

Exercise is prescribed according to all of the information that has been gathered. See chapter 5 for further details on how to prescribe exercise for patients in every phase of cardiac rehabilitation. Much additional information is available and should be read, and it is also helpful if the person writing the exercise prescription has a thorough understanding of exercise physiology.

Self-Monitoring Skills

Self-monitoring skills involve teaching the patient to ''listen to'' and ''read'' the body and its responses to exercise. The first skill needed is learning to take a pulse accurately (see chapter 5). Second, the patient needs to be able to rate how hard he is working. Ask him to listen to his breathing: Is it smooth, gasping, harsh, heavy, medium, light? He should also evaluate the stress he feels in his muscles while he is exercising: Are they hurting? Do his limbs shake as they try to perform work? Is there fatigue as the muscles contract? How is the patient sweating in response to exercise? Is sweating excessive (e.g., shirt becomes soaked and there is water running off the face, head and neck)? Does he feel pleasantly energized as he exercises? Does his skin have a healthy pink color? Is he experiencing dizziness, shortness of breath, nausea, any chest pain? When the exercise is over and the patient has relaxed for an hour or two, he should have sensations of having worked out a bit but should not be fatigued, have muscle soreness, or feel the need to take a nap to recover.

The patient should also know what you want him to do if he experiences any problem while exercising (call the doctor, go to the emergency room, call the therapist over, back off of the exercise, sit down and rest, etc.) Whatever the response is, the patient should thoroughly understand what to do if a given problem occurs during, or following, exercise.

Patient Education

The main thrust of Phase III/Phase IV—maintenance—also applies to the educational aspects. The objective is to help the participant maintain lifestyle changes and possibly fine tune them as new findings are published in the research literature. Many Phase III programs allow participants to access lectures or seminars provided through Phase II or through a hospital's education or health promotion department. Other programs may use existing educational classes offered in the community through the American Heart Association, American Lung Association and American Cancer Society. They may also refer participants to registered dieticians, Weight Watchers, or other programs for ongoing problems with management of diet and weight problems. Education is an important part of the program and should be provided. Weekly lectures, one-page information handouts, free brochures, videos, guest speakers, and question boxes are all good methods to ''sell information.'' The question box is available for participants to drop their questions into; a staff member then writes a brief answer, which then may stimulate more questions. Being innovative and creative never hurts in getting participants involved. Two of the most successful weight loss programs I have seen were at the La Crosse Exercise Program Phase III/Phase IV program. These programs were run for 3 months each in successive years. The rules for weight loss followed American Dietetic Association guidelines. The first one was entitled ''The Adios Adipose Contest'' and the second program was the ''La Crosse Exercise Nobelly Prize Program.'' One involved a measure of pounds lost over 3 months, which was checked with diet diaries and pre- and postprogram weigh-ins. The other involved circumferential measurement, pre- and postprogram. Prizes were solicited from business and industry, and people had a great time participating.

In all cases of risk factor information and lifestyle change I encourage you to apply the techniques and methods that are outlined in chapter 2. This is one of the most current and easily applied descriptions of how to help the participant become her own change agent.

One aspect of the educational component that is truly the nuts and bolts of participant growth is the one-on-one relationship between the participant and the case manager. Talking, walking together, recording daily information, and reviewing medication changes and exercise test results creates a trust between the staff member and the participant. This is the education that makes the program. The lack of form and structure is not a detraction but an enhancement. This allows the program to meet individual needs within a group setting.

Critical to this individual programming is the area of instruction concerning medical management and medication adherence. Participants should be instructed on the use of the medication, what its action is, what possible side effects may occur, why compliance is important, and how regularity in time is important. Often the participant only knows he takes the green pill three times a day and the white pill two times a day. This is not enough; the participant must be responsible for his own medical regimen.

Emergency Procedures and Program Safety

Exercise of any type and in particular aerobic exercise carries with it a certain degree of risk. For people who have cardiovascular disease, their risk is increased particularly when the following related conditions exist:

Increased age

Increased severity of disease

Symptoms of angina

History of sudden death syndrome

Left ventricular dysfunction

Existence of other medical conditions such as diabetes, renal failure, COPD

Psychological instability

Cigarette smoking

Outpatient cardiac rehabilitation has been demonstrated to be very safe, with one arrest occurring per 111,996 patient-hours, one myocardial infarction per 293,990 patient-hours, and one fatality per 783,972 patient-hours of exercise (Van Camp & Peterson, 1986). Typically, participants who demonstrate an increased risk for arrest or myocardial infarction are in a high-risk category and should not be in a Phase III/Phase IV program unless the following conditions are stable or resolved (Van Camp & Peterson, 1989):

A history of chronic heart failure

Prior cardiac arrest

A history of ventricular tachycardia by ECG or Holter with exercise sessions

Poor exercise capacity

ST depression at heart rate of <120 bpm

A peak systolic blood pressure <120 mm Hg

Exertional hypotension ≥10 mm Hg drop

Ventricular tachycardia

What precautions and training are necessary for the operation of a Phase III/Phase IV program? The AHA provides the recommended training and certification levels for staff working in Phase III/Phase IV cardiac rehabilitation (Fletcher, Froelicher, Hartley, Haskell, & Pollock, 1990). Once again I refer you to the information in chapter 7 relative to staff. If the program policies and procedures determine that there is to be an emergency drug cart with a defibrillator present, then a staff member who is licensed and certified to provide ACLS and carry out standing orders must be present and in visual contact with the participants during exercise. In view of the expense of the defibrillator and cart (more than $6,000) and the expense of a staff

nurse, paramedic, or physician ($26 to $50 per hour), I suggest that you follow the recommendations of the AACVPR (1991) and AHA (1990): Keep appropriate records, obtain appropriate exercise prescriptions and evaluations, and be sure the program is supervised by trained exercise personnel.

Those who supervise and manage the exercise program and sessions should perform mock codes on a regular monthly basis, testing all of the emergency procedures that have been outlined by the medical advisory board. At the University of Wisconsin–La Crosse Phase III/Phase IV program, all exercise leaders were required to submit a monthly cardiopulmonary resuscitation (CPR) strip from a resuscitation doll, and the strip was to be judged perfect within the accepted parameters; additionally, practice codes and drills were performed monthly. Last, a well-designed and coordinated plan that involves the emergency transportation or paramedic emergency medical technician (EMT) service that you will call in the case of emergency should be reviewed every 3 to 6 months.

Just as it is essential for the staff to be prepared for an emergency situation, participants must be prepared as well. They should be instructed on a regular basis on what to do should a code occur. You and your staff should have well-constructed instructions and should teach participants how to follow them. Additionally, participants and their family members should have the opportunity to learn and certify in basic life support instruction. This is an important and integral part of the education program.

Innovations in Programming

Phase III and Phase IV provide the broadest base for setting up innovative and creative programs. Traditionally, cardiac rehabilitation programs and participants could win the world championships at treadmill walking at 3 miles per hour at a 5% grade. We need to remind ourselves on a regular basis that people stop being active when their regimes become boring.

If your program is in a multipurpose facility, use all of the available equipment. Encourage participants to swim or to learn to swim. Badminton, paddle ball, and volleyball can be played for fun, not competitively; basketball, bowling, and golf are also good activities. Remember, Blair et al. (1989) indicated that activity is essential to ensure lowered morbidity and mortality. And DeBusk et al. (1990) demonstrated that health benefit may occur with short bouts of exercise interspersed with rest.

At Allegheny General Hospital we have three cardiac special events each year and are working on establishing more. We have a winter bowling tournament, a May golf outing, and a July fun run and walk. The objective is to emphasize participation in activities that the patient can do for a lifetime. The Christ Hospital in Cincinnati has a "Fall Into Step" 2-mile walk and low-fat picnic and a "Spring Forward" afternoon at a local park for all graduates of the rehabilitation programs.

Allegheny General has a very large park across the street from the hospital, and on nice spring and fall days we walk and run with our Phase III/Phase IV patients in the park. We are looking for a way to ride bikes and teach bicycle safety.

William Beaumont Hospital, in Royal Oak, Michigan, uses many of the areas of a renovated elementary school for its programs, which include swimming, weight training, volleyball, and an innovative program called "On the Ball" (Franklin, Oldridge, Stoedefalke, & Loechel, 1990), which uses balls for flexibility and rhythmic exercise. This hospital also uses the more traditional bicycle ergometer, treadmill, rowing, and exercise programming.

Occasionally at Allegheny General we have set up our exercise room in a circuit activity program. Patients are given a score card and while staying within their prescriptions have to walk 10 min on a treadmill, shoot 20 Nerf ball baskets, ride for 10 min on a bicycle, throw 20 darts at a dart board, row 500 yd on the Concept II rowing machine, and putt into three indoor putting traps for number of holes-in-one with three tries at each hole. On other occasions we have done video low-impact aerobics.

The objective is to reintroduce any activity that a participant may have done before her cardiac incident and wishes to do again, or to explore new activities. Staff members should concentrate on helping participants find out what they are able to do, rather than telling them what they cannot do.

Conclusion

Cardiac rehabilitation has been an integral part of community facilities for more than 30 years. These programs have successfully provided participants with group exercise, camaraderie, and education for thousands of participant-hours without in-creased risk for sudden death and reinfarction. There is a need for facilities that are able to provide exercise and education for high-, medium-, and low-risk status patients who have stabilized and wish to continue exercise in a supervised setting. As health care costs continue to rise, the number of people who do not carry insurance increases. Also, the burden is becoming too large for Medicare programs to handle. We must develop low-cost programs that can provide surveillance and guidance as cardiac patients recover and reenter active lifestyles. Community programs have already proven their worth and may become one of the answers to increasing the provision of rehabilitation at lower costs.

Additionally, these programs provide family and social supports for the participant and may as a result positively influence the family at risk for heart disease. Creative programming, staffing, and support structures are required for the community facilities to support such ventures; however, programs operating over the last 30 years have demonstrated that these ventures are possible.

References

American Association of Cardiovascular and Pulmonary Rehabilitation. (1991). *Guidelines for cardiac rehabilitation.* Champaign, IL: Human Kinetics.

Blair, S.N., Kohl, H.W., Paffenbarger, R.S., Clark, D.G., Cooper, K.H., & Gibbons, L.W. (1989). Physical fitness and all-cause mortality. *Journal of the American Medical Association, 262*(17), 2395-2401.

DeBusk, R.F., Blomqvist, C.G., Kouchoukos, N.T., Luepker, R.V., Miller, H.S., Moss, A.J., Pollock, M.L., Reeves, T.J., Selvester, R.H., Stason, W.B., Wagner, G.S., & Willman, V.L. (1986). Identification and treatment of low-risk patients after acute myocardial infarction and coronary-artery bypass graft surgery. *New England Journal of Medicine, 314*(3), 161-166.

Fletcher, G.F., Froelicher, V.F., Hartley, L.H., Haskell, W.L., & Pollock, M.L. (1990). Exercise standards: A statement for health professionals from the American Heart Association. *Circulation, 82,* 2286-2322.

Franklin, B.A., Oldridge, N.B., Stoedefalke, C.G., & Loechel, W.E. (1990). *On the ball.* Carmel, IN: Benchmark Press.

Grais, S., Franklin, B.F., Bonzheim, K.A., & Gordon, S. (1991). Value of surveillance data on building medical/surgical interventions. (Abstract). *Medicine and Science in Sports and Exercise*, **23**(4), 5-26.

National Center for Health Services Research and Health Care Technology Assessment. (1987). *Health technology assessment reports, cardiac rehabilitation services* (DHHS Publication No. PHS 88-3427). Rockville, MD: U.S. Department of Health and Human Services. 1-89.

Naughton, J. (1973). The effects of acute and chronic exercise on cardiac patients. In J. Naughton & H.K. Hellerstein (Eds.), *Exercise testing and exercise training in coronary heart disease* (pp. 337-346). New York: Academic Press.

Pyfer, H.R., & Doan, B.L. (1973). Aspects of community exercise programs. In J. Naughton & H.K. Hellerstein (Eds.), *Exercise testing and exercise training in coronary heart disease* (pp. 365-374). New York: Academic Press.

Van Camp, S.P., & Peterson, R.A. (1986). Cardiovascular complications of outpatient cardiac rehabilitation programs. *Journal of Cardiopulmonary Rehabilitation*, **256**(9), 1160.

Van Camp, S.P., & Peterson, R.A. (1989). Identification of the high risk cardiac rehabilitation patient. *Journal of Cardiopulmonary Rehabilitation*, **9**, 103.

Wenger, N.A. (1984). Early ambulation after myocardial infarction: Rationale, program components, and results. In N.K. Wenger & H.K. Hellerstein (Eds.), *Rehabilitation of the coronary patient* (pp. 97-114). New York: Wiley.

Wilson, P.K., Fardy, P.S., & Froelicher, V.F. (1981). *Cardiac rehabilitation, adult fitness and exercise testing*. Philadelphia: Lea & Febiger.

Chapter 5

Exercise Prescription for Cardiac Patients

Linda K. Hall, PhD

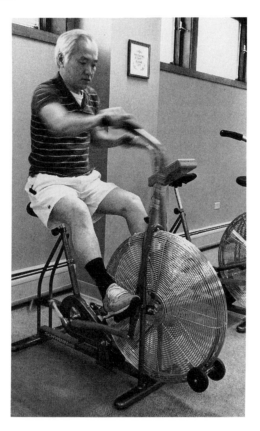

Writing an exercise prescription for cardiac patients requires knowledge of the body's physiological responses to progressive work loads in a state of wellness as well as a state of disease. To write prescriptions, you must understand exercise physiology and pathophysiology, fields that help you understand the exertional continuum achievable by people in various stages of health and disease (AACVPR, 1991). This chapter outlines steps and procedures for prescribing exercise for patients in the four phases of cardiac rehabilitation.

Learning Objectives

1. To understand the principles of returning cardiac patients to optimum activity levels

2. To learn and understand the tools for prescribing exercise intensity, mode, duration, and progression

3. To understand the continuum of recovery of energy, activity, and return to optimal functional capacity

4. To understand the use of weight training as a tool for reconditioning the cardiac patient

---

No single formula will give you the magic exercise prescription for each cardiac patient referred to your program. People differ physically and physiologically, and the changes caused by coronary artery disease and its concomitant problems such as left ventricular dysfunction, myocardial ischemia, and arrhythmias make it even more important to individualize each patient's exercise protocol. It is essential to consider the following relative to each patient as you develop exercise prescriptions: age, sex, clinical status, related medical problems, past physical activity patterns, musculoskeletal status, and the results of a graded exercise test. You can glean all of this information, with the exception of the graded exercise test, from the patient's files and by interviewing the patient.

Exercise Prescription

The primary purpose of Phase I is to prevent deconditioning of the inpatient and to prepare the patient to go home. The Phase II objective is to recondition the patient to an active and recreative physiology. For the Phase III/Phase IV program, the objective is the continued emphasis on activity as a habitual part of lifestyle. The Centers for Disease Control (1987) have emphasized that inactivity is a major risk factor for coronary artery disease, equal in causative weight to high cholesterol levels, cigarette smoking, and high blood pressure. Regular activity appears to have a protective effect with accompanying drop in blood pressure, decrease in triglycerides, increase in high-density lipoproteins, augmentation of weight reduction, and positive psychological effects (AHA, 1990). Additionally, Blair and associates (1989) enumerated the positive reductions in morbidity and mortality for people who maintain moderate fitness levels with moderate daily activity. Thus the most important part of an exercise prescription is to help the participant increase activity as a part of daily living (e.g., by taking the stairs when possible, parking farther away from stores and walking the extra distance, gardening, and walking around the neighborhood in nice weather).

When you write a formal exercise prescription, you should address five main features: frequency, intensity, duration, mode, and progression.

Frequency

Traditionally, cardiac rehabilitation programs have established a 3-day-a-week program for exercise and education, usually a Monday/Wednesday/Friday schedule. Some program directors feel that compliance to exercise is enhanced when the Friday session is substituted with a Thursday session, because Friday is a signal to people that the week has ended, and getting home or going away on a weekend trip is more important than exercise sessions. Even though the program is structured for 3 sessions a week, this does not mean participants should be limited to 3 days of exercise a week. Encourage participants to accept the responsibility for an alternate-day program with family and friends and to use different modes of exercise.

Intensity

The graded exercise test acts as a guide for setting the intensity of exercise for outpatient programs.

Graded Exercise Test

Table 5.1 presents cumulative exercise test data on a patient as he progressed from 1988 to 1990 through Phases II, III, and IV of an exercise program. The data presented in the exercise test allow for determination of exercise prescription heart rates. Several factors are evident from the graded exercise test results. For all four tests, a maximal heart rate and a maximal functional capacity were attained. Maximal functional capacity is that point in the exercise test—as measured by MET level, heart rate, rating of perceived exertion, and rate pressure product—at which the first symptom of overexertion appears. For the four tests reported in Table 5.1, the symptom was ST segment depression of 1.0 mm, at heart rates of 121, 116, 121, and 128 beats per minute. This is where the red line or limit of exercise heart rate should be drawn for this patient; the patient's exercise prescription should be written for each test at a rate lower than that at which symptoms occurred.

Notice, however, that the patient continued to exercise in all four exercise tests to heart rates of 171, 149, 160, and 150 bpm, which is considered to be his maximal exercise heart rate. An additional point of interest is that although his maximal heart rate was different for each test and his maximal systolic blood pressure was different also, his rate pressure product (RPP) at the time of ST depression

Table 5.1 Graded Exercise Testing Results

Date	11/30/88	11/22/89 (thallium)	11/1/90	12/20/90
Cardiac medications	Inderal LA 80 mg/qid	Tenormin 50 mg/bid	Tenormin 25 mg/tid	Cardizem 30 mg/qid
	Aspirin qid	Nitropatch 20 mg/qid		NTG patch 5 mg/qid
		Xanax 0.25 mg/qid		
		Ecotrin qid		
Test protocol	Bruce	Bruce	Bruce	Bruce
Test duration (min:s)	9:56	9:00	7:43	8:01
Termination criteria	Fatigue	ST depression	ST depression	ST depression
Maximal speed (mph) and grade (%)	4.2/16	3.4/14	3.4/14	3.4/14
Maximal HR attained (bpm) and predicted maximum HR (%)	171/107	149/94	160/101	150/95
Maximal BP attained (mmHg)	164/86	162/88	182/86	154/84
Symptoms	None	None	None	None
Functional capacity (METs)	10	9	8	8
Fitness level	Above Average	Average	Average	Average
Onset 1.0 mm ST Depression, lead V5 (bpm)	121	116	121	128
RPP at 1.0 mm ST Depression	–	18,096	18,876	18,432

Note. The November 1988 graded exercise test was probably a truly maximal evaluation, because it was terminated due to fatigue. Subsequent tests were more functional evaluations, because they were stopped due to ST segment criteria. BP = blood pressure; HR = heart rate; RPP = rate pressure product; qid = four times a day; tid = three times a day; bid = two times a day.

onset was relatively the same for each test. Rate pressure product is an expression of the oxygen demand made by the myocardium; you can obtain this value by multiplying systolic blood pressure times the heart rate obtained at the same point in the test. Usually exercise training affects at what point in time, speed, grade, or all three that ischemia appears; however, the RPP at which ischemia appears usually remains the same. We will return to these results further on in this chapter as we get into the actual heart rate calculations.

Intensity during exercise sessions is monitored in several ways; however, it must never exceed the level of intensity demonstrated on the exercise test that was clear of any clinically determined or patient-determined signs and symptoms. The heart rate at which a clinically determined or patient-determined sign or symptom appears is the absolute cutoff point. In the example presented in Table 5.1, the patient's most current functional maximal heart rate is 128 bpm, which is the heart rate at which 1.0 mm ST segment depression occurred.

Intensity Calculations

Because of the nature of cardiac illness, the intensity of activity needed to improve physical condition will vary greatly according to the amount of

disability and the period of time over which the disability developed. For example, inpatients improve each day, first getting out of bed, then moving from chair to across the room, then eventually walking in the hall. This is very low-intensity work; however, the patient perceives it as very hard at the time she is doing it. Using the exercise stress test as a measure of functional capacity, we find that some individuals increase physical capacity with as little as 50% of maximal functional capacity as the intensity prescription. There is a relationship between the intensity of exercise and the length of the exercise bout. Lower intensity exercise requires longer bouts, whereas higher intensity exercise requires shorter bouts to achieve the same results. Low- to moderate-intensity exercise has less likelihood of producing negative side effects such as overuse tendon, muscle, and ligament injury; foot and ankle problems; and excessive fatigue. Low-intensity activity may be considered as ⩽40% of $\dot{V}O_2$max, whereas moderate exercise intensity is categorized as 60% of $\dot{V}O_2$max (AHA, 1990). A study by DeBusk, Stenestrand, Sheehan, and Haskell (1990) showed that multiple short bouts of moderate-intensity exercise training can significantly increase peak oxygen uptake. Multiple short bouts may fit into busy schedules better than longer bouts and are sufficient to

---

FIGURING HEART RATE

The patient represented in Table 5.1 exercised to a symptom-limited heart rate of 128 bpm. This means that symptoms appeared at a heart rate of 128 bpm, so the patient should exercise at a percentage of heart rate below 128 bpm. ACSM (1991) and AHA (1990) recommend that training will occur between 50 and 80% of maximal symptom-limited heart rate. Using simple multiplication, you will arrive at heart rates between 64 and 102 bpm.

To use the Karvonen method, you need to know the resting heart rate (RHR), which was 74 bpm for the patient in Table 5.1. Subtract RHR from the maximal symptom-limited heart rate.

Maximal symptom-limited heart rate	=	128
minus resting heart rate	=	−74
		54

Multiply the result by 50% and 80%.

$54 \times .50 = 27$

$54 \times .80 = 43$

Add these results to the RHR to determine the HR range for exercise.

$27 + 74 = 101$

$43 + 74 = 117$

The HR range is 101 to 117 bpm. Notice the difference between the straight percentage heart rates (64 to 102) and the Karvonen heart rates (101 to 117), despite the fact that the percentages used for calculations were 50% and 80%. Dressendorfer and Smith (1984) reported that the Karvonen calculation may overestimate the heart-rate intensity early in the cardiac patient's recovery, although for healthy people it is very accurate as an intensity indicator. The Karvonen formula is used for the patient represented in Table 5.1, because he is in a Phase IV class.

rehabilitate patients. You can determine training intensity for the participant by using heart rates as predictors of intensity.

The ACSM (1991) guidelines provide three different methods of calculating heart rate: linear plotting, Karvonen formula (Karvonen, Kentala, & Mustala, 1957), or simple multiplication of percentage desired times maximal achieved heart rate. The most frequently used methods for calculating heart rate prescriptions are the Karvonen formula and the heart-rate percentage formula.

Although exercise heart rate is prescribed at percentages of maximal oxygen uptake or maximal functional heart rate, it is difficult for patients to understand what a percentage is when determining how hard they must work. Also, if people are able to continue to condition at low heart rates, it is not important to give them heart rate cutoffs below which they should not exercise, only to give heart rates above which they should not exercise. There are many ways to help the patient self-monitor. This is critically important, because when data were examined relative to cardiac emergencies in rehabilitation programs, they showed that incidents usually occurred because patients had exceeded their target heart rates or exercise prescriptions (Haskell, 1978). In the case we have discussed, the patient's absolute cutoff is 117 bpm. If the patient counts his own heart rate for 10 seconds, there is a cushion for a margin of error that could be as much as 6 beats in a 10-s count. Give the patient a peak heart rate above which he or she must not go. Do not give a bottom heart rate.

Using Intensity Monitors

Heart Rate: Teaching a patient to find her pulse and then to count it while watching a clock is no small task. The most common places to locate pulse are the inside thumb side of the wrist (radial artery pulse), to the right or left of the Adam's apple in the neck (carotid artery pulse), or over the heart. Counting for 10 s and multiplying by 6 is an easy method. Refer to Table 5.2 for a conversion from a 10-s count to heart rate for 1 min.

Counting pulse begins with zero as a mark of the first beat counted. Teach participants other parameters with which to check the intensity of their work.

Ratings of Perceived Exertion: It is traditional in the United States to rate things. We are always saying things such as, "On a scale of 1 to 10, how would you rate this dinner?" Interestingly, people instinctively know what each number on the rating scale represents. Borg (1962) introduced the idea of measuring the "feeling" relative to the degree of effort that is exerted during exercise. Since the introduction of the Borg Scale, also called the Rating of Perceived Exertion Scale (RPE), many studies have validated its use as a measure of exercise intensity. Study this particular methodology, and then use it when teaching your participants how to quantify the intensity of their exercise. Maresh and Noble (1987) discussed its use quite thoroughly and provided pointers for its application. Table 1.5 gives the most commonly used form of the Borg Rating of Perceived Exertion Scale. Generally, moderate exercise on the low end will start at 12 and extend on the high end to a rating of 16 (ACSM, 1991). Use 10 to 14 as the range with Phase II and Phase III patients. An RPE of 10 to 12 generally is prescribed for patients with low functional capacity or more extensive pathophysiology; 12 to 14 for higher functioning patients.

Table 5.2 Heart Rate Chart

Beats in 10 s × 6 = heart rate/min

8 × 6 = 48	17 × 6 = 102
9 × 6 = 54	18 × 6 = 108
10 × 6 = 60	19 × 6 = 114
11 × 6 = 66	20 × 6 = 120
12 × 6 = 72	21 × 6 = 126
13 × 6 = 78	22 × 6 = 132
14 × 6 = 84	23 × 6 = 138
15 × 6 = 90	24 × 6 = 144
16 × 6 = 96	25 × 6 = 150

"Talk, Sing, Gasp" as an Intensity Measure: This method teaches patients that if they are able to speak in full sentences while they exercise, they are achieving the correct intensity. If they can sing while exercising, they can increase the intensity. If they are gasping, they are working too hard and need to back off.

The participant needs to become familiar with other signs in order to monitor the intensity of her exercise. How does she feel? Is she perspiring comfortably and not excessively? Is her skin pink? When pressed does it go white and then turn pink quickly? Does she have any pain in the chest, leg, any muscle, or back? When she finishes exercise does she feel pleasantly exhilarated? If the participant is slightly fatigued after exercise, she should recover within an hour or so. Encourage the participant to check the next day for muscle soreness; excessive amounts indicate she is exercising too hard.

All of these signals become a part of the patient's arsenal for determining how hard he should work. As he becomes predictable at reaching appropriate heart rate, rhythm, and blood pressure responses and begins to achieve conditioning, give the patient a target heart rate or RPE that he should not exceed. However, allow him to play with intensity below that target and don't force him to adhere to one heart rate, one speed, and one grade.

Duration

Traditionally we have told exercisers that they must exercise at least 30 min per session to achieve fitness, that is, to improve maximal oxygen uptake. Research has now shown that short bouts of 10 min each two or three times per day produce substantial increases in maximal oxygen uptake (DeBusk et al., 1990) and that modest levels of fitness that are obtainable by most adults appear to protect against early mortality (Blair et al., 1989). Essentially, we are now finding that it is important to discuss with the patient just exactly how much time she is willing to spend and start from there. Most Phase II, Phase III, and Phase IV programs operate on an hourly basis with 10 to 15 min set aside at the beginning for warm-up activities and 10 to 15 min at the end for cooling down, which leaves 30 to 40 min for bouts of aerobic activity. The AACVPR (1991) recommends as few as 1 or as many as 36 visits for Phase II patients, 4 to 6 months of visits for Phase III patients, and an indefinite number of visits for Phase IV patients.

Mode

What's the best way to get fit? A better question is, What does the patient like to do, and what will she do regularly, for a lifetime? Any activity that may be done for 20 to 60 minutes at a moderate pace is appropriate. Walking, bicycling, water walking, swimming, and using stair climbers, cross-country ski machines, arm/leg ergometers, and rowing machines are all appropriate. The exercise must be something the patient is willing to do; must not produce injuries, pain, or discomfort; must be enjoyable; and must be financially affordable.

Progression

Participants may progress in duration, intensity, and mode within the limitations of the parameters

of heart rate, blood pressure, ectopic rhythms, ischemia, angina, and signs and symptoms set by the exercise test. To extend these parameters, you can retest the participant to establish new limits. Most often Phase III and Phase IV participants habituate themselves to a specific number of minutes duration and to intensities that are quite often tempered daily by how participants feel, which means checking out all of the sensations going on in their bodies. There really is no better guideline than how participants feel. I currently have a participant who exercises to "three Oreo cookies." He is not done until he burns the cookies (300 kcal), which for him requires 30 min of brisk walking and intermittent jogging.

When you write the exercise prescription and set up the plan for the exercise sessions, address the patient's recreational and vocational needs. What kind of activities does he do or would he like to do? Does he canoe, camp, hike, fish, mow grass, or play golf? What kind of work will he return to; what muscle groups will that involve; what types of lifting or carrying will he do; and what type of physical labor does the job require? What kind of muscle strength does the patient have right now, and what will he need to do to meet his job's demands? And finally, will the patient be able to return to his former type of work? Once you have assessed all of these areas, set up the program to get the patient back into condition to return to work, and report your results and impressions to his physician. This brings us to another area that is relatively new to exercise training with cardiac patients: weight training.

Weight Training

For many years weight training was believed to be contraindicated for heart disease patients, but strength training is now accepted as an important part of the rehabilitative process. Hickson, Rosenkoetter, and Brown (1980) found that strength training can increase endurance time in bicycle and treadmill exercise even though there is no concomitant effect on $\dot{V}O_2$max. Further studies by Goldberg, Elliot, Schutz, & Kloster (1984) demonstrated increases in HDL and decreases in LDL as a result of strength training. Specific guidelines are elucidated in the AACVPR (1991) guidelines and should be followed when you set up a program for a patient. Table 5.3 lists the steps recommended for developing the weight programs for cardiac patients.

Little information is available about the amount of weight a Phase II patient should work with or the number of repetitions she should perform.

Table 5.3 Recommended Steps for Developing Weight Training Programs for Cardiac Patients

1. Define the purpose of prescribing strength training for the patient.
2. Define the type of program that will be prescribed:
   (a) dynamic, static, isokinetic, or
   (b) strength, endurance, power.
3. Evaluate and identify the muscle groups to be developed.
4. Emphasize symmetrical movement, specifically for the upper body.
5. Include exercises that develop the agonist and the antagonist to maintain muscular balance.
6. Determine the appropriate starting loads for each exercise.
7. Develop guidelines for progression of weight overloads.

Start with an overall evaluation of the patient when she first enters the program: past history, nursing notes, Phase I assessment, and graded exercise test. Then talk with the patient; the most important questions you should ask concern activities she wants to return to recreationally and vocationally. The answers will give you an idea of the patient's fitness level before the cardiovascular incident. Next ask about her current activities.

1. How many times a day does she go up and down the stairs?
2. Has she been lifting and carrying anything? Ask her to list items no matter how light or heavy they are, such as laundry baskets, grocery bags, garbage bags, exercise clothing bags, shoes, boots, shovels, and hoses. The answers will tell you how much weight the patient has been moving.

A patient who goes up and down stairs three times a day is lifting his body weight for three sets of 12 lifts (for an average flight of stairs) daily, so questions about whether weight lifting is safe really aren't relevant. An average pair of shoes weighs 2 to 4 lb, and an average grocery bag is from 8 lb (paper products) to 15 lb (cans and solids). So asking questions about daily activity helps you know what starting weight is reasonable for a Phase II patient.

Additionally, consider what the patient needs in the way of muscle work; the questions in Table 5.3 will help you. Generally work from one of two starting points with the patient: Either he is so debilitated that he has muscle atrophy and needs to build muscle (pure strength, low repetitions), or he has muscle but no endurance (weight training, higher repetitions).

Generally, with uncomplicated patients with no arrhythmias who were fairly active before their cardiac incidents, start women with 5-lb dumbbells and men with 8-lb dumbbells. For the 1st week work on form, making sure that eccentric and concentric contractions are done properly.

Require patients to stretch before they exercise. Figure 5.1 gives examples of general body stretching patients can do before exercise and weight training. Table 5.4 lists the specific exercises for upper body and arm strengthening. Hand weights, Heavy Hands, and dumbbells are all appropriate for increasing strength and in some cases increasing training load during aerobic exercise.

CASE STUDY: 53-YEAR-OLD WOMAN
WITH MULTIPLE VALVE REPLACEMENTS

A 53-year-old woman was referred to our Phase II program for rehabilitation. She said she had been told at age 16 that she had valvular disease and was never to do anything strenuous in her life. With no definition of *strenuous*, she managed to do as little daily work and activity as possible. Subsequent deterioration, infections, and faulty valves brought about three mitral valve replacements and an aortic valve replacement in a period of 14 years. Upon discharge from the hospital to her own home, she was so debilitated that she required home health care in order to turn on the bath water faucets. We started her out with 1-lb dumbbells in each hand, which produced tremor on effort. We prescribed five repetitions twice during her exercise session, one set at the beginning and one set at the end. She "perceived" the exercise at a 14 or 15 at the beginning and grumbled that we were slave drivers. But she was building strength. Today this woman is taking care of all her daily household and lifestyle needs with no assistance for the first time since she was 16.

Instructions

A. Hold the stretch for 15 to 30 s.

B. Achieve the stretch position gently; do not bounce.

C. The stretch should feel tight but never painful.

D. Do all the exercises on both sides of the body.

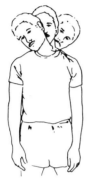

1. **Neck stretch:** Keep shoulders back. Tilt head to shoulder; reverse to other side.
◄

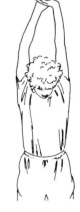

2. **Neck and back stretch:** Tuck chin to chest. Press upward with hands.
►

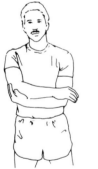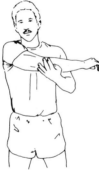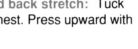

3. **Elbow cross:** Grasp elbow from underneath; pull arm slightly downward and across the chest. Do not shrug shoulders.
◄

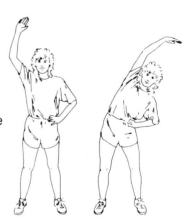

4. **Hip and waist stretch:** Keep knees slightly flexed. With one arm reaching overhead, bend directly to the opposite side.
►

(continued)

Figure 5.1 Cardiac rehabilitation stretching program.
Note. From Allegheny General Hospital. Reprinted by permission.

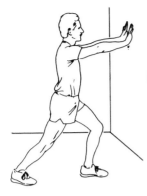

5. **Calf stretch:** Use a wall for balance. With toes facing wall, shift weight forward until stretch is felt in back leg. Keep back foot down.
◀

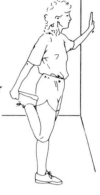

6. **Quadricep stretch:** Use a wall for balance. Grab ankle with hand; keep bent leg vertical. Push forward with hips to feel stretch.
▶

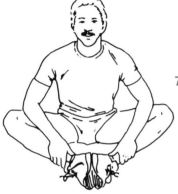

7. **Groin stretch:** With hands on ankles, push down gently on legs with elbows. Keep back straight; lean forward from hips.
◀

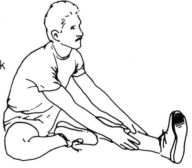

8. **Hamstring stretch:** Keep back straight; lean forward from hips until stretch is felt.
▶

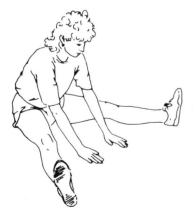

9. **Inner thigh/low-back stretch:** Keep toes pointed up. Lean forward from hips, keeping back straight.
◀

Figure 5.1 *(continued)*

Table 5.4 Sample Exercises for Muscle Groups Specific to Upper Body Strength Training

Shoulder flexors Shoulder adductors Elbow extensors	Bench press
Shoulder extensors Shoulder adductors Elbow flexors	Lateral pull-down Arm curl
Shoulder flexors Shoulder abductors Elbow extensors	Standing press
Elbow extensors	Triceps extension
Shoulder girdle elevators	Shoulder shrugs
Shoulder abductors Elbow flexors	Upright row

At the Phase III and Phase IV levels, regular weight training programs that use Nautilus, Universal Gym, or even free weights are appropriate. Usually weights equal to between 40 and 60% of maximal lifting capacity are recommended. Make sure the participant understands these basic rules: (a) don't strain, (b) stay within an RPE of 10 to 13, (c) don't hold your breath, and (d) pay attention to warning signs and symptoms. Unless the Phase III/Phase IV patient is subject to noted restrictions, approach her weight training program the same way you would for a non–cardiac patient of her age, weight, height, and exercise capacity. Design the program specifically toward what the patient wants to achieve.

There is no accounting for the experience and intuition of the person writing the exercise prescription. I have two or three staff members with whom I have new interns and staff people work. These experienced people know pathophysiology, ask the right questions of patients, and mix intuition with knowledge and experience. They follow accepted guidelines; however, their prescriptions are creative, giving the patient a feeling of involvement and thus self-control. So learn from someone who has experience, after you have done your reading. Watch her, question her, and have her critique your sample prescriptions.

RECREATIONAL CASE STUDY

A 39-year-old man who had undergone coronary artery bypass surgery with three grafts and who was 2 months into his Phase III program came to us proposing a canoeing trip to the Boundary Waters in northern Wisconsin. His physician said that if we would assess the patient's ability to meet the demands of the trip and simulate physiological parameters, such as heart rate, blood pressure, heart rhythms, and exertion, that looked normal, the physician would approve. We set up a month's training program in which the patient tipped and righted a canoe in our swimming pool, paddled with a staff member on the local river, lifted and carried for portage, packed and packaged his medicines (two sets plus 5 extra days, one for him to carry and one for a person to carry in another canoe), and removed his clothes and swam 500 yd using sidestroke and backstroke. He passed all of the measures with no problems. His physician said go, and he did. The worst problem he encountered in the whole 5 days was a horrendous case of poison ivy. However, he demonstrated a tremendous sense of self-confidence as a result of completing the trip.

VOCATIONAL CASE STUDY

A postal service employee who underwent bypass surgery wanted to return to his job, which involved handling mailbags that weighed 60 to 90 lb. We prescribed treadmill walking and arm and leg ergometers. Also, we worked him progressively throughout his rehabilitation. He lifted and carried empty bags first, then he carried bags with 5, 10, and 20 lb in them, until by the end of his rehab he was mimicking his work at the post office. We sent the results to his physician with ECG strips, blood pressures, and a written impression of his progress. The man is back at work.

Conclusion

There are many facets of prescribing exercise, and possibly the most important is the preparation of the information you glean from medical records and the exercise test. Talking with the patient and determining his or her needs, desires, and selected end points will assist you also. Last, reading research journals and talking with experienced professionals who have worked with and know the disease and its impact on the myocardium, physiology, and anatomy are excellent ways to increase your ability to prescribe optimally for your patients' health and safety.

Further Reading

American College of Sports Medicine. (1988). *Resource manual for guidelines for exercise testing and prescription*. Philadelphia: Lea & Febiger.

American College of Sports Medicine. (1991). *Guidelines for exercise testing and prescription* (4th ed.). Philadelphia: Lea & Febiger.

American Heart Association. (1990). Exercise standards: A statement for health professionals from the American Heart Association. *Circulation*, **82**(62), 2286-2322.

Franklin, B.A., Hellerstein, H.K., Gordon, S., & Timmis, G.C. (1989). Cardiac patients. In B.A. Franklin, S. Gordon, & G.C. Timmis (Eds.), *Exercise in modern medicine* (pp. 44-80). Baltimore: Williams & Wilkins.

References

American Association of Cardiovascular and Pulmonary Rehabilitation. (1991). *Guidelines for cardiac rehabilitation*. Champaign, IL: Human Kinetics.

American College of Sports Medicine. (1991). *Guidelines for exercise testing and prescription* (4th ed.). Philadelphia: Lea & Febiger.

Blair, S.N., Kohl, H.W., Paffenbarger, R.S., Clark, D.G., Cooper, K.H., & Gibbons, L.W. (1989). Physical fitness and all-cause mortality. *Journal of the American Medical Association*, **262**(17), 2395-2401.

Borg, G.A.V. (1962). *Physical performance and perceived exertion*. Lund, Sweden: Gleerup.

Centers for Disease Control. (1987). The protective effect of physical activity on coronary artery disease. *Morbidity, Mortality Weekly Report*, **36**, 426-430.

DeBusk, R.F., Stenestrand, U., Sheehan, M., & Haskell, W.L. (1990). Training effects of long versus short bouts of exercise in healthy subjects. *American Journal of Cardiology*, **65**, 1010.

Dressendorfer, R.H., & Smith, J.L. (1984). Predictive accuracy of the maximum heart rate reserve method for estimating aerobic training intensity in early cardiac rehabilitation. *Journal of Cardiopulmonary Rehabilitation*, **4**, 484-489.

Fletcher, G.F., Froelicher, V.F., Hartley, L.H., Haskell, W.L., & Pollock, M.L. (1990). Exercise standards: A statement for health professionals from the American Heart Association. *Circulation*, **82**, 2286-2322.

Goldberg, L., Elliot, D.L., Schutz, R.W., & Kloster, F.E. (1984). Changes in lipid and lipoprotein levels after weight training. *Journal of the American Medical Association*, **252**, 504-506.

Haskell, W.L. (1978). Cardiovascular complications during exercise training of cardiac patients. *Circulation*, **57**, 920.

Hickson, R.C., Rosenkoetter, M.A., & Brown, M.M. (1980). Strength training effects on aerobic power and short-term endurance. *Medicine and Science in Sports and Exercise*, **12**, 336-339.

Karvonen, M., Kentala, K., & Mustala, O. (1957). The effects of training on heart rate: A longitudinal study. *Annales Medicinae Experimentalis et Biologiae Fenniae*, **35**, 307-315.

Maresh, C.M., & Noble, B.J. (1987). Utilization of perceived exertion ratings during exercise testing and training. In L.K. Hall, G.C. Meyer, & H.K. Hellerstein (Eds.), *Cardiac rehabilitation: Exercise testing and prescription* (pp. 155-174). Champaign, IL: Life Enhancement Publications.

Chapter 6

High-Risk and Special Populations

Kathy Berra, BSN, FAACVPR
Cindy Lamendola Rudd, BSN, FAACVPR

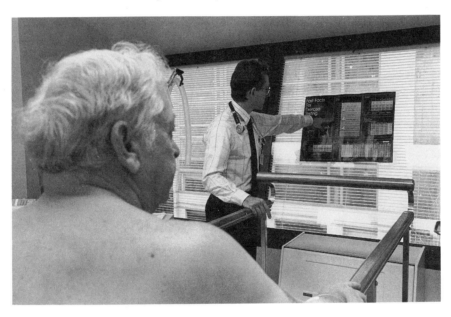

The preceding five chapters have provided a comprehensive perspective on what cardiac rehabilitation is and to whom we are now applying it. What of the future? Is the cardiac rehabilitation model applicable to high-risk cardiac patients and to other patient populations, such as those with chronic obstructive pulmonary disease (COPD) and chronic renal failure? If so, what adjustments to process and procedure will need to be made? Chapter 6 addresses these questions. It identifies and discusses moderate- to high-risk cardiovascular patients and others who can potentially benefit from cardiac rehabilitation interventions (including patients with advanced cardiovascular disease manifested by severe left ventricular dysfunction, heart failure, valvular heart disease, and serious arrhythmias). It also identifies additional patient populations that can be served by the cardiac rehabilitation model.

Learning Objectives

1. To understand future challenges of the cardiac rehabilitation model

2. To define patient populations that may benefit from the therapeutic model of cardiac rehabilitation

3. To develop a strategy to meet the safety issues that arise in applying cardiac rehabilitation therapy to diverse patient populations

4. To review current knowledge and learn new theory in applying the cardiac rehabilitation model to diverse patient populations

---

The authors gratefully acknowledge the invaluable assistance of Marilyn Ellis, Medical Data Exchange in Los Altos, CA, in the preparation of this manuscript.

The Challenge

The management of cardiovascular disease is a challenging and compelling focus in the care of the cardiac patient. Options for care today are vastly different from those of 20, 10, or even 5 years ago. Patients can be critically evaluated and, based upon these evaluations, can be offered important medical and surgical interventions. These interventions are designed to decrease morbidity and enhance survival and quality of life. Patients can be instructed to lose weight, exercise regularly, stop smoking, alter their eating habits, and manage the stress in their lives while being evaluated or treated with the following:

- Antithrombolytic therapy—the use of certain medications designed to prevent and/or treat blood clots.
- Atherectomy—Surgical removal of atheromatous plaque from the inside of the artery wall via a catheter that has a rotary blade on its tip.
- Automatic implantable cardioverter defibrillator (AICD)—A device implanted in the abdomen that is attached, via electrode patches and sensors, to the heart muscle. The device senses life-threatening abnormal rhythms and automatically sends an electrical discharge (defibrillation) to terminate the rhythm.
- Cardiac transplantation—The surgical removal of a terminally diseased or damaged heart and replacement with a donor heart.
- Coronary artery bypass surgery—Surgery designed to improve the supply of blood to the heart muscle. Veins and mammary arteries are used to allow blood flow to bypass blocked sections of the coronary arteries.
- Cryoablation—Localized application of cold to specific areas of the heart muscle as a means of terminating irregular heart rhythms.
- Echocardiography—A test which utilizes sound pulses transmitted into the body. Echoes returned from the surfaces of the heart are plotted electronically to measure various heart functions, such as the contractility of the heart muscle.
- Electrophysiologic studies (EPS)—Studies of the electrical conduction system of the heart.
- Endocardial resection—Surgical removal of small portions of heart muscle thought to be causing life-threatening abnormal heart rhythms.
- Exercise test—A test usually performed on a bicycle ergometer or a treadmill, which gradually stimulates the cardiovascular system by increasing work loads. The purpose of the test is to evaluate and measure the functional capacity of the cardiovascular and pulmonary systems as well as to detect any abnormalities in blood flow to the heart or irregular heart rhythms that may occur during exercise.
- Holter monitor—An ambulatory continuous recording (12 to 24 hr) of the electrocardiogram.
- Intravascular stent—A small device placed inside the artery wall that is designed to keep the artery open.
- Laser therapy—The use of laser energy to dissolve a blockage in the vascular system.

- Percutaneous transluminal coronary angioplasty (PTCA)—A procedure used to open narrowed arteries. A catheter with an uninflated balloon on its tip is passed into a narrowed artery segment. The balloon is then placed in the area of the narrowing and is inflated. This widens the narrowed segment.
- Thallium scan—A radioisotope that when used in conjunction with exercise testing measures blood flow to the heart muscle.

What, if anything, can help us integrate such technological maneuvering with the human being that houses the heart? Cardiac rehabilitation, perhaps, can be the facilitator and the counterbalancing effect of cardiovascular technology for the patient.

Cardiac rehabilitation implies a comprehensive plan for recovery. It implies a commitment to the inclusive management of known coronary risk factors to lessen future cardiovascular morbidity and mortality. Cardiac rehabilitation includes health education designed to inform patients and their families about medical and surgical procedures, outcomes, and their future health. It provides guidance in the areas of emotional recovery, medication management, smoking cessation, dietary habits, stress management, return to work, sexual activity, and usual sports and leisure activities. To most patients, however, cardiac rehabilitation means simply "getting into shape" through a regular exercise program. The exercise component of the rehabilitation program is often what patients enjoy the most and are most likely to participate in, and it is the component that generally gives the most immediate sense of reward. What remains a challenge to people with coronary artery disease and to health care professionals is development and maintenance of new behaviors beyond exercise that promote "heart-healthy living" over a lifetime. These new behaviors are numerous for some patients and not as numerous for others. They include the following (Berra, 1992):

- Taking medications daily for an indefinite period of time, which often involves complex regimens
- Remaining smoke-free for life
- Being aware of the impact of certain foods on cholesterol, triglycerides, blood sugar, sodium, and weight, and monitoring intake of those foods for life
- Exchanging old, comfortable food habits for new and healthier food habits for life
- Learning new ways to respond during times of acute stress and learning how to manage stressful situations

- Taking an active role in an often confusing and frustrating health care system
- Accepting the importance of regular aerobic exercise and finding exercise routines that are enjoyable, safe, and effective
- Evaluating the signals received from the body, especially the heart, and knowing when to ask for help
- Seeing oneself as a partner in health care, along with the physician, family, and friends

The cardiac rehabilitation model involves multiple and diversely trained health care professionals who facilitate these important lifestyle changes. Their professional expertise and management of patients during the rehabilitation process enhance the speed of recovery and the success of long-term lifestyle interventions (Hamalainen, Luurila, & Kallio, 1989; Kallio, Hamalainen, Hakkila, & Luurila, 1979; Oldridge, Guyatt, Fischer, & Rimm, 1988). Because of the multidisciplinary model, cardiac rehabilitation programs can easily diversify their efforts to meet the needs of other chronically ill patient populations.

Defining the Patient Population

Dr. Nanette Wenger described new cardiac rehabilitation patients of the 1990s as those patients previously excluded from programs, such as

- patients with cardiac enlargement;
- patients with compensated heart failure;
- patients with implanted pacemakers/cardioverter/defibrillators;
- patients with residual myocardial ischemia;
- patients with significant arrhythmias;
- elderly, more complicated cardiac patients;
- patients experiencing multiple complex medical therapies; and
- patients taking multiple cardiac and other medications (Wenger, 1987; Wenger & Alpert, 1989).

The new cardiac rehabilitation patient of the 1990s is, in two words, "high risk." High-risk patients are generally defined as those who, because of alterations in cardiac function due to myocardial ischemia or damage, are at a higher risk of suffering future coronary events or sudden cardiac death. As early as 1962, Peel and associates (Peel, Semple, Wang, Lancaster, & Dall, 1962) described a method of grading the severity of infarction and thus developed the early coronary prognostic index. In 1983, the Multicenter Post-Infarction Research Group reported that four variables that assess physiologic measurement of heart function can predict greater than average mortality after myocardial infarction (MI). These variables include the following:

1. An ejection fraction of less than 0.40 at 1 week post-MI
2. Ventricular ectopy of 10 or more depolarizations per hour
3. Advanced New York Heart functional class (II to IV) prior to infarction (generally indicating prior MI)
4. Rales in the upper two-thirds of the lung fields at 24 to 48 hr post-MI, early rales being an indicator of poor left ventricular ejection fraction (LVEF) at Day 7 post-MI

The data from this study (Multicenter PostInfarction Research Group, 1983; see Figures 6.1 and 6.2) also indicate that as the numbers of these identified risk factors increase, so does cardiac mortality. In addition, the study found a progressive increase in cardiac mortality as the ejection fraction (EF) fell below 0.40 and as the frequency of premature ventricular contractions (PVCs) rose above one per hour.

In this study, EF had a considerably stronger effect on the increase in mortality compared to PVCs. It is interesting to note that in this study, angina, prior to patients' hospital discharge, did not significantly discriminate between survivors and nonsurvivors.

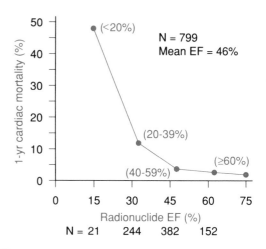

Figure 6.1 Cardiac mortality rate and ejection fraction (EF) radionuclide angiography.
Note. Adapted from "Risk Stratification and Survival After Myocardial Infarction," by the Multicenter PostInfarction Research Group, 1983, *New England Journal of Medicine,* **309,** pp. 331-336. Copyright 1983 by the *New England Journal of Medicine.* Adapted by permission.

In a review of sudden cardiac death, Kremers, Black, and Wells (1989) reported that although postinfarction survivors with arrhythmias are at increased risk for sudden cardiac death, this risk is only about 5% in the 1st year and has not been shown to be improved by conventional antiarrhythmic drugs. The authors cite small study size, variability, ill-defined end points, and proarrhyth-

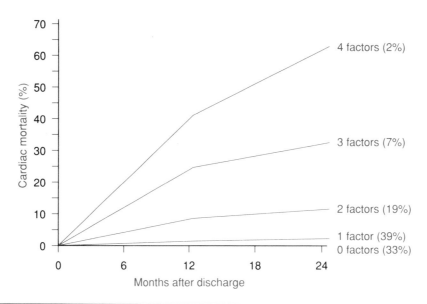

Figure 6.2 Mortality curves after discharge and zones of risk according to numbers of risk factors.
Note. Adapted from "Risk Stratification and Survival After Myocardial Infarction," by the Multicenter PostInfarction Research Group, 1983, *New England Journal of Medicine,* **309,** pp. 331-336. Copyright 1983 by the *New England Journal of Medicine.* Adapted by permission.

mia (causing or stimulating arrhythmia) as partial explanations of the apparent lack of efficacy of drug therapy. They compared the Multicenter PostInfarction Program (MPIP), the Multicenter Limitation of Infarction Size Study (MILIS), and the Beta Blocker Heart Attack Trial (BHAT) to determine the prognostic value of arrhythmia after a myocardial infarction (see Table 6.1). They showed that in patients recovering from acute MI, the presence of ventricular arrhythmias identifies a subset of patients at increased risk of death due to ventricular arrhythmia. These studies also showed that the frequency of arrhythmias declines at Days 3 to 5 following acute MI and increases again at Weeks 6 to 12 of the recovery period. There have been problems identifying patients who will have the 6- to 12-week recurrence of ventricular arrhythmia. The problems relate to poor correlation between arrhythmias that occur during the acute phase of the MI and either subsequent outcome or arrhythmias that occur long term. Twenty-four hour ambulatory ECG monitoring between Weeks 6 to 12 of high-risk patients (those with poor left ventricular function or those who have previously experienced sustained ventricular tachycardia/VT, or sudden death at the time of the acute MI) may be helpful in this problem of identification. Also, participation in cardiac rehabilitation programs, which provide additional

arrhythmic monitoring, can facilitate identification of this higher risk group (Fletcher, Froelicher, Hartley, Haskell, & Pollock, 1990; McHenry et al., 1990; Van Camp & Peterson, 1989).

However, myocardial function remains the single best predictor of total mortality following acute MI. The MPIP study showed that LVEF of less than 30% was associated with a 3-1/2-fold increase in mortality (Multicenter PostInfarction Research Group, 1983). Poor LVEF plus complex arrhythmias has become a significant marker for the high-risk coronary patient. It is essential that health care workers evaluate multiple clinical parameters in addition to the presence and severity of arrhythmias in setting the course of therapeutic interventions. The impact on quality of life due to adverse side effects from many of the antiarrhythmic medications often leads to a problem of compliance and further complicates the management of ventricular arrhythmia and poor left ventricular function (Croog, Levine, & Testa, 1986).

Benefits and Risks

Can cardiac rehabilitation programs offer benefits to high-risk patients, and do these benefits outweigh the increased risk patients may experience by participation in such programs?

The benefits for patients are both psychological and physiological; they include the following:

1. The patient is closely monitored for changing patterns of cardiovascular signs and symptoms, such as angina, ventricular ectopics, and shortness of breath.
2. The patient receives regular evaluation of ventricular function, myocardial ischemia, atrial and ventricular arrhythmias, and functional capacity via treadmill exercise testing and other noninvasive evaluations.
3. The patient is frequently assessed regarding the influences of coexisting metabolic and orthopedic problems that may interfere with compliance in the cardiac rehabilitation routine. Often CAD is not the primary concern for a patient who has chronic renal failure or severe COPD.
4. The patient is regularly evaluated for medication adherence, efficacy of medication, and medication side effects that may negatively influence quality of life and compliance.
5. The group environment provides support and motivation for patient, spouse, and family.

Table 6.1 Prognostic Value of Arrhythmias After Myocardial Infarction

Feature	MPIP	MILIS	BHAT
Number of patients	819	533	1,640
Arrhythmia	>3 PVC/hr	>10 PVC/hr	Multiple
Follow-up (yr)	2	1.5	2.1
Total mortality (%)	11.2	11.4	10
Annual SCD with arrhythmia (%)	6	8.5	3.8-5.1
Relative risk of SCD with arrhythmia	2.5	3.0	2.3-2.7

Note. MPIP = Multicenter PostInfarction Program; MILIS = Multicenter Limitation of Infarction Size; BHAT = Beta Blocker Heart Attack Trial; SCD = sudden cardiac death; PVC = premature ventricular contraction.

6. The patient learns self-monitoring skills.
7. The patient is assessed as to readiness to return to work, sexual activities, and social functions as she improves both physically and emotionally.
8. The patient can monitor and aggressively manage their coronary risk factors.
9. The patient who may have a limited sense of reward from physical activity and coronary risk factor interventions learns to identify positive achievable goals.
10. The patient is enabled to positively impact self-efficacy as it relates to physical tasks, lifestyle changes, and the maintenance of new health behaviors (Berra, 1992).

What do we know about the effects of exercise training in patients with left ventricular dysfunction? David Cody and his co-workers in Sydney, Australia (Cody, Dennis, & Ross, 1983), looked at exercise training and mortality in patients with severe left ventricular dysfunction. They reported an annual mortality of 9% in the exercise training group versus an expected mortality of 35 to 40% in a similarly matched population of patients who were not exercising.

Squires of the Mayo Clinic reported an annualized mortality of 8% ± 4% in a follow-up interval of 29 months in a group of patients with severe ischemic ventricular dysfunction who participated in an exercise training program (Squires, Lavie, Brandt, Gau, & Bailey, 1987). His results were very similar to those expressed by Cody et al. (1983). Duke University researchers Sullivan, Higgin-

bothom, and Cobb (1988) looked at exercise responses before and after physical conditioning in patients with severely depressed left ventricular function. In a comparison of patients matched for age and LVEF, the authors noted no increase in mortality in the exercise group; see Table 6.2.

Hoffman, Duba, Lengyel, and Majer (1987) reported similar findings in the *European Heart Journal*. They found no increased mortality or morbidity in an exercising group versus a control group of men with impaired LVEF following acute MI.

Although the numbers of studied subjects are small, the clear implication is that exercise training greatly enhances functional capacity, does not appear to increase the risk of sudden death, and does not affect LVEF at rest or with exercise. In all of these studies, the authors stress that using a change in LVEF as a marker of improved cardiovascular function is not reliable in this population. It is also important to note that poor LVEF has not been shown to correlate with exercise capacity or the ability to improve functional capacity with exercise training. Improvements in cardiovascular function in this population are more accurately measured by the following:

1. Increased maximal oxygen consumption ($\dot{V}O_2$max) with treadmill exercise testing, that is, increased MET capacity (1 MET = 3.5 ml/kg/min of oxygen consumed)
2. The ability of a patient to perform submaximal physical tasks at a lower heart rate and mean arterial blood pressure
3. A decrease in peripheral vascular resistance

Table 6.2 Comparison of Exercise Studies in High-Risk Cardiac Patients

Author	Number of patients	Age	Mean resting LVEF at rest (%)	Length of training	Deaths in exercise program	Changes in functional capacity (METs)	Changes in LVEF after training
Cody	32	53 ± 13	18 (10-22)	12 months	0	3.7 ± 13 to 7.0 ± 1.8	0
Sullivan	12	54 ± 10	24 ± 10	16 to 24 weeks	0	4.7 ± 1.0 to 5.8 ± 1.6	0
Squires	20	53 ± 8.7	20.9 ± 3.1	8 weeks	0	6.5 ± 2.5 to 8.9 ± 2.5	0
Conn	10	57.5 ± 13.5	<27 (13-26)	minimum 2 months; average 12.7 months	0	7.0 ± 1.9 to 8.5 ± 2.9	0

Note. LVEF = left ventricular ejection fraction.

due to vasodilitation during dynamic exercise, with a resulting fall in afterload (the amount of blood in the ventricles after contraction)

4. Biochemical and morphologic adaptations of skeletal muscles in response to habitual and familiar exercise
5. A widening of the arteriovenous oxygen difference with exercise (Sullivan et al., 1988).

Exercise Testing

Knowing that poor LVEF is a marker of poor prognosis, what do we know about the prognosis of patients with arrhythmias? Young, Lampert, Graboys, and Loron (1984) at Brigham and Women's Hospital in Boston evaluated the safety of maximal exercise testing in patients at high risk for ventricular arrhythmia (Table 6.3). They compared 263 patients referred for treatment of malignant ventricular arrhythmia to 3,444 cardiac patients referred for routine exercise testing. Of the 263 high-risk patients, 9.1% experienced a complication, compared to 0.12% of the low-risk group. There were no deaths in either group. When the authors evaluated a total of 1,377 treadmill tests in the high-risk group, they found that life-threatening complications—defined as sustained arrhythmia or cardiac arrest that warranted the therapeutic intervention of CPR or cardioversion or the administration of antiarrhythmic or other drugs to restore sinus rhythm—occurred in just 2.3% of the high-risk group. Among the 8,221 maximal exercise tests performed on the 3,444 low-risk patients, the incidence of life-threatening complications was .05%. Self-terminating arrhythmias, including VT, were not designated as complications in this study. This study confirms the low event rate in properly supervised settings even

with high-risk patients. This low event rate has also been found in cardiac rehabilitation programs due (we believe) to close medical supervision provided by these programs (Van Camp & Peterson, 1986).

The exercise test has become the "gold standard" for the development of the exercise prescription and for the determination of the intensity of monitoring in cardiac rehabilitation programs. This evaluation is critical in patients with known arrhythmia or left ventricular dysfunction.

For inpatient rehabilitation, an exercise test is often not performed until just prior to discharge or very soon thereafter. The following criteria have been developed by the ACSM (1991) to guide the monitoring of patients who have recently had coronary events.

The ACSM recommends that inpatient exercise be terminated if the patient experiences the following:

1. Unusual fatigue
2. Light-headedness, ataxia, confusion, pallor, cyanosis, dyspnea, nausea, or any peripheral circulatory insufficiency
3. The onset of angina with exercise, especially low-level exercise
4. Symptomatic supraventricular arrhythmia
5. VT (3 or more consecutive PVCs)
6. ST displacement (3 mm) horizontal or downsloping from resting ECG
7. Exercise-induced left bundle branch block
8. Onset of second- or third-degree atrioventricular (AV) block
9. Any R on T PVCs (a PVC between the R and T waves occurring during ventricular repolarization)
10. Multifocal PVCs greater than 30% of the total complexes
11. Increase in heart rate over 20 bpm above standing resting heart rate for MI patient (adjusted upward for coronary artery bypass graft or heart-transplant patient)
12. A drop of 20 mm Hg or more in systolic blood pressure (SBP); exercise hypotension
13. Excessive blood pressure rise: SBP $\geq$ 220 or diastolic blood pressure (DBP) $\geq$ 110
14. Inappropriate bradycardia with an increase in work or no change in work load (drop in heart rate $\geq$ 10 bpm)
15. Failure of the monitoring system

Table 6.3 Safety of Maximal Exercise Testing in Patients at High Risk for Ventricular Arrhythmia

	High risk	Low risk
Number of patients	263	3,444
Total number of TET	1,377	8,221
Life-threatening events (%)	2.3	0.05
Number of deaths	0	0

Note. TET = treadmill exercise test.

These guidelines are appropriately conservative and can be adjusted as to intensity, frequency, and heart rate as individual patients appear to tolerate the exercise well or begin to have cardiovascular difficulties.

Following the patient's discharge, the exercise test again becomes the critical guide in the development of the exercise prescription. It takes on greater importance with patients who have more complications. The American College of Cardiology has recommended guidelines, which are based upon the exercise tests and other clinical criteria, for more intensive monitoring of cardiac patients during cardiac rehabilitation (Parmley, 1986). Patients who require such monitoring include the following:

1. Patients with severely depressed LVEF (less than 30%)
2. Patients with resting complex ventricular arrhythmia (Lown type 4), repetitive PVCs in pairs or runs, and Lown type 5-PVCs which occur early in the repolarization of the normal sinus complex (Lown & Wolf, 1971)
3. Patients with ventricular arrhythmia appearing or increasing with exercise
4. Patients who experience a decrease in SBP with exercise
5. Survivors of sudden cardiac death
6. Patients with complicated myocardial infarction, such as congestive heart failure (CHF), cardiogenic shock or serious ventricular arrhythmias
7. Patients with severe coronary artery disease or marked exercise ischemia
8. Patients who cannot self-monitor heart rate due to physical or mental impairment

It is vitally important that when performing the exercise test in preparation for entry into a cardiac rehabilitation program, the patient take all medications at the same time before the treadmill test as will be taken before the cardiac rehabilitation exercise session. This allows for a more accurate estimate of heart rate guidelines and greatly diminishes the frustration patients may feel when beginning their exercise programs. Patients will have fewer problems in achieving or staying at the recommended heart rate guidelines if the treadmill exercise test truly represents their exercise medication levels.

Safety Issues

The safety of patients participating in rehabilitation programs is a primary concern of all health care professionals involved. Careful adherence to nationally endorsed guidelines, such as those published by AACVPR (1990), Fletcher, Froelicher, Hartley, Haskell, and Pollock (1990), and ACSM (1991), provides an atmosphere of safety for all program participants.

Van Camp and Peterson (1986) have done extensive research in the area of safety. Their research describes the unique characteristics of patients who suffer cardiac arrest while participating in cardiac rehabilitation programs. They found the following:

1. Historically, features of importance were

   • a history of CHF,
   • prior cardiac arrest, and
   • a history of ventricular tachycardia (as measured by ECG or Holter) during an exercise session.

2. Clinically, features of importance were

   • poor exercise capacity (less than 4.5 min of the Bruce protocol, <6 METs),
   • ST depression beginning at a heart rate less than 120 bpm with exercise,
   • a peak systolic blood pressure with exercise of less than 120 mm Hg,
   • exertional hypotension of equal to or greater than 10 mm Hg drop in SBP with exercise, and
   • ventricular tachycardia.

3. Cardiac catheterization findings of importance were

   • LVEF of less than 40%, and
   • left main or three-vessel CAD.

These authors also reported the total number of cardiac arrests, myocardial infarctions, and fatalities in 167 randomly chosen cardiac rehabilitation programs. The programs reported 51,303 patients entering from January 1980 to December 1984. All 167 programs provided data regarding serious events that occurred during this 4-year period. During this time, there occurred 21 cardiac arrests (CA), or 8.9 per one million hr of exercise; three fatalities, or 1.3 per one million hr of exercise; and eight myocardial infarctions (MI), or 3.4 for one million hr of exercise.

This encouraging study demonstrated a very low rate of complications related to exercise in cardiac rehabilitation programs. Additionally, there was a very high rate of successful resuscitation. This study is comparable to an earlier one by Dr. William Haskell of Stanford (1978). What we can learn from these studies is that serious cardiovascular events are rare in cardiac rehabilitation programs. Additionally, it makes sense that patients believed to be at higher risk of experiencing complications will most likely derive the greatest benefit from the supervision offered by cardiac rehabilitation programs.

It is important to note that in Van Camp's study, 86% of the programs included in the study reported no major cardiovascular complications (either cardiac arrest [CA] or MI) during this 4-year period.

There is a group of high-risk patients who, because of the severity of their disease, should not participate in therapeutic exercise programs (ACSM, 1991). This group includes patients with

- unstable angina pectoris,
- recurrent VT,
- severe left ventricular outflow tract obstruction (aortic stenosis),
- dissecting aneurysm,
- active thrombophlebitis,
- recent systemic or pulmonary embolus,
- severe uncontrolled high blood pressure,
- uncontrolled diabetes mellitus,
- severe heart failure,
- moderate to severe pulmonary congestion,
- uncontrolled peripheral edema, or
- severe orthopedic limitations.

Other medical conditions which warrant careful consideration include patients currently undergoing chemotherapy and those with moderate to severe anemia.

Exercise Training

Exercise prescription and exercise training for high-risk patients include careful cardiovascular evaluation, low-level sign- or symptom-limited treadmill testing, and regular medical supervision. In addition to the safety techniques applied to all adults who undertake an exercise prescription, other considerations for this population should include the following (Squires et al., 1987):

1. The patient should undertake slow, progressive aerobic exercise lasting 5 to 10 min, 4 to 5 times per week, at 50 to 60% of maximal heart rate, onset of angina, onset of blood pressure abnormality, or clinically concerning shortness of breath.

2. The patient should increase these intervals to 30 to 40 min, 4 to 5 times per week, as tolerated based on signs or symptoms using the same heart rate and symptom-limiting guidelines found in item 1.
3. Standard warm-up and cool-down exercises are recommended for this population.

Lipkin, Scriven, Crake, and Poole-Wilson (1986) described a 6-min walk test as a simple and inexpensive means to serially monitor the effects of the exercise program in more complicated pulmonary patients. This 6-min walk test, which can easily be used for cardiac patients, is a means of measuring the appearance of symptoms such as angina, arrhythmias, or clinically significant shortness of breath during a 6-min walk. Like a treadmill test, this test can correlate with improvement in function or deterioration in function.

In addition to low-level, short-duration, frequent bouts of exercise, a few other features of the exercise prescription are important to consider.

1. The use of prophylactic nitrates prior to exercise
2. The proper timing of the exercise routine in relation to all medications
3. The use of supportive exercise equipment such as stationary bicycles
4. Frequent positive physiological feedback to enhance motivation and compliance to the program and to determine the safety and assess the efficacy of the exercise prescription
5. Setting small achievable goals in order to maximize the patient's sense of accomplishment
6. The provision of a psychologically supportive and carefully monitored program environment

The scientific evidence suggests that exercise training in certain high-risk cardiovascular patients with left ventricular dysfunction or arrhythmias can be achieved safely and with no apparent increase in morbidity and mortality. The data also suggest that these improvements can enhance quality of life in a population that has generally been given very limited guidelines for physical activities. By carefully monitoring their cardiovascular signs and symptoms, medication, and exercise guidelines, this group of patients can look forward to a potentially greater life expectancy and a greater likelihood of return to usual work, social, and family roles.

Educational Needs for High-Risk Patients

As cardiovascular technology advances with resultant decreases in hospital stays and admissions (Burek, Kirscht, & Topol, 1989; Topol et al., 1988), our ability to ''capture the cardiovascular audience'' is constantly being challenged. The need to provide intensive rehabilitation, especially risk factor intervention, remains. However, with earlier return to work and to a normal lifestyle, the cardiovascular patient needs options that include home rehabilitation, rehabilitation at the work site, and community-based rehabilitation. Our ability to risk-stratify patients has enabled us to move patients into rehabilitation models that can provide a comprehensive long-term approach to exercise and risk factor intervention. As patients are referred into cardiac rehabilitation programs, we can assess functional capacity and risk. Higher risk patients can be placed in rehabilitation sessions designed to offer closer medical supervision through a higher staff-to-patient ratio. As the stability of signs and symptoms is assessed and patients gain confidence in their abilities to self-monitor, they can then be graduated into other programs as appropriate. The reality we face today is that complicated patients are living full and relatively normal lifestyles. If cardiac rehabilitation programs can offer consistent supervision of self-monitoring skills and can help patients know when to avail themselves of the health care system, morbidity and mortality statistics may be reduced, and quality of life may be greatly enhanced. Self-monitoring skills are a fundamental safety feature for all coronary patients. Self-monitoring skills can also be lifesaving skills. These skills enable patients to know when to call their physicians about concerns and when to seek immediate medical attention. Self-monitoring skills can be divided into those for anginal symptoms and those for heart rate and arrhythmias. Self-monitoring skills for anginal symptoms include the following questions (Berra, 1992; Fry & Berra, 1981):

1. What does my usual angina feel like? (tightness, heaviness, fullness, banding)
2. Where is it usually located? (in the chest, neck, jaw, arm, back)
3. How often do I usually experience angina? (once a week, twice a day)
4. What are my usual triggers/causes? (eating, severe emotional upset, exposure to cold or exertion)
5. How severe is my usual angina? (Grades 1 through 4, Grade 1 being onset and Grade 4 being the most severe)
6. What usually relieves my angina? (rest, nitroglycerine, other intervention)
7. Does my angina ever wake me from my sleep, or does it occur at rest or without provocation? (If *yes*, how often does this occur, how long does it last, how severe is it, and what intervention is necessary to relieve the angina?
8. Am I taking any medication to control my anginal symptoms? If *yes*, what are they?

Self-monitoring skills for heart rate and arrhythmia assessment include the following questions (Berra, 1992; Fry & Berra, 1981):

1. What is my usual resting heart rate? (taken in the morning)
2. Do I have irregular heartbeats normally? If so, how many do I usually have in a 3-min period?
3. What heart rate guidelines has my doctor given me for my exercise program?
4. Do I have trouble achieving this heart rate, or do I go over my heart rate very easily while exercising?
5. Do I have increased numbers of irregular heartbeats while exercising?
6. Am I taking any medications that may alter my usual heart rate in response to exercise? If so, should I take these medicines before exercising?
7. When I have irregular heartbeats, do I ever feel dizzy or as if I am going to faint?
8. Does my doctor want me to call him or her if I develop new or worsened irregular heartbeats?

When you provide thorough analyses of physical and emotional status, develop comprehensive exercise and cardiovascular risk reduction programs, and provide safe and caring environments in which patients can learn and practice new and healthier lifestyle techniques, cardiovascular patients and other patients with chronic disease can actively manage their health and hopefully live longer and more productive lives.

Assessing and Treating Special Populations

For the past 20 to 30 years, the care of the hospitalized cardiac patient has evolved from 6 weeks of bed rest to ambulation within 24 hours to beginning a walking, swimming, or biking program 2 to 3 weeks following hospital discharge. Principles of rehabilitation that were applied to patients with neuromuscular and musculoskeletel problems in the 1940s led to further research that positively impacted the recovery of patients with coronary artery disease.

As the benefits of rehabilitation were realized in cardiac patients, researchers began to evaluate similar programs for diverse chronically ill patient populations. By reviewing the specific guidelines for patients with chronic obstructive pulmonary disease (COPD) and end stage renal disease (ESRD) we can see how the cardiac rehabilitation program model benefits these patients.

Much has been written about rehabilitation of the patient with COPD, although only a moderate amount of literature is available about the rehabilitation of ESRD patients. Nationwide, directors of cardiac rehabilitation programs have found it feasible, safe, and rewarding to expand their models to provide services to these special patient populations.

Hellerstein and Franklin (1984) stated that exercise should be treated like a drug, and they emphasized the implications, the dosage, and the contraindications. When offering rehabilitative services to any special patient population, you must thoroughly understand the disease process, potential health problems associated with rehabilitation, special educational needs, and contraindications to exercise. Although each special population will have specific needs, certain guidelines that are necessary for safety and success are common to all groups. What are these common guidelines?

1. Is this patient appropriate for rehabilitation? (Are there unstable medical conditions present?)
2. What is the best way to evaluate

   - functional capacity,
   - benefits from exercise,
   - emotional needs,
   - educational needs, and
   - patient goals?

3. Which assessment tools should you use in developing a safe and effective exercise prescription?
4. What type of exercise format will work best for this patient and will allow for success?
5. What type of exercises will be most beneficial?
6. What are realistic short-term and long-term goals for this patient?
7. What are appropriate outcome measures?

The most important step in the process is proper patient selection, for which physician referral information becomes the guide. The physician refer-

ral provides the necessary medical information to establish medical history, current medication therapies, results of diagnostic testing, and special concerns. Establishing appropriate communication with referring physicians is a critical link to successful rehabilitation. During the course of the program you must regularly communicate information with the referring physician. In this way, rehabilitation becomes an integral part of patient care, and the referring physician is continually apprised of her patient's progress or difficulties.

It is recommended that a thorough medical history be collected and a physical exam performed on the patient prior to entry. This exam may uncover potential problems that could prohibit or delay the patient from entering the rehabilitation program. This exam can be performed by the medical director of the program or by the patient's personal physician. It should be performed within a week or two of the patient's entry into the program to assure the patient's medical stability and readiness to participate. At this time, other members of the rehabilitation team should evaluate the patient's needs and begin the goal-setting process. Educational needs, psychosocial needs, medication compliance, nutritional assessment, and functional capacity are fundamental to the initial assessment.

There are several ways to assess functional capacity in these special populations. In deciding which method is best to use, consider the information needed to correctly evaluate the particular population group. Such information includes but is not limited to the following:

1. Is the patient at risk for cardiovascular disease?
2. Are heart rate or blood pressure responses to exercise altered by the disease state?
3. What are the effects of current medications on hemodynamic responses, dyspnea, and fatigue with exercise?
4. Is there a potential for the patient to develop significant arrhythmias?
5. Is the patient at high risk for oxygen desaturation during exercise?
6. Is the patient limited by peripheral vascular disease?
7. Which is the best tool to utilize in the development of an accurate exercise prescription?

Because many patients have led sedentary lives as a result of their chronic illness, these questions cannot be answered until a functional capacity evaluation is performed. Sign- or symptom-limited exercise testing in which the patient uses a treadmill or bicycle ergometer is useful in the evaluation of functional capacity. You can evaluate underlying problems such as new or unstable angina, congestive heart failure, arrhythmias, abnormal heart rate and blood pressure responses, or medication complications at this time (ACSM, 1991).

Exercise Evaluation

The protocol you choose for the exercise evaluation will depend upon many factors, including age, previous exercise history, orthopedic limitations, cardiovascular symptoms, current medication therapy, present activity level, and psychological status (Pollock, Wilmore, & Fox, 1984).

Research has established the safety of exercise testing in the cardiac patient who has a low functional capacity or serious arrhythmias. Similar guidelines have been established for patients with pulmonary disease and ESRD (Belman, 1986; Belman, 1989; Goldberg et al., 1980; Hagberg, 1989; Hodgkin, 1987; Miller & Morley, 1987; Painter, Nelson-Worel, et al., 1986). Most patients, because of their disease processes, deconditioned status, or both, must begin the exercise test at very low work loads. You can use modifications of the Naughton or Balke protocols, and incremental changes in work load can be as small as .5 MET (Miller & Morley, 1987). An additional way to evaluate the functional capacity of special populations is through the use of the 12-min walk test (Belman, 1986; Belman, 1989; McGavin, Gupta, & McHardy, 1976). This test is a simple and non-threatening means of assessing the individual's functional capacity and exercise tolerance and is useful in developing the exercise prescription. Additionally, you can use the 12-min walk test to evaluate progress.

McGavin and co-workers (1976) found a significant correlation between the distance covered in the 12-min walk and $\dot{V}O_2$max during treadmill testing in patients with COPD. Because walking is a familiar skill, the walk test is an ideal method for exercise testing. To perform the test, have the patient walk a measured distance, or any part of that distance, in 12 min. At the end of the 12-min, take three measurements: the patient's heart rate, rate of perceived exertion (RPE), and level of perceived dyspnea. During the 12-min walk test the patient may stop and rest if needed, but the clock keeps going. Make it clear to the patient that this is not a race against time; 12 min is a randomly picked time frame. Research has also shown that 3- or 6-min walk tests are equally effective (Lipkin et al., 1986). Using a smaller time increment may

help the patient to feel more successful, especially one who has a very low functional capacity or has significant anxiety regarding exercise. If you use telemetry monitoring during the test, you can also evaluate the patient for arrhythmias. If a patient has little or no risk for cardiovascular disease, the walk test may be an ideal measurement. Studies have suggested repeating the test one to three times to obtain an accurate baseline (Belman, 1986).

Prescribing Exercise

Following evaluation of functional capacity, you can prescribe exercise guidelines. The exercise prescription must be individualized for each patient. Factors to consider are cardiovascular responses to exercise, age, disease process, precautions or contraindications to exercise, exercise history, current medications, orthopedic problems, and the patient's psychological status (Skinner, 1987b). Because many special population groups have different physiological responses to exercise, tools such as the RPE scale, the Karvonen formula, and the dyspnea scale may be used alone or in combination when you develop an exercise prescription.

A well-known scale for measurement of perceived exertion was developed by Borg (1982). The scale enables the exerciser to rate the exertion she perceives while performing a given amount of exercise (see Table 6.4). The RPE scale will help you develop the exercise prescription when you obtain ratings with heart rate and $\dot{V}O_2$max during exercise testing, or with heart rate during standardized exercise tests for which the energy costs are known. Once the patient perceives the effort associated with various exercise intensities, she may better understand appropriate intensities associated with different levels of exercise. After training regularly at a prescribed intensity, the patient can then transfer the subjective feelings to other activities (e.g., to estimate fatigue and varying intensities associated with games or other non-steady state activities) (Skinner, 1987a). For patients with lower levels of functional capacity, a modified scale of perceived exertion may be more useful in the development of the exercise prescription. Prior to exercise testing, familiarize the patient with the RPE scale to be used, emphasizing the measures of light effort, moderate effort, moderate to hard effort, and significantly hard effort.

The Karvonen formula for heart rate guidelines is very helpful for patients with low functional ca-

Table 6.4 Ratings of Perceived Exertion (RPE)

Original RPE	New rating scale	
6	0	Nothing at all
7 Very, very light	0.5	Very, very weak
8	1	Very weak
9 Very light	2	Weak
10	3	Moderate
11 Fairly light	4	Somewhat strong
12	5	Strong
13 Somewhat hard	6	
14	7	Very strong
15 Hard	8	
16	9	
17 Very hard	10	Very, very strong
18		
19 Very, very hard		
20	•	Maximal

Note. The original RPE scale and the revised ratio scale may be used in exercise testing or exercise programs.

From "Psychophysical Basis of Perceived Exertion," by G.V. Borg, 1982, *Medicine and Science in Sports and Exercise,* **14,** pp. 377-387. Copyright 1982 by American College of Sports Medicine. Reprinted by permission.

Table 6.5 American College of Sports Medicine Dyspnea Scale

1. Mild—noticeable to patient but not to observer
2. Some difficulty—noticeable to observer
3. Moderate difficulty—but patient can continue
4. Severe difficulty—patient cannot continue

Note. From *American College of Sports Medicine: Guidelines for Exercise Testing and Prescription,* 4th ed. Philadelphia, Lea & Febiger, 1991. Reproduced with permission.

pacities. This formula takes into consideration the peak heart rate (PHR), the resting heart rate (RHR), and a percentage of the exercise intensity as factors in the equation (Hodgkin, 1988; Karvonen et al., 1957). Thus if a person has an atypically high or low RHR, this will be taken into consideration as a factor in the exercise prescription equation. (See chapter 5, page 74 for further discussion regarding methods for exercise prescription.)

You can use the ACSM Dyspnea Scale (Table 6.5) as an additional guide for exercise intensity in conjunction with the RPE scale and heart rate guidelines. This scale of 1 to 4 is a subjective measure of dyspnea ranging from *mild* to *severe difficulty.*

When prescribing exercise, you must also consider the type, intensity, frequency, and duration. Beginning a patient at an appropriately low level of exercise for which frequency and duration can be adjusted at regular intervals will more likely assure safety and a sense of success for the patient.

The format of the exercise class will be similar to that used in cardiac rehabilitation programs. It should include warm-up, aerobic, and cool-down exercises along with relaxation training. In considering appropriate warm-ups and aerobic exer-

cises, you should be familiar with specific medical problems resulting from the specific disease process. Many chronically ill patients have difficulty with nutritional balance and, like aging adults, experience decreases in muscle mass and increases in body fat (Hodgkin, 1988; Skinner, 1987b). Adrian (1981) reported that cartilage, tendon, and ligaments become stiffer and more rigid with age. Smith and Serfass (1981) stated that disuse and aging each accounted for about one-half the normal functional decline occurring from ages 30 to 70. These findings mean that the older adult is less able to adjust and recover from physiologic stimuli. This can be translated into a need to provide longer warm-up and cool-down periods. An appropriate warm-up including the use of light weights can be designed to last for 25 or 30 min. Some patients will be unable to manage floor exercises for warm-up routines (because of muscle wasting or decreased quadricep strength). Such patients should perform warm-up exercises sitting in chairs. The aerobic portion can include walking, swimming, rowing, bicycle ergometry, or very low level nonimpact aerobic movement. Jogging is not recommended secondary to low functional capacities and orthopedic complications. Begin with familiar exercises, exercises that patients like, and exercises that are easy and comfortable to perform. Familiarity and ease of performance may help to relieve anxiety and ensure success. You can also incorporate the use of very low level weights and weight training. Enhancing muscle strength can greatly improve the patient's ability to perform activities of daily living with much less fatigue (Hodgkin, 1987; Mahler & O'Donnell, 1991).

Health Education

In addition to exercise, health education plays an important role in the rehabilitation of chronically ill patients. Educational needs will vary, and some can be met by existing programs such as diet and nutrition, smoking cessation, and stress management. Other educational topics for special populations include the following:

- The disease entity and treatment modalities
- Realistic and achievable goals for exercise programs
- Early warning signs and symptoms that should be reported to their health care providers
- Self-monitoring and self-reporting skills
- Energy conservation and adaptive techniques for activities of daily living
- Medication, including its therapeutic uses and side effects
- Special dietary needs
- Sexuality
- Adapting to chronic illness

Guidelines for COPD Patients

In 1974, the American College of Chest Physicians defined pulmonary rehabilitation as

an art of medical practice wherein an individually-tailored multidisciplinary program is formulated which through accurate diagnosis, therapy, emotional support and education stabilizes or reverses both the physio- and psychopathology of pulmonary diseases and attempts to return the patient to the highest possible functional capacity allowed by his pulmonary handicap and overall life situation. (Hodgkin, 1988)

In the United States, COPD—including emphysema, chronic bronchitis, and related conditions—ranked as the fifth leading cause of death in the 1980s. The mortality for COPD increased 71% from 1966 to 1986 (Ries, 1991). Pulmonary rehabilitation programs have the potential to positively impact this significant rate of mortality from COPD.

Any patient with respiratory symptoms, abnormal spirogram, or COPD may benefit from a pulmonary rehabilitation program (Hodgkin, 1988; Ries, 1991). This includes those diagnosed with chronic emphysema, chronic bronchitis, and asthma. Entrance into an exercise program should include careful assessment, as previously described. In addition, this assessment should include pulmonary function testing and an evaluation of oxygen saturation during exercise. It is important to establish oxygen saturation levels at rest and with exercise to determine the need for possible supplemental

oxygen therapy (see Figure 6.3). Bicycle ergometry or treadmill testing using measurement of oxygen saturation may be preferred initially over the 12-min walk test, to assess both cardiac and pulmonary status (Hodgkin, 1987). Goals should be realistic and should be based on impaired pulmonary function, exercise performance, and oxygen saturation. If the patient has unrealistic expectations regarding potential improvement, disappointment and hostility may result (Hodgkin, 1988).

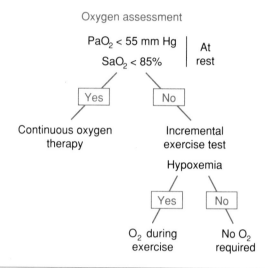

Figure 6.3 Exercise testing protocol for use of supplementary oxygen.
Note. From ''Exercise in Chronic Obstructive Pulmonary Disease'' by Michael J. Belman. In *Exercise in Modern Medicine* (pp. 175-193) by B.A. Franklin, S. Gordon, & G. Timmis (Eds.), 1988, Baltimore, MD: Williams & Wilkins. Copyright 1988 by Williams & Wilkins. Reprinted by permission.

In developing the exercise prescription, you must include specific considerations. Although patients with COPD are usually able to exercise to heart rates within the prescribed range (50 to 70%), their heart rates do not necessarily provide a reliable guide to exercise intensity. These patients often have a more rapid rise in heart rate with exercise than is normal, probably resulting from a reduced stroke volume response. Pulmonary patients experience a higher ventilatory requirement for the rate of work performed. There is a greater than normal rise in oxygen consumption of the ventilatory muscles with hyperpnea (abnormal increase in the depth and rate of respiration), resulting in less oxygen available for the exercising limbs (Belman, 1989). Therefore, in developing the exercise prescription, use a combination of the rate of perceived exertion, a dyspnea scale, and the

Karvonen formula for heart rate guidelines (Belman, 1989; Hodgkin, 1988).

Aerobic activities can include bicycle ergometry, walking, water exercise, rowing, swimming, and use of light weights. The duration of exercise can begin with increments as small as 30 s to 1 min with a frequency of 5 to 10 repetitions. A 1-min rest interval between each exercise bout usually provides adequate rest. The frequency can begin at three to four 30-min sessions per week. As the patient improves, increase duration, frequency, or both. A cool-down and relaxation period of 10 to 15 min with each exercise session will allow the patient to learn relaxation techniques that should be useful in daily life.

Incorporate breathing exercises into the warm-up, aerobic session, and cool-down. Pursed-lip breathing and prolonged exhalation time increase arterial oxygen saturation, decrease respiratory rate, decrease panic breathing, and reduce alveolar-arterial oxygen difference (Belman, 1986; Belman, 1989; Hodgkin, 1988).

The benefits of pulmonary rehabilitation are many. Some of them, however, are controversial, and further studies are necessary. Sinclair and Ingram (1980) found improvement with 8 to 12 months of exercise training; Mungall and Hainsworth (1980) found no improvements in 12 weeks of training. Long-term endurance training may be necessary in order for patients with pulmonary disease to show improvement. It is still unclear as to how the benefits of exercise training are accomplished in some pulmonary patients. Hodgkin (1979, 1981) showed that subjects who exercise experience decreases in heart rate and in minute ventilation; he also showed an increase in survival rate, but this may be due to better comprehensive care (Hodgkin, 1988). For some patients, although they obtain appropriate heart rates with exercise, the intensity of exercise may not be high enough for them to show actual training benefits (Belman, 1989). If there is an improvement in skill performance, this can be translated to improved activities of daily living. Research at Loma Linda University has shown a decrease in hospital stays from 19 to 6 days in an 8-year follow-up of pulmonary patients participating in a rehabilitation program (Hodgkin, Branscomb, Anholm, & Gray, 1984).

Guidelines for ESRD Patients

Less is known about the benefits of rehabilitation in the patient with ESRD. It is believed, however, that most patients with ESRD will benefit from a rehabilitation program. This includes patients pre- and post–kidney transplant, those on hemodialysis, and those on chronic ambulatory peritoneal dialysis (CAPD). With advanced medical technology the ESRD patient's life span may be prolonged but not without complications. Hypertension, elevated triglycerides, decreased HDL, glucose intolerance, and insulin resistance make this patient a high-risk candidate for cardiovascular disease. Other complications include anemia with hemoglobin and hematocrit levels approximately 50% of normal, peripheral neuropathies, osteoporosis, multiple blood chemistry abnormalities, and depression (Goldberg et al., 1980; Hagberg, 1989; Painter, Messer-Rehak, Hanson, Zimmerman, & Glass, 1986; Painter, Nelson-Worel, et al., 1986).

As with all special populations, the intake evaluation should include a thorough history and physical as well as exercise testing to evaluate for possible underlying coronary artery disease, arrhythmias, or abnormal hemodynamic blood pressure responses to exercise. Hagberg (1989) recommended avoiding exercise testing if the patient's potassium level is greater than 5 meq/L. If the patient is on hemodialysis, you must decide whether to test pre- or postdialysis. Barnea et al. (1980) found no significant difference in subjects' physical work capacity before or after dialysis, but you should consider how the patient feels as well as his blood pressure response to dialysis. The $\dot{V}O_2$max is lower for patients with ESRD (except for post–kidney transplant patients), sometimes as much as one-half of that compared to age- and sex-matched healthy sedentary individuals (Painter, Messer-Rehak, et al., 1986). Therefore, to avoid starting the patient at close to his $\dot{V}O_2$max, use a low-level exercise testing protocol.

To develop an exercise prescription for patients with ESRD, you should understand some of their atypical physiologic responses to exercise. The maximum heart rate of the hemodialysis and peritoneal dialysis patient can be 20 to 40 bpm lower than that found in healthy individuals (Painter, Nelson-Worel, et al., 1986). This is thought to be due to abnormalities within the sympathetic nervous system. The heart rate response during exercise is also somewhat abnormal secondary to autonomic dysfunction known to exist in these patients (Hagberg, 1989). With these variables in responses to exercise, the ESRD patient may benefit the most when you use a combination of the Karvonen Formula and the RPE scale when developing an exercise prescription. Because the Karvonen formula uses both the patient's resting and maximal heart rates, the abnormal responses of heart rate to exercise are thereby taken into account. Target heart rates may be lower and will be appropriate for individual patients. The RPE scale considers the patient's ''actual'' sense of fatigue at a given work load, whether this is secondary to abnormal heart rate response, chronic anemia, deconditioning, or other factors. Using these two scales in combination allows for the differences in physiologic responses to exercise; therefore patients will enjoy more success in exercising because they will be given more appropriate guidelines.

Prescription of low-level exercise intensity can also enhance the long-term efficacy and safety of the exercise routine. In the warm-up phase, due to muscle wasting and muscle weakness, some patients may need to sit in chairs. Others may be able to get up and down from floor mats. The CAPD patient generally exercises with fluid in the peritoneal cavity; this patient should avoid exercises that place her on her hands and knees because of the additional stress this causes on the abdominal muscles. Exercise modes can include walking, biking, rowing, swimming, low-level nonimpact aerobic movement, and low-level weight training. Because the bicycle ergometer allows the user to establish a very constant work rate and provides non-weight-bearing exercise, it is an excellent exercise modality for this patient population (Hagberg, 1989).

Potential problems with exercise for ESRD patients may include hypotension, hypertension, angina, arrhythmias, muscle cramps, bone fractures, and congestive heart failure. It is important that you evaluate the patient's medical stability prior to each exercise session. Concerning changes include a sudden weight gain, a sudden increase in blood pressure, low blood pressure, or new shortness of breath.

What are the benefits for the ESRD patient in a rehabilitation program? Much research remains to be done; however, some benefits have been shown, including the following (Barnea et al., 1980; Carney et al., 1983; Carney, Wetzel, Hagberg, & Goldberg, 1986; Goldberg et al., 1980; Hagberg, 1989; Hagberg et al., 1983; Painter, Nelson-Worel, et al., 1986; Shalom, 1984):

1. Increase in $\dot{V}O_2$max as much as 20 to 30%.
2. Increase in serum hemoglobin and hematocrit
3. A more normal response of blood pressure to exercise

4. Better control of serum triglyceride, very low density lipoproteins (VLDL), and high density lipoproteins (HDL)
5. Decrease in fasting serum insulin levels
6. Decrease in depression
7. Increase in self-confidence and motivation.

Conclusion

It is exciting to consider the potential for special populations to benefit from rehabilitation based on the cardiac rehabilitation model and modified to the specific needs of the individual. To ensure a safe and successful program, you should follow several important guidelines. First, carefully evaluate the patient's medical condition. Second, be sure there is a personal commitment from the patient and support from family and friends. Third, develop realistic and achievable goals and periodically review and update these goals to provide motivation for continued participation. Fourth, keep the exercise routines simple and diversified and allow individuals to work at their own pace. Fifth, provide expert knowledge in the specific disease entity, appropriate protocols and emergency procedures, and competent and caring medical supervision. Last, and most important, offer constant feedback, praise, and encouragement for motivation. Measurements of positive physiologic adaptations as a result of rehabilitative efforts are of critical importance to the patient. Equally important, however, are improvements in quality of life and an increased sense of independence, which may have a significantly greater impact on the patients for whom we care.

References

Adrian, M.J. (1981). Flexibility in the aging adult. In E.L. Smith & R.C. Serfass (Eds.), *Exercise and aging: The scientific basis* (pp. 45-58). Hillside, NJ: Enslow.

American Association of Cardiovascular and Pulmonary Rehabilitation. (1990). *Guidelines for cardiac rehabilitation*. Champaign, IL: Human Kinetics.

American College of Sports Medicine. (1991). *Guidelines for exercise testing and prescription* (4th ed.). Philadelphia: Lea & Febiger.

Barnea, N., Drory, Y., Iaina, A., Lapidot, C., Reisin, E., Eliahou, H., & Kellermann, J.J. (1980). Exercise tolerance in patients on chronic hemodialysis. *Israeli Journal of Medicine and Science*, **16**, 17-21.

Belman, M.J. (1986). Exercise in chronic obstructive pulmonary disease. *Clinics in Chest Medicine*, **7**(4), 585-595.

Belman, M.J. (1989). Exercise in chronic obstructive pulmonary disease. In B.A. Franklin, S. Gordon, & G. Timmis (Eds.), *Exercise in modern medicine* (pp. 175-193). Baltimore: Williams & Wilkins.

Berman, L.B., & Sutton, J.R. (1986). Exercise for the pulmonary patient. *Journal of Cardiopulmonary Rehabilitation*, **6**, 52-61.

Berra, K. (1992). Community resources for rehabilitation. In N.K. Wenger & H.K. Hellerstein (Eds.), *Rehabilitation of the coronary patient* (pp. 543-565). New York: Churchill Livingstone.

Borg, G.V. (1982). Psychophysical basis of perceived exertion. *Medicine and Science in Sports and Exercise*, **14**, 377-387.

Burek, K.A., Kirscht, J., & Topol, E.J. (1989). Exercise capacity in patients 3 days after acute, uncomplicated myocardial infarction. *Heart & Lung*, **18**, 575-582.

Carney, R.M., McKevitt, P.M., Goldberg, A.P., Hagberg, J., Delmex, J.A., & Harter, H.R. (1983). Psychological effects of exercise training in hemodialysis patients. *Nephron*, **33**, 179-181.

Carney, R.M., Wetzel, R.D., Hagberg, J., & Goldberg, A.P. (1986). The relationship between depression and aerobic capacity in hemodialysis patients. *Psychosomatic Medicine*, **48**, 143-147.

Cody, D.V., Dennis, A.R., & Ross, D.A. (1983). Early exercise testing, physical training and mortality in patients with severe left ventricular dysfunction. *Journal of the American College of Cardiology*, **2** (Suppl. 1), 718.

Conn, E.H., Williams, R.S., & Wallace, A.G. (1982). Exercise responses before and after physical conditioning in patients with severely depressed left ventricular function. *American Journal of Cardiology*, **49**, 296-300.

Croog, S.H., Levine, S., & Testa, M.A. (1986). The effects of antihypertensive therapy on the quality of life. *New England Journal of Medicine*, **314**(26), 1657.

Fletcher, G.F., Froelicher, V.F., Hartley, L.H., Haskell, W.L., & Pollock, M.L. (1990). Exercise standards: A statement for health professionals from the American Heart Association. *Circulation*, **82**, 2286-2322.

Fry, G., & Berra, K. (1981). *YMCArdiac therapy:*

Community based cardiac rehabilitation, **2**, 429-511. San Francisco: Carolyn Bean.

Goldberg, A.P., Hagberg, J., Delmez, J.A., Carney, R.M., McKevitt, P.M., Ehsani, A.A., & Harter, H.R. (1980). The metabolic and psychological effects of exercise training in hemodialysis patients. *American Journal of Clinical Nutrition*, **33**, 1620-1628.

Hagberg, J.M. (1989). Patients with end-stage renal disease. In B.A. Franklin, S. Gordon, & G. Timmis (Eds.), *Exercise in modern medicine* (pp. 146-155). Baltimore: Williams & Wilkins.

Hagberg, J.M., Goldberg, A.P., Ehsani, A.A., Heath, G.W., Delmez, J.A., & Harter, H.R. (1983). Exercise training improves hypertension in hemodialysis patients. *American Journal of Nephrology*, **3**, 209-212.

Hamalainen, H., Luurila, O.J., Kallio, V. (1989). Long-term reduction in sudden deaths after a multifactorial intervention programme in patients with myocardial infarction: 10-year results of a controlled investigation. *European Heart Journal*, **10**, 55.

Haskell, W.L. (1978). Cardiovascular complications during exercise training of cardiac patients. *Circulation*, **57**, 920.

Hellerstein, H.K., & Franklin, B.F. (1984). Exercise testing and prescription. In N.K. Wenger & H.K. Hellerstein (Eds.), *Rehabilitation of the coronary patient* (pp. 197-284). New York: Wiley.

Hodgkin, J.E. (1979). Current concepts in diagnosis and comprehensive care. In J.E. Hodgkin (Ed.), *Chronic pulmonary disease* (p. 34). Park Ridge, IL: American College of Chest Physicians.

Hodgkin, J.E. (1981). Pulmonary rehabilitation. In D.H. Simons (Ed.), *Current pulmonology* (p. 361). New York: Wiley.

Hodgkin, J.E. (1987). Exercise testing and training. In J.E. Hodgkin & T.L. Petty (Eds.), *Chronic obstructive pulmonary disease current concepts* (pp. 120-127). Philadelphia: Saunders.

Hodgkin, J.E. (1988). Pulmonary rehabilitation: Structure, components, and benefits. *Journal of Cardiopulmonary Rehabilitation*, **11**, 423-434.

Hodgkin, J.E., Branscomb, B.V., Anholm, J.D., & Gray, L.S. (1984). Benefits, limitations, and the future of pulmonary rehabilitation. In J.E. Hodgkin, E.G. Zorn, & G.L. Connors (Eds.), *Pulmonary rehabilitation: Guidelines to success* (pp. 403-414). Boston: Butterworth.

Hoffman, A., Duba, M., Lengyel, M., & Majer, K. (1987). The effect of training on the physical working capacity of MI patients with left ventricular dysfunction. *European Heart Journal*, **8** (Suppl. G), 43-49.

Kallio, V., Hamalainen, H., Hakkila, J., & Luurila, O.J. (1979). Reduction of sudden deaths by a multifactorial intervention programme after acute myocardial infarction. *Lancet*, **2**, 1091-1094.

Karvonen, M., Kentala, K., & Mustala, O. (1957). The effects of training on heart rate: A longitudinal study. *Annales Medicinae Experimentalis et Biologiae Fenniae*, **14**, 406.

Kremers, M.S., Black, W.H., & Wells, P.J. (1989). Sudden cardiac death: Etiologies, pathogenesis, and management. In R.C. Bone (Ed.), *Disease a month*, **35**, 385-435. Chicago: Yearbook Medical.

Leon, A.S., Certo, C., & Comoss, P. (1990). Scientific evidence of the value of cardiac rehabilitation services with emphasis on patients following myocardial infarction. Section 1: Exercise conditioning component. *Journal of Cardiopulmonary Rehabilitation*, **10**(3), 79.

Lipkin, D.P., Scriven, A.J., Crake, T., & Poole-Wilson, P.A. (1986). Six minute walking test for assessing exercise capacity in chronic heart failure. *British Medical Journal*, **292**, 653-656.

Lown, B., & Wolf, M. (1971). Approaches to sudden death from coronary heart disease. *Circulation*, **44**, 130-142.

Mahler, D.A., & O'Donnell, D.E. (1991). Alternative modes of exercise training for pulmonary patients. *Journal of Cardiopulmonary Rehabilitation*, **11**, 58-63.

McGavin, C.R., Gupta, S.P., & McHardy, G.J. (1976). Twelve-minute walk test for assessing disability in chronic bronchitis. *British Medical Journal*, **1**, 822-823.

McHenry, P.L., Ellestad, M.H., Fletcher, G.F., Hartley, H., Mitchell, J.H., & Froelicher, E.S. (1990). A position statement for health professionals by the committee on exercise and cardiac rehabilitation of the council on clinical cardiology, American Heart Association. *Circulation*, **81**(1), 396.

Miller, H.S., & Morley, D.L. (1987). Low functional capacity. In J.S. Skinner (Ed.), *Exercise testing and exercise prescription for special cases* (pp. 281-290). Philadelphia: Lea & Febiger.

Multicenter PostInfarction Research Group. (1983). Risk stratification and survival after myocardial infarction. *New England Journal of Medicine*, **309**, 331-336.

Mungall, I.P.F., & Hainsworth, R. (1980). An objective assessment of the value of exercise training to patients with chronic obstructive airways disease. *Quarterly Journal of Medicine*, **49**, 77-85.

Oldridge, N., Guyatt, G., Fischer, M., & Rimm, A. (1988). Cardiac rehabilitation after myocardial infarction: Combined experience of randomized clinical trials. *Journal of the American Medical Association*, **260**, 945.

Painter, P., Messer-Rehak, D., Hanson, P., Zimmerman, S.W., & Glass, N.R. (1986). Exercise capacity in hemodialysis, CAPD, and renal transplant patients. *Nephron*, **42**, 147-151.

Painter, P., Nelson-Worel, J.N., Hill, M.M., Thornbery, D.R., Shelp, W.R., Harrington, A.R., & Weinstein, A.B. (1986). Effects of exercise training during hemodialysis. *Nephron*, **43**, 87-92.

Parmley, W.W. (1986). President's page: Position report on cardiac rehabilitation. *Journal of the American College of Cardiology*, **7**(2), 451-453.

Peel, A.A., Semple, T., Wang, I., Lancaster, W.M., & Dall, J.L. (1962). A coronary prognostic index for grading the severity of infarction. *British Heart Journal*, **24**, 745-760.

Pollock, M.L., Wilmore, J.H., & Fox, S.M. (Eds.) (1984). Medical screening and evaluation procedures. In M.L. Pollock, J.H. Wilmore, & S.M. Fox (Eds.), *Exercise in health and disease* (pp. 155-243). Philadelphia: Saunders.

Ries, A.L. (1991). Pulmonary rehabilitation: Rationale components, and results. *Journal of Cardiopulmonary Rehabilitation*, **11**, 23-28.

Shalom, R., Blumenthal, J.A., Williams, R.S., McMurray, R.G., & Dennis, V.W. (1984). Feasibility and benefits of exercise training in patients on maintenance dialysis. *Kidney International*, **25**, 958-963.

Sinclair, D.J.M., & Ingram, C.P. (1980). Controlled trial of supervised exercise training in chronic bronchitis. *British Medical Journal*, **1**, 519-521.

Skinner, J.S. (1987a). General principles of exercise prescription. In J.S. Skinner (Ed.), *Exercise testing and exercise prescription for special cases* (pp. 21-30). Philadelphia: Lea & Febiger.

Skinner, J.S. (1987b). Importance of aging for exercise testing and exercise prescription. In J.S. Skinner (Ed.), *Exercise testing and exercise prescription for special cases* (pp. 67-75). Philadelphia: Lea & Febiger.

Smith, E.L., & Serfass, R.C. (Eds.) (1981). *Exercise and aging: The scientific basis* (pp. 11-17). Hillside, NJ: Enslow.

Squires, R.W., Lavie, C.J., Brandt, T.R., Gau, G.T., & Bailey, K.R. (1987). Cardiac rehabilitation in patients with severe ischemic left ventricular dysfunction. *Mayo Clinic Proceedings*, **62**, 997.

Sullivan, M.J., Higginbothom, M.B., & Cobb, F.R. (1988). Exercise training in patients with severe left ventricular dysfunction. Hemodynamic and metabolic effects. *Circulation*, **78**(3), 506-515.

Topol, E.J., Burek, K., O'Neil, W.W., Kewman, D.G., Kander, N.H., Shea, M.J., Schork, M.A., Kirscht, J., Juni, J.E., & Pitt, B. (1988). A randomized controlled trial of hospital discharge three days after myocardial infarction in the era of reperfusion. *New England Journal of Medicine*, **318**(17), 1083-1088.

Van Camp, S.P., & Peterson, R.A. (1986). Cardiovascular complications of outpatient cardiac rehabilitation programs. *Journal of the American Medical Association*, **256**(9), 1160-1163.

Van Camp, S.P., & Peterson, R.A. (1989). Identification of the high risk cardiac rehabilitation patient. *Journal of Cardiopulmonary Rehabilitation*, **9**, 103.

Wenger, N.K., (1987). Editorial: Future directions in cardiovascular rehabilitation. *Journal of Cardiopulmonary Rehabilitation*, **7**, 168-174.

Wenger, N.K., & Alpert, J.S. (1989). Rehabilitation of the coronary patient in 1989. *Archives of Internal Medicine*, **149**, 1504-1506.

Young, D.Z., Lampert, S., Graboys, T.B., & Loron, B. (1984). Safety of maximal exercise testing in patients at high risk for ventricular arrhythmia. *Circulation*, **70**(2), 184-191.

Part II

Program Implementation and Operation

When preparing to set up a program in a hospital, you must incorporate a number of basic strategies, components, and preprogram surveys to ensure there is a market for the program. It is important that you examine certain questions and answers before investing money in development.

Learning Objectives

---

1. To develop a plan for preimplementation review of needs and strategies

---

2. To recognize who are the most important people on your organization and implementation team

---

3. To understand program structure and advisory board composition in the preliminary stages of program development

---

Quite often, when asked to assist a hospital in setting up a cardiac rehabilitation program I am surprised to find that the hospital administrators and the program development team have not investigated whether a program is feasible. There are many questions to ask, some surveys to conduct, and brainstorming to do before you form a conceptual model of a program. You may discover that a cardiac rehabilitation program is not financially or operationally feasible and may decide not to start a program.

Predevelopment Homework

From the outset, you must be realistic in the preliminary questions you ask. The main questions that you must ask are, Who is asking for a program, and why are they asking? The *who* is particularly important because this is the driving force for the program. If the people behind the program development are physicians or a physician group that has a huge referral base at the hospital, clinic, or medical office complex, then the program will be successful. However, it is necessary that the number of supporting physicians be large, that they desire the program, and that they will support the program with patient referrals. If the people behind the program development are the hospital administrators, then again the program will be successful. The administrators are the fiscal officers and will control the money to develop and run a program. If the people behind the movement are nurses, physical therapists, occupational therapists, exercise physiologists, or a similar professional group, they will have to be excellent salespeople because they are not financial or patient gatekeepers.

Substantiating the Benefits

When examining reasons for developing a cardiac rehabilitation program, consider the following:

1. A cardiac rehabilitation program provides excellent public relations for the hospital and for physicians who refer to the program. The program at the TCH receives from its patients an average rating of 4.5 on a 1-5 Likert Scale for three areas: ''Learned a lot from the program,'' ''The program was very valuable,'' and ''All cardiac patients should have

this program'' (1 = very poor, 5 = excellent). The opinions of patients are very important, because these people will provide repeat business (33% of total business each year).

2. A cardiac rehabilitation program is not a revenue generator. Such programs will be even less profitable in the next 10 to 20 years. Many programs do not make money when direct revenues are the only revenues counted; the majority of programs barely make their bottom line. However, there are several indirect revenue sources that the wise department director may include or may claim a share of when figuring the department's bottom line. For example, any pre- and postexercise tests performed on patients as they enter cardiac rehabilitation generate revenue, as do any catheterizations, thallium stress tests, or other invasive procedures done while patients are undergoing cardiac rehabilitation.

Additionally, about 33% of all cardiovascular patients require some interventional or ''re-do'' procedures within 10 years postdischarge. If those patients are a part of cardiac rehab, you can claim that their loyalty to the hospital was enhanced in the cardiac rehabilitation center. Thereby you can claim revenue from the cardiovascular invasive procedure labs and surgery areas for those repeat procedures and additional invasive procedures on people who are former patients of cardiac rehabilitation. This

---

DOING THE HOMEWORK

When The Christ Hospital (TCH) in Cincinnati, Ohio, began to explore the need to set up a cardiac rehabilitation program, it was because of the expressed wish of the director of the cardiothoracic surgery group. TCH is a large tertiary care hospital in downtown Cincinnati and has been marketed as ''The Heart Hospital.'' The cardiothoracic surgery group was the only surgical group that performed cardiothoracic surgeries at TCH, and the group traveled to three other local hospitals as well. As a result this group held a great deal of power in the TCH administration because of its strong financial infusion into the hospital's bottom line.

After the surgical director asked for a cardiac rehabilitation program to be developed, no survey was conducted to see who would refer to the program. In the first 5 years after the program was developed it experienced very difficult financial struggles, because the greatest referral sources were two cardiologists who had large practices but only captured about one-quarter of the potential market. Ironically, the surgical director did not become a good referral source until 2 to 3 years after the program was up and running. It is critical that you establish referral bases before you begin to spend money.

strategy is acceptable in the current market-driven plan of hospital programming (Coddington, Keen, Moore, & Clarke, 1990).

Allegheny General Hospital (AGH) has the largest inpatient program in the nation and bills for each inpatient visit. Although other insurers do reimburse for inpatient therapy, Medicare billing is no more than a paper chase. The AGH administration chooses to give the paper value of revenue generated to the cardiac rehabilitation cost center. *Paper chase* means that Medicare gives a specific amount of money for each major diagnostic procedure code that is documented.

At AGH, when we include in our 1989-1990 budget all areas of the program such as stress testing, employee fitness, diet programs, and outpatient programs, we show a profit of $150,000 (cost = $625,000 and revenue = $775,000). When compared to profits of other departments in the hospital, this profit is just a drop in the bucket; however, the program is not a loser and is looked upon with favor. Cardiac rehabilitation programs are expensive to operate, and the largest overhead expense is personnel.

3. Practicing cardiac rehabilitation is practicing good medicine; for several reasons, it has been proven efficacious (National Center for Health Services Research and Health Care Technology Assessment, 1987; O'Connor et al., 1989; Oldridge, Guyatt, Fischer, & Rimm, 1988). Patients feel better when they undergo rehab, and although for the long term the results are equivocal between those who have rehabilitation and those who do not, short term there are significant differences between functional improvement and psychological well-being for the cardiac rehabilitation participants.

Examining the Numbers

Investigation of potential inpatient and outpatient numbers is crucial to determining the need for a cardiac rehabilitation program. What is the size of the hospital (number of beds, number of intensive care beds) and the number of cardiology admissions per year? Does the hospital do cardiothoracic surgery, and if so, how many procedures? Are transplants and cardiological research a part of the hospital's mission? Is it a tertiary care hospital? Are

the majority of patients local or do they live out of the area?

It is difficult to predict the actual numbers of patients who will enter cardiac rehabilitation, but some guidelines can be followed. Suppose that you are in a tertiary care hospital that performs 1,000 bypass surgeries a year. If inpatient rehabilitation is a standing order procedure this will generate between 850 and 900 patients per year with about five visits per patient. Thus from the surgical group there will be roughly 4,500 inpatient visits a year. The hospital also treats about 350 cardiology patients per year with about a 50% referral order census (this is a fairly accurate estimate of the percentage of cardiologists, internists, and family practice physicians who write referral orders). Of the 350 patients, about 300 are eligible; however, just 150 are referred and they average five visits per patient. The total cardiology visits are 750 plus the 4,500 surgical visits, for a total of about 5,250 visits in the inpatient program. Because you are part of a tertiary care hospital, you will probably capture 30% of the cardiology patients and about 10 to 15% of the surgical patients for your outpatient program, or altogether 150 patients who will average 18 visits each over a 6- to 8-week period.

Suppose that you are not a tertiary care hospital but are a 350-bed community hospital that does about 300 surgeries a year and has about 250 to 300 cardiology admissions per year. Depending upon the standing orders and physician interest you are likely to have about 1,200 inpatient visits from the surgical and about 700 from the medical. Depending upon physician interest and support, your potential outpatient program is about 150 patients in the year for 18 visits each, spread out over a 6- to 8-week period.

As you can see from these examples, essential questions are, Who wants the program? Who will refer patients and how many patients? and Where does the program support come from? Generally, large tertiary care hospitals have the potential for sizable inpatient programs and small outpatient programs. Sometimes the tertiary care programs' hardest job is referring patients to appropriate programs in their hometowns upon discharge, because it is essential that they know what such programs entail and how good they are. Smaller hospitals in the 250- to 400-bed range will have fairly well-balanced numbers of patients from cardiology and surgical consults; however, it is important that the physicians want the rehab program, believe it is valuable, and will support it with patient referrals and vocal support to the administration.

Survey all of the potential referring physicians—cardiologists, internists, family practice physicians, and cardiovascular surgeons—and ask them the following questions:

1. Do you believe that cardiac rehabilitation is a viable program for your patients after MI, angioplasty, surgery, or valve replacement?
2. Do you believe that rehab will reduce the risk of sudden death postevent during the recovery period?
3. Will you refer patients who would benefit from a comprehensive cardiac rehab program to a program at this hospital?
4. Are there specific components that you wish to see in the cardiac rehabilitation program?
5. What will prevent you from referring patients to a cardiac rehabilitation program?

It is essential to ask these and any other questions to which you seek answers before making the decision to start a program. In order to sell a program, you have to ask the potential buyer what he will buy, when he will buy it, and how often.

After you have asked all of these preliminary questions, you should have an idea whether the number of potential patients will support a program and what size the program will be. The new AACVPR (1991) guidelines recommend a 1:5 staff-to-patient ratio for outpatient Phase II rehabilitation. There must also be an observer to assist in emergencies; this person may be a secretary, a data entry person, an intern from a university, a part-time staff member—essentially anyone who is trained in the appropriate emergency procedures protocol. A small outpatient program might meet three times a week for 1 hr each time. It might have 2 or 3 classes a week which represents 6 to 9 contact hours a week. The staff could then do inpatient education and exercise therapy during the other half of the day. A comprehensive program can exist with a staff of one nurse-physiologist, a medical director, and an intern/secretary or part-time assistant. In a large center you can end up with a staff of 15 because your inpatient and outpatient demand can equal 15,000 patient contacts per year.

Another predevelopment concern is the reimbursement picture in your city. Reimbursement mandates are regional, each insurance provider has different coverages, and specific diagnoses are not covered in all policies. (See chapter 12 for direction on obtaining reimbursement.) This is an area that you should investigate before the program is started.

Location and Administration

Once you have determined that there will be a cardiac rehabilitation program, there are more crucial questions to ask.

In What Administrative Division Shall Cardiac Rehabilitation Reside?

The cardiac rehabilitation program should become a division unto itself and should reside in the Department of Cardiology or Division of Cardiovascular Surgery. The program should report to an administrative officer directly. Cardiac rehabilitation should not become a part of nursing, physical therapy, or occupational therapy, although it could be placed in a division of rehabilitation and stand as a department of rehab, the same as physical therapy and occupational therapy. The main reason for this is reimbursement: it is important to establish that cardiac rehab is not just a part of nursing or physical therapy care but is a specific treatment/intervention applied by trained professionals.

Who Shall Direct the Program?

The person who is selected for the director/manager should have a comprehensive knowledge of cardiac rehabilitation. This professional should meet the specifications outlined in the AACVPR (1991) guidelines. This person must also have budget, personnel, and other management skills and must know how to develop programs and business plans and evaluate performance. An applicant who has earned a master's degree in business or has completed some of the course work for a master's degree will likely have these abilities.

Will the Program Be Headed by a Medical Director or by a Medical Steering Committee?

This question is a difficult one to answer because either way there are pros and cons. A medical director can make decisions more easily, and the program can establish medical and interventional policies much faster and with less hassle. However, the medical director must have no ulterior motives (e.g., increasing practice size or recruiting other physicians' patients) and should be comfortable with and not offensive to any other physician or physician group. A steering committee allows all practices involved in referring patients a chance to give input, which can generate new ideas and create a more balanced program. A committee does make decision making cumbersome, it means rotating supervisors, and it will slow the administrative process by days, weeks, and sometimes even months. I have worked with both and I favor the medical director, ideally one who does not have a private practice, who is salaried by the clinic/hospital, and whose primary responsibility is to the rehab program. Having a medical director allows for a closer relationship with the staff members (because they need to interface with only one person) and for a more informal process of official paperwork; plus, communication is reduced by three or four steps.

Your physician/medical director and your administrative officer will help you to make inpatient cardiac rehabilitation a standing orders procedure. Most often the surgical team will establish this procedure because surgeons know cardiac rehabilitation facilitates healing and shortens length of stay. The standing orders mechanism can work through scheduling such that when the patient enters the hospital for presurgical testing and teaching, the cardiac rehabilitation staff is consulted at that time and enters the patient into the rehabilitation continuum. Medical referrals can occur when admissions notifies the department that a patient whose physician has established referral patterns and who is an appropriate candidate for cardiac rehabilitation has checked in. Your program will be much more successful if you can establish standing order and referral procedures, because you will not spend as much time trying to enroll patients. To achieve these procedures, you must provide state-of-the-art rehabilitation, use your physician medical director, and practice good politicking.

Will the Program Be Considered in Its Entirety or as Separate Phases?

Many times Phase I is part of the nursing department, Phase II is part of the cardiology department, and Phase III is administered by the local community college, high school, or YMCA. Three cost centers, three directors, three philosophies, and three different sets of policies and procedures produce a great deal of confusion as well as poor transitions and referral for the patients. This sort of separation can work if there is good communication among all leaders, but the usual result is chaos, jealousy, and a loss of potential patients and revenue. Thus I recommend that the department be its own entity from the inhospital Phase I to the outpatient Phase III and IV program. The department should have one director, one medical director, and a staff that works in and through all phases.

Conclusion

Other questions will arise as you go through the preliminary question/answer work. One of the best approaches you can take when setting up a program is to find a program in another hospital/setting that is similar to your hospital/setting. Make sure the program is well founded and state of the art. Make a site visit, observe how the program operates, and ask plenty of questions. Sometimes you may have to pay a fee, but you can also gather many answers that will save you money in the long run.

Finally, use all of the departments in your hospital to help you set up the preprogram planning and decision making. Write a business plan, and work with the marketing department for your market research. Talk with the medical committee and the director of medicine in your hospital. Good preplanning, questioning, and laying foundations are inherent in knowing when and how the establishment of a cardiac rehabilitation program may prove efficacious.

Further Reading

Fardy, P.S., Yanowitz, F., & Wilson, P.K. (1988). *Cardiac rehabilitation, adult fitness and exercise testing*. Philadelphia: Lea & Febiger.

Pashkow, F., Pashkow, P., & Schafer, M. (1987). *Successful cardiac rehabilitation*. Loveland, Colorado: HeartWatchers Press.

References

American Association of Cardiovascular and Pulmonary Rehabilitation. (1991). *Guidelines for cardiac rehabilitation*. Champaign, IL: Human Kinetics.

Coddington, D.C., Keen, D.J., Moore, K.D., & Clarke, R.L. (1990). *The crisis in health care*. San Francisco: Jossey-Bass.

National Center for Health Services Research and Health Care Technology Assessment. (1987). *Health technology assessment reports, cardiac rehabilitation services* (DHHS Publication No. PHS 88-3427, pp. 1-89). Rockville, MD: U.S. Department of Health and Human Services.

O'Connor, G.T., Buring, J.E., Yusuf, S., Goldhaber, S.Z., Olmstead, E.M., Paffenbarger, R.W., & Hennekens, C.H. (1989). An overview of randomized trials of rehabilitation with exercise after myocardial infarction. *Circulation,* **80**, 234-244.

Oldridge, N.B., Guyatt, G.H., Fischer, M.E., & Rimm, A.A. (1988). Cardiac rehabilitation after myocardial infarction: Combined experience of randomized clinical trials. *Journal of American Medical Association,* **260**, 945-950.

Wittels, E.H., Hay, J.W., Gotto, A.M. (1990). Medical costs of coronary artery disease in the United States. *American Journal of Cardiology,* **65**, 432-440.

Chapter 7

Staffing the Program

Linda K. Hall, PhD

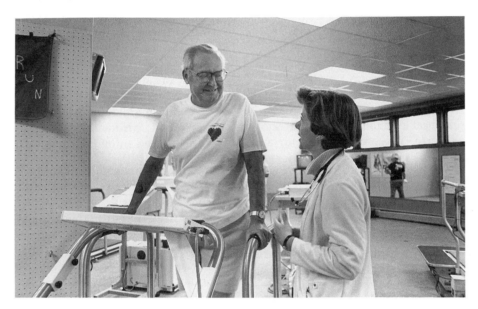

Planning your Phase I, II, or III/IV program is one small part of the job. The next biggest task that management faces is hiring staff members with the skills, knowledges, and personalities to make the program a success. Often, the staff is the first interface with patients, physicians, and family in the application of cardiac rehabilitation. Because of this, staff is your major marketing tool to ensure success of your program. This chapter discusses task analysis, job descriptions, and staffing qualifications to effect good program application.

Learning Objectives
1. To ascertain what positions you will need to fill to operate your program
2. To understand the writing and evaluation of performance objectives to assist in optimum job performance
3. To understand the basis of writing job descriptions to fulfill the needs of your department

People often ask me who the best person is to deliver cardiac rehabilitation: a nurse, a physical therapist, an exercise physiologist, or some other professional. My answer is the person who has the professional training, skills, and abilities that fit the job description and who presents a personality that fits the job you are seeking to fill. You should consider a number of things as you staff your cardiac rehabilitation center. This chapter will cover staffing concerns such as task analysis, job descriptions, performance objectives, performance evaluation, and the various professionals who make up the cardiac rehabilitation team and their recommended qualifications.

Selecting the Appropriate Person for the Job

Initially, you need to fill three positions in order to operate a cardiac rehabilitation program: These positions are medical director, program director, and registered nurse. The program director and the registered nurse may be the same person. AACVPR (1991) has delineated required qualifications for each of these positions, and you should ensure at least the minimum qualifications for each person you hire.

A number of programs are directed by nurses or exercise physiologists, and the majority of the personnel that make up departments come from the nursing and exercise physiology fields. In the past, medical doctors or administrators have started departments by appointing a critical care unit or intensive care unit nurse as director of cardiac rehabilitation and also as program developer. Such a nurse knows the disease process and medical interventions, is familiar with emergency procedures, and knows the pathophysiology. However, this nurse may lack a number of skills and knowledges related to exercise physiology, teaching, psychological and health strategies for risk factor modification, and basic management principles. AACVPR (1991) has established a baseline statement:

> The collective knowledge base of the person or persons assigned to the patient service must include a comprehensive and up-to-date understanding of cardiovascular diseases, cardiovascular nursing, cardiovascular emergency procedures, nutrition, exercise physiology, health psychology and medical and educational strategies for CAD risk factor management. (p. 34)

Additionally, qualifications required for the nurse and/or director of the department are the following (AACVPR, 1991, pp. 35-36):

- Bachelor's degree in an allied health field such as exercise physiology, or licensure in jurisdiction as a registered nurse
- Advance knowledge of exercise physiology, nutrition, risk-factor modification strategies, counseling techniques, and uses of educational programs and technologies as applied to cardiovascular rehabilitation services
- Certification, experience, and training equivalent to those specified for an exercise specialist by ACSM or the advance specialty in cardiopulmonary rehabilitation of the American Physical Therapy Association
- Experience in coordination of staff and delivery of cardiovascular rehabilitation services to patients
- Certification in basic life support (BLS) or advanced cardiac life support (ACLS) (if registered nurse)

With the delineation of these specific requirements, the specialty of the cardiac rehabilitation professional has arrived.

As you start to form the structure, policies, and procedures of the department, job characteristics and descriptions will begin to take form. In order to write the job description for a position you should have some idea of the skills required for the position. Table 7.1 provides a series of job requirement characteristics and the tasks that are usually a part of those job characteristics. These will help you establish the job descriptions. Also, you should determine the types of certifications or licenses that the job will require, such as nursing and physical therapy licensure or ACSM certifications. Appendix B provides examples of job descriptions for the director, exercise specialist, and clinical nutritionist. Usually your hospital human resources department will have a special form or method that you should follow when writing a job description. Each year the job description should be reviewed by you and by those staff members who fill the position to see if the description needs adjustment.

A word of budgetary prudence is necessary here and will be discussed further in the budget chapter (chapter 13). When you are setting up your department and hiring personnel, make sure that you hire people who fill the program's needs and do not hire overqualified people. For example, you do not need to hire a person with administrative

Table 7.1 Job Characteristics and Tasks

Manage information and utilize computers

Maintain appropriate records
Provide data for procedure manuals
Prepare daily work schedules
Identify and submit quality assurance data
Submit data and information for long-term planning
Operate audiovisual equipment

Perform keyboard functions
Input new data into the computer
Search/review patient files
Edit reports
Retrieve reports, profiles, and statistics

Maintain appropriate ethical practices

Follow medical/legal standards
Obtain patient authorization
Follow policies and procedures relative to patient
  confidentiality

Protect patient confidentiality
Maintain appropriate professional demeanor

Recognize emergency situations

Maintain Basic Life Support/Advanced Cardiac Life
  Support
Identify and report potential hazards
Recognize life-threatening arrhythmias

Activate institution's emergency medical system
Identify emergencies appropriately
Refer emergencies appropriately
Report/record incident forms

Perform testing procedures

Prepare and operate equipment
Recognize equipment malfunctions
Record/collect appropriate data
Record electrocardiograms
Take blood pressures
Perform graded exercise tests

Interpret and analyze data
Instruct the patient about the testing procedure
Administer informed consent
Prepare the patient
Comply with facility and other regulatory agency
  procedures and policies

Identify normal and abnormal pathophysiology

Apply basic anatomy and physiology concepts
Identify and correlate circulatory system

Recognize abnormal physiologic response
Identify normal/abnormal heart rhythms

Use good communication skills

Follow verbal and written directions
Present and speak well
Use technical writing skills
Recognize and use medical terminology
Conduct patient interviews

Explain test procedures/results
Recognize body language
Allay patient anxieties
Read and interpret results/charts

(continued)

113

Table 7.1 *(continued)*

Practice patient relations and integration

Coordinate and integrate all pertinent patient
  information
Apply appropriate principles of exercise physiology
  to individual patients
Coordinate patient recovery and reentry into
  activities of daily living

Assist in lifestyle change efforts
Listen actively
Establish trust
Show empathy
Encourage the patient
Display a sense of humor

Maintain professional development

Attend workshops and seminars
Use self-assessment techniques
Visit other work sites
Participate in professional interaction
Affiliate with local, state, regional, and national
  professional organizations

Read current journals, books, and papers
Integrate what is new and worthwhile
Continuously examine current practices

Note. From *The Generic Cardiac Rehabilitation Task Analysis* by Carol Robbins, 1988, Morristown, NJ: National Board of Cardiovascular Testing. Copyright 1988 by Carol Robbins. Adapted by permission.

---

secretarial skills ($10.34 per hour) to do billing and data entry ($7.50 to $8.50 per hour), because that will increase your budget by as much as $5,000 per year. It is better to hire people who are a bit underqualified but who are eager to learn.

Questions you may ask when considering job skills and qualifications include these: What are the strengths of the current department staff? What are the department's weaknesses? What skills are needed in the future? Is this a part-time or full-time position? In all cases fill the needs, skills, and knowledges your department staff lacks and do not hire full-time when part-time will do. It is easier to justify increasing staff (see chapter 14) than firing or letting people go because of budgetary overruns.

Performance Objectives and Evaluation

If quality care of the patient is compromised, this is probably due to one of three reasons: The staff does not have the knowledge to do the job, the staff has attitude and behavior problems, or there is a breakdown in the systems. The knowledge question is discussed in chapter 10 and the systems question is covered in chapter 13; attitudes and behavior will be discussed here. The process

of writing performance objectives and also evaluating performance is the specific area where you can manage attitude and behavior problems. If an employee knows how you expect him to perform his job and the timelines for the completion of certain tasks, then there should be no difficulty in the way he performs his work. When problems arise with an individual employee, do an impromptu midyear performance check. Go over the performance objectives with the employee and see if the difficulty is with the job. If it is, look at the objectives or the job description and negotiate a rewrite. If the difficulty is not with the objectives or the job description, direct the employee toward counseling or an agency to help with the problem. Remember, you wrote the performance objectives in order to remove obstacles that prevent optimum work performance. The key to optimum performance is an up-to-date job description and a set of performance objectives describing what optimum performance is.

Performance Objectives

Once you have hired personnel, the way you guide and assist them toward optimum performance is a major determinant of your department's success. I have observed that no matter how wonderful the facilities and equipment or how fancy the paper educational materials, if a staff is not professional, knowledgeable, and good with people, the program will fail. You can ensure good performance from employees by using many tools, not the least of which are good, modern management techniques (see chapter 10). It is equally important that staff members have comprehensive job descriptions and know how they will be evaluated and rewarded for doing their jobs.

Establishing performance objectives is an excellent way for you and the employee to establish goals, objectives, and outcome measures. When writing the performance objectives for staff members, use the following guidelines.

1. Write performance objectives around the job description. Do not include things that are not in the description unless the employee includes them as "growth" objectives.
2. Write goals as nonspecific statements with a global perspective. Example: I wish to become a published author. This is a statement of a goal because it does not specify what I wish to write, when, or for what type of audience. An example of a goal in cardiac rehabilitation may be this: Perform the responsibilities for the job of exercise specialist in the department of cardiac rehab. Once again there is no specific delineation of how, when, or where the stated goal is accomplished.
3. Write objectives so they specifically enumerate how the goals are to be achieved. There are many guidelines for writing objectives; however, I favor using the mnemonic SMART (Miller, 1988).

S — Specific: The objective specifies the job skill or duty that is to be evaluated.

Example: Complete performance of Phase II exercise specialist as assigned: paper work, billing, education, charting, exercise prescriptions.

M — Measurable: The way in which you judge whether the objective is met and can be checked off, counted, quantified, and qualified.

A — Appropriate: The objective is functional. It makes sense and is a suitable way of evaluating the activity.

R — Reasonable: The information being sought is available and will not require additional work or steps.

T — Timely: There is a specific date for the objective to be met.

The following is an example of performance objectives for a clinical coordinator in an outpatient program.

PERFORMANCE OBJECTIVES

I. To perform optimally the duties and responsibilities outlined in my (the clinical coordinator) job description

Measurable parameters:

A. Every 6 months a random examination of staff charting procedures within the Phase II program
 1. Three to four charts per staff
 2. All staff reviewed one time within 6 months
 3. Reviewed for completeness, documentation, and follow-up
 4. Report includes
  a) Who were reviewed (staff)
  b) Evaluation (rating scale 1 to 5, 5 being excellent)
  c) Variance found
  d) Action taken
 5. First report due December

B. Every 6 months a performance evaluation of staff members in their duties in Phases II and III, to include the following:
 1. Patient interaction, communication skills, educational expertise, and one-on-one and group skills
 2. First evaluation due in December

C. A quarterly summary report written on the following:
 1. Number of intake interviews and exit interviews done by you (numbers only)

  How many in: MET level, risk factors, body weight

  How many out: MET level, risk factors, body weight

  Brief summary statement

 2. Number of patients in exercise training; total month and outpatient evaluations (Quality Assurance information)
 3. A summary report on Phase II education program:
  a) Number of people attending
  b) Staff performing the program
 4. First quarterly report due September 30, 1989

D. Annually evaluate the staff relative to performance in program areas that you supervise

Measurable parameters

1. Write a performance objective for staff relative to each area you supervise that includes methods of evaluation and parameters. Submit to the department director by September 30 each year (See SMART principles, page 115)
2. Submit the evaluation of each staff member relative to those parameters according to hospital evaluation standards by May 15

II. To serve as chairperson of the committee to rewrite and revise the policies and procedures relative to Phases II and III. These policies include but are not limited to patient referral, pre-entry testing, intake interview, exercise prescription, exercise prescription revision, progress evaluation, charting, educational materials, exit criteria, exit interview, monitoring/nonmonitoring parameters, psychological consults, and others

Measurable parameters

A. Submit first drafts to the department for review and approval as developed. Complete first drafts on all areas by December 30, 1989. Complete project May 31, 1990.
   1. *Complete* means signed by department directors and hospital administrator
B. A plan for yearly review and revision

III. To serve actively on all other committees as assigned

IV. New projects and review of other areas
A. Participate in the work to totally restructure the Phase II and Phase III programs

Measurable parameter

1. Write material as asked for: Specific literature search of discharge, graded exercise testing, immediate post-discharge, predischarge, within 3 to 4 weeks postevent for MI, CABG, and angioplasty
   a) Written summary of following:
      1) Morbidity/mortality
      2) Specific protocol—symptom limited, HR limited, or MET limited
      3) General conclusions: Due September 30, 1989
B. Develop a plan to increase referral of Phase I patients to the Phase II (exercise program), specific to higher risk patients

Measurable parameter

1. Review literature relative to risk stratification and efficacy of exercise intervention
   a) Bibliography
   b) Summary of the literature
      1) Emphasis on prescription: duration, intensity, and mode of exercise
      2) Monitoring: duration
   c) Due October 31, 1989
C. Assist with in-services to nursing, occupational therapy, physical therapy

V. Pursue professional growth:
A. Attend and participate in national meeting
B. Become an ACSM fellow
C. Complete research as designated

BEHAVIORAL OBJECTIVES

I. Participate as an active leader within all functions of the department
A. Attitude appropriate to management perspective
   1. Language and communication style: verbal and nonverbal
   2. Constructive support of department objectives and mission
B. Support the department medical director and director in administrative decisions and leadership
   1. Advise and consent
   2. Constructive input

After you have designed the performance objectives for an employee, give the objectives to the employee to adjust, change, add to, or agree with. The objectives should be a tool upon which you and the employee mutually agree. Thus, when the employee is evaluated, she knows with what parameters she will be evaluated, and there are no surprises.

Evaluating the Employee's Performance

The Joint Commission on Accreditation of Healthcare Organizations (JCAHO) as well as AACVPR recommend or expect a review of performance as a part of Quality Assurance and yearly efficacy evaluations. There are numerous reasons why evaluating employees on an annual basis is a good management technique. It helps you and the employee to answer the following:

- Is she fulfilling the job as described and the agreed upon performance objectives?
- Does she know and understand what is expected in the job description and performance objectives?
- Is she working to her highest potential, with peak performance?
- Is she using good work habits and performing to a high standard?
- What strengths can be enhanced?
- What areas of performance deserve recognition?
- Is there a potential for advancement as a result of performance?
- What areas need to be improved, and what avenues are available for improvement?

A performance evaluation should be a joint effort between you and the employee, not a confrontation that is viewed with apprehension. If you have had good, open communication throughout the year, the employee should have no surprises on her evaluation. Following are some suggestions to make the evaluation process a "healthy," eagerly anticipated event.

1. Inform the employee of the evaluation at least a month before the evaluation date. Ask him to submit in writing a summary of his own performance and to highlight as a reminder the "plus" activities for the past year.
2. Make notes and keep letters, programs, and any other documentation of the employee's performance in his file during the year (e.g., programs from symposia or workshops the employee attended or spoke at, published articles, and patient thank-yous and recognition notes).
3. Review the performance objectives and job description and tally those criteria that are measurable relative to performance. Characteristics that you may describe include quality of work, consistency of performance, work effort, job knowledge, cooperation, attitude, loyalty to the company, and interaction with fellow employees. Follow the same format for each evaluation: Identify the objective and then consider the employee's performance and methods for improvement, if improvement is needed. We use the following designations at Allegheny General Hospital when evaluating personnel:

EA = Exceeds all expectations: 100% of plan objectives exceeded

EE = Exceeds most expectations: Greater than 90% of plan objectives and job responsibilities met and or exceeded

ME = Meets expectations: Greater than 80% of plan objectives and job responsibilities met or exceeded

BE = Below expectations: Less than 80% of plan objectives and job responsibilities met or exceeded

4. Write up the performance evaluation and arrange an appointment with the employee for the review and a discussion of the evaluation. This is an important meeting; take your phone off the hook and give the employee the impression that you value this meeting time with her and that she has your undivided attention.
5. During the meeting it is important that you do the following:
   - Put the employee at ease.
   - Give the employee an opportunity to express how he views the job, the climate, and his performance.
   - Provide a summary of the employee's performance from an interpersonal, technical, and administrative point of view.
   - Point out and praise desirable behaviors.
   - Point out opportunities for improvement (no more than two, and work-related items only).
   - Create a mutually agreed upon plan of improvement.
   - Discuss opportunities for advancement, pay increases, and career directions.
   - Conclude the evaluation on a pleasant and constructive note.
6. Give the employee the opportunity to present any additional information that he believes may improve the evaluation.

It is critically important that personnel information remains confidential; it should be available only to you, the employee, and designated people in administration and personnel. If there is negative information in the employee's file, be sure the employee is aware of how she can "clear the record." Once a negative behavior has been corrected, it is removed from the record. It is also of utmost importance that professional accomplishments and achievements are made known to peer staff and administrative staff. This tells the employee that you are interested in her and working on her behalf.

Developing the Rehabilitation Team

I have alluded to the AACVPR *Guidelines for Cardiac Rehabilitation Programs* (1991) several times in this chapter, and at this time I refer you to chapter 4 for general comments relative to staffing, staffing ratios, and competencies of personnel who should or may be involved in a cardiac rehabilitation program. The specific required as well as preferred qualifications are especially important to adhere to as you involve different professional groups in your team. Chapters 8 and 9 discuss related information specific to the dietitian, social worker, and pastoral care counselor; these positions have been singled out because they can cross many of the other professions and make up a large part of your team.

Who Does What

Anyone who has been trained to be a cardiac rehabilitation professional is able to do inpatient and outpatient rehabilitation. The staff at Allegheny General Hospital, for example, is made up of nurses, exercise specialists, a dietitian, a psychologist, and a medical director. Some of the nurses worked step-down (the postcoronary care unit) and others worked critical care unit, emergency, and nursing staff development before being hired to the cardiac rehab department. The exercise physiologists come with a myriad of past experience such as physical therapy work-evaluation units, and fitness in business and industry. They go through a very extensive in-service training program before they are alone with the patients: They are taught, they observe, they are observed, they work with someone, and then they are on their own with spot checks. Every staff member works inpatient, carrying a patient load of about seven patients per day on a case management basis. They work with another therapist in one outpatient Phase II class per day, carrying a load of no more than four patients for each therapist per class with a case management perspective. Each staff member has an integral role in the entire outpatient pro-

gram, rotating responsibility of phase supervision every 3 months. They are also trained to manage the technician's role in exercise testing. Each of them brings knowledge to the job that they share with one another, through training, working together, going to meetings, having in-services, and participating in continuing education. They share an incredibly large body of knowledge, and there is no one professional background that lends itself to cardiac rehabilitation better than another. However, cardiac rehab specialists possess a unique body of knowledge and skill that the ordinary nurse, exercise specialist, and physical therapist do not have.

At the 1984 Exercise and Health Symposium in La Crosse, Philip K. Wilson of the La Crosse Exercise Program said this: "When you are spending your money on building and maintaining your program, put your biggest dollars into your staff. Your staff—their education, personal qualities, and professionalism—is your biggest marketing and public relations tool." Wilson was correct. There is no machine or fancy exercise room that will do a better job than a personable, intelligent, enthusiastic employee who makes patients believe they are the most important people in the world.

Further Reading

American College of Sports Medicine. (1991). *Guidelines for exercise testing and prescription* (4th ed.). Philadelphia: Lea & Febiger.

Fardy, P.S., Yanowitz, F., & Wilson, P.K. (1988). *Cardiac adult fitness and exercise testing* (2nd ed.). Philadelphia: Lea & Febiger.

Pashkow, F., Pashkow, P., & Schafer, M. (1987). *Successful cardiac rehabilitation*. Loveland, CO: HeartWatchers Press.

References

American Association of Cardiovascular and Pulmonary Rehabilitation. (1991). *Guidelines for cardiac rehabilitation programs*. Champaign, IL: Human Kinetics.

Miller, T. (May, 1988). Spring workshop on long-range planning, AACVPR board of directors meeting. Dallas, Texas.

Wilson, P.K. (October, 1984). Administrative concerns in cardiac rehabilitation. La Crosse exercise and health symposium, La Crosse, WI.

Chapter 8

Use of a Registered Dietitian

Karen E. Luffey, RD

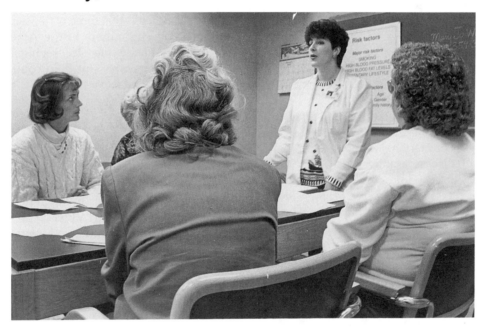

Most reference books on cardiac rehabilitation include a chapter on the educational information the cardiac patient should receive about diet and nutrition. Any registered dietitian has the basic knowledge of cholesterol-lowering, low-fat, low-salt diets. This chapter approaches the situation from a different angle. What skills beyond nutrition knowledge should your dietitian have? What kind of training beyond a registered dietitian's program should she have undergone? What is the best way to use the dietitian in your program?

Learning Objectives

1. To obtain guidelines for selecting the right dietitian for your program

2. To develop responsibilities and functional expectations for a dietitian in cardiac rehabilitation

3. To establish policies and procedures for using dietary services in cardiac rehabilitation

Nutrition education is not only vital information for every stage of life but is crucial in the prevention, treatment, and rehabilitation of cardiac-related health problems. Despite recent advances in these areas, heart disease remains the number one killer of Americans. Since 1968, however, the death rate for heart disease in Americans has continued to decline. Researchers have concluded that reducing the serum cholesterol level is the single largest contributor to improved cardiac health (Grundy, 1989). Generally, a 1% reduction in total serum cholesterol causes a 2% reduction in heart attack risk (Grundy, 1989).

An elevated serum cholesterol level is firmly established as one of the major risk factors in the development of coronary heart disease and in the progression of disease among those with diagnosed atherosclerosis (Gotto, 1989). In addition to high levels of total blood cholesterol, high levels of the LDL cholesterol fraction have been established as a major coronary heart disease risk factor (Grundy et al., 1982). Blankenhorn, Johnson, Mack, El Zein, and Vailas (1990) reported an increase in the risk of new lesions in human coronary arteries for each quartile of increased consumption of total fat and polyunsaturated fat. Diet is the first recommendation for treatment of patients with high blood cholesterol levels (Expert Panel, 1988).

Diet Intervention

The rationale for diet intervention becomes more and more impressive as scientific data from experimental animal studies, epidemiologic studies, and clinical trials provide highly suggestive evidence that particular dietary habits affect coronary heart disease risk (Grundy, 1982). For many years, the AHA has recommended modification of risk factors as a safe and effective way of reducing coronary heart disease. Although the range of serum cholesterol levels in Americans is large and may be influenced to a certain extent by genetic factors,

the relatively high mean is thought by many to be due to dietary patterns (Grundy, 1982). Because Americans in general have relatively high cholesterol levels, which appear to increase risk for coronary heart disease, AHA recommends a specific dietary plan designed to reduce serum cholesterol to a safer level for the general public (AHA, 1984b). AHA recommends that those with diagnosed hyperlipidemia strictly adhere to the American Heart Association diet while also seeing a registered dietitian for intensive nutrition counseling.

Prescribing the Diet

The specific dietary components shown to influence serum lipid levels are total fat, saturated fat, dietary cholesterol, total calories, alcohol, and fiber (Frank, 1988). Dietary modifications to reduce serum cholesterol levels in the general public, as recommended by the AHA Phase I program (AHA, 1984b), include the following: Lower the percentage of total daily calories obtained from fat to below 30%. From the 30% fat calories, obtain less than 10% from saturated fat, 10% from polyunsaturated fat, and 10% from monounsaturated fat. Lower intake of dietary cholesterol to below 300 mg per day. Reduce intake of calories to achieve and maintain ideal body weight, and increase complex carbohydrate foods, particularly those containing soluble fiber. For those requiring specific dietary therapy for hypercholesterolemia, AHA (1984b) recommends a progressive reduction in the percent of calories as fat to 20%, as well as reduction of cholesterol intake to 100 to 150 mg per day.

Reducing body weight to within one's ideal body weight range and decreasing intake of simple carbohydrates, alcohol, and total fat are primary modes of therapy for hypertriglyceridemia (Expert Panel, 1988). Weight loss decreases production of VLDL, thus lowering triglycerides and possibly raising HDL. The effect of weight loss on levels of LDL is variable in patients with hypertriglyceridemia; weight loss may reduce LDL levels in hypercholesterolemia patients. A reduction in saturated fat, total fat, and dietary cholesterol to lower LDL is important to affect high triglyceride levels (AHA, 1984b).

The coexistence of other medical conditions may affect the overall diet prescribed. Patients with renal failure may need to restrict protein; hypertensive patients may need to restrict sodium. The AHA diet is currently consistent with the diabetic diet recommended by the American Diabetes Association (AHA, 1984a). When drug therapy is indicated for some patients, diet therapy should continue and should be used in combination because the effects of both therapies are additive (Expert Panel, 1988).

Changing the Diet

The importance of having a nutritious, appetizing diet cannot be overemphasized. A well-balanced diet will promote good health aside from the modifications in fat intake. Because high blood cholesterol frequently has a familial component, the patient's family members should also eat diets low in total fat, saturated fat, and cholesterol (AHA, 1984a). This provides important support to the patient and sets a good example as well. *The American Heart Association Cookbook* (1984a) and *The American Heart Association Low-Fat, Low-Cholesterol Cookbook* (Grundy & Winston, 1989) are excellent references for patients and their families. *The New American Diet* (Connor & Connor, 1986) is also a very good resource. There are no harmful effects known to the general public for the dietary modifications recommended by AHA. These dietary recommendations seemingly will benefit all family members above the age of 2 years.

Although coronary heart disease is a disease of multifactorial etiology, diet has been documented numerous times as affecting coronary heart disease risk. All of the existing data point to the importance of truly effective nutrition counseling for hyperlipidemic patients and their families.

Diet is one of the risk factors that the patient can affect, yet diet modification is difficult. Literature shows that people are willing to make temporary dietary changes, but they do not follow these recommendations long term. This proves the need for an extensive follow-up program to support and encourage new eating habits.

One of the reasons diet is such a difficult area to permanently change is that food holds such strong emotional and social meanings. Actual hunger is one of the least common reasons people eat.

Most often people eat in response to environmental and internal stimuli such as the sight, sound, or smell of food; television commercials; time of day; social gatherings; and such emotional cues as boredom, stress, sadness, anger, and happiness. In addition, some individuals use food as comfort and as reward. A person's beginning in life, the mother-infant bond, revolves around food. Later in life, food continues to be the center of life for many people. Choosing when, what, how much, and what to eat gives people the sense of control.

Major dietary changes can uproot a person's life and change many aspects of daily living. In our society, nearly every social gathering is centered around food, which adds to the difficulty of changing eating habits. Dietary change is social change for many patients and families. Professional, social, and family support are necessary and crucial to ensure long-term eating habit change. Equally important is the patient's desire and degree of motivation to improve her eating habits.

The terms *diet, American Heart Association diet,* and *heart diet,* often associated with those nutrition recommendations for cardiac patients, connote deprivation, suffering, and torture to many people. This type of thinking can set a person up for failure at the very beginning of a program. Many heart patients and dieters believe a "good diet" will take away all favorite, good-tasting foods and leave a bland, boring, unpalatable, unsatisfying life and diet. These beliefs about diet are myths that need to be dispelled. Through proper nutrition education by a qualified registered dietitian, people will learn about and learn to follow a healthier eating style.

Nutrition Education

Effective and appropriate nutrition education is interesting, and it encourages patients to take advantage of the wide variety of foods available; it emphasizes what a person can eat instead of what to avoid. It is important that patients know what they should not eat, but accentuating the positive by concentrating on foods patients should eat is practical and enhances patients' chances of following recommended dietary guidelines.

A registered dietitian is the best qualified professional to provide nutrition counseling. Because sound nutrition and diet education is a cornerstone in cardiac rehabilitation, choosing the best qualified nutrition educator is essential for successful rehabilitation. A registered dietitian's major responsibilities are effectively communicating diet recommendations and following a patient for as long as necessary to support and guide the patient toward self-sufficiency and toward maintenance of dietary changes.

Choosing a Registered Dietitian

There are major differences between a registered dietitian and a nutritionist. Most importantly, there are no educational or professional requirements for a nutritionist. Anyone can claim to be a nutritionist with or without nutrition expertise or a credible background. To become a registered dietitian (RD), an individual must earn a degree in nutrition or a related field from a college or university accredited by the American Dietetic Association, complete an internship or special work experience approved by the American Dietetic Association, pass the American Dietetic Association National Registration Examination, and participate in continuing education reviewed yearly by the American Dietetic Association.

In addition to education and professional credentials, a registered dietitian must possess a number of important knowledge and practice skills to function effectively in a cardiac rehabilitation setting.

- In order to set a good example, have an empathetic understanding, and really know what he is talking about, the registered dietitian should live the lifestyle and recommendations he professes. Practicing and believing in exercise and diet as a healthy combination are essential.
- This role model should be able to convincingly describe how satisfying and tasteful a healthy, nutritious diet is, so as to dispel the negative images of *diet* or *heart diet*.
- A pleasant and sincere personality and an ability to develop an open, friendly, honest rapport are essential for effective communications. Patience and an understanding attitude tempered with appropriate assertiveness enhances diet compliance.
- The registered dietitian must have proficient nutrition counseling skills; such skills help the patient understand the diet and also help the registered dietitian know how well the patient will comply with the diet.
- Additional training in psychology enhances weight loss nutrition counseling.
- Behavior modification training and experience are essential to promote permanent eating habit changes. The dietitian should know and

understand lifestyle modification concepts to better facilitate long-term behavior change.
- Excellent written and oral communication skills are vital requirements, because the registered dietitian will depend on these valuable skills to effectively perform many responsibilities. In chart reporting or developing nutrition handouts, the registered dietitian will need a polished writing ability. When speaking to groups or individuals, the dietitian needs good oral communication skills to impress important information on the audience and to hold the audience's attention. Formal training in oral presentations and public speaking is required, and experience, comfort, and ease in group talking are vital.
- The ability to work productively without supervision is important because the registered dietitian completes the majority of her responsibilities independently. Dependability and reliability are also important employee traits.

In addition to being a trained professional, a registered dietitian needs these knowledge and skill characteristics to function to his utmost capabilities, to perform most effectively in a cardiac rehabilitation setting, and to effectively disseminate nutrition and diet education to guide patients toward self-sufficiency and maintenance of recommended dietary change.

Responsibilities and Functions

The capabilities of a registered dietitian to perform effectively in a cardiac rehabilitation setting are limited only by time and money. Imagination and creativity along with a self-motivated personality can make nutrition education an enjoyable, memorable learning experience. The following section describes the broad range of responsibilities and functions of a registered dietitian.

Counseling Services

The registered dietitian can provide individual nutrition counseling for cardiac patients on intensive, intermediate, and brief levels. Individual nutrition counseling can be designed to meet the needs of patients in each progressive phase, as well as in each patient's developmental recovery stage. This is more personalized care, and it may effectively enhance short- and long-term dietary compliance, especially if it includes follow-up meetings.

Group nutrition counseling classes designed for specific groups (e.g., spouses, family members, and employees) or on specific topics may be held by the registered dietitian. These classes may include one or more sessions depending on the audience and topic. Teaching group classes is a time-efficient method of dietary counseling, enabling the registered dietitian to see more patients in a day than can be seen individually. For some patients, but not all, group nutrition counseling may be equally as effective as individual counseling. Group counseling enables patients to learn basic change strategies by helping and learning from other group members. Important and necessary support and reinforcement are provided by the group as members solve mutually important problems.

Staff Interactions and Rehabilitation Phases

The registered dietitian must display good interpersonal and team skills, because she must interact with the cardiac rehabilitation staff on a regular basis to facilitate the patient's nutritional care plan. To inform a referring physician and the cardiac rehabilitation staff of the patient's diet instruction and progress, the registered dietitian should chart progress notes in the patient's chart or mail the physician a progress letter.

The registered dietitian may be required to develop specific nutrition protocols for patient visitation in each progressive phase for standard department procedure documentation and to inform other medical staff personnel. The registered dietitian may need to be involved in the policy and procedure developmental process as it relates to the nutritional care of patients.

The registered dietitian is responsible for diet instruction of all types. Most commonly requested diets include low-calorie, low-cholesterol, low-fat, low-sodium, and diabetic diets; the dietitian must also provide nutritious eating habit counseling. Nearly all nutrition counseling should be based on the principles set forth by the American Diabetes Association, the American Dietetic Association, and AHA. The registered dietitian must be capable of detailed diet analysis and instruction that are individualized for the patient's lifestyle and preferences. Follow-up care to determine a patient's understanding and compliance to dietary recommendations is vital to support long-term behavior and diet change. The goals of nutrition counseling and of the counselor are to tailor a diet plan to fit an individual's lifestyle and needs, effectively

communicate diet recommendations, and guide the patient toward self-sufficiency and the ability to make and maintain dietary changes.

Diet Analysis and Education Materials

Computerized nutritional analysis can be an effective educational and assessment tool in nutrition counseling; it is also an efficient and practical way of evaluating current dietary status and dietary adherence. Proficiency in operating one of the many software packages developed for nutritional analysis aids in effective job performance. A brief overview of nutrition analysis software can be found on pages 25-26.

Development of nutrition education materials is an important responsibility because such materials enable the registered dietitian to disseminate written nutrition/diet information to patients to reinforce what is verbally discussed. For example, if a patient requests information on fiber, it is very effective for the dietitian to discuss a chart showing the amount of dietary fiber in different food groups and to give a copy of the chart to the patient for future reference along with oral and written suggestions for increasing dietary fiber intake. A nutrition education file of handouts either developed in-house or purchased commercially is a valuable asset. Should the need or interest arise, the registered dietitian may choose to develop and write a weekly or monthly nutritional handout/newsletter. Because nutrition and new recipes are such popular, never-ending topics, a creative and imaginative presentation will be of great interest to a nutrition-conscious public.

The registered dietitian may participate as part of the editorial staff in a cardiac rehabilitation department collaborative effort to develop and market an educational, multipurpose cardiac rehabilitation newsletter. Current nutrition topics, diet information, recipes, and book reviews are several areas the registered dietitian may be well suited to write about.

The registered dietitian may participate in a cardiac rehab speaker referral service. Speaking to community, church, and other groups raises public consciousness of the diet–heart disease relationship; the dietitian may present on a cardiac-related nutrition topic or other nutrition topic as needed by a particular group.

A registered dietitian who develops a professional resource network with professional peers—organizations such as the local dietetic association, American Dietetic Association, American Heart Association, and National Dairy Council; the local health department; and local area hospitals—is better informed and better able to obtain current and varying information for patients.

The registered dietitian may create, develop, and administer a number of nutrition education programs such as weight loss and weight maintenance courses; heart-healthy cooking classes (e.g., Culinary Heart Kitchen by the American Heart Association); low-fat and low-cholesterol seminars; diabetic eating and cooking workshops; specialty cooking classes (e.g., low-fat French cooking, low-fat and low-sodium Italian cooking); balanced, nutritious eating programs; special nutrition programs for couples, children, and spouses; and many other topics pertinent to good nutrition and heart-healthy eating. These programs may consist of one, two, or more sessions to suit the particular topics and group dynamics. The audience targeted may be a particular patient population, employees, or public/community groups. Along with developing the program, the registered dietitian may help develop advertising and marketing schedules for each program. The registered dietitian can be a valuable resource as well as participant and author in the collection and publication of research data. Assisting in the education and training of student interns may be another responsibility of the registered dietitian.

Although serving primarily as an expert in food, nutrition, and diet, the registered dietitian is required to perform a wide array of duties. Imagination, motivation, cooperation, and flexibility allow the registered dietitian to function as an active and valuable member of the cardiac rehabilitation team.

Utilizing the Registered Dietitian

Many options are available for using a registered dietitian. The registered dietitian may be a full-time employee, a part-time employee, or a consultant, depending on the size of the department, the budget, the number of patients, the type of programs planned, and other variables.

The degree of the registered dietitian's involvement with the patient in Phases I, II, and III is important to consider. For the part-time or consulting registered dietitian, prioritizing patients and responsibilities is especially crucial for time management. One interpretation of how to best meet the needs of the patient and most effectively use the registered dietitian is as follows.

Phase I—Inpatient Dietary Counseling

In Phase I, hospitalized patients, alerted to the seriousness of their situations, may be receptive to dietary instruction; however, because some are experiencing many physical discomforts and psychological adaptations, they may only be expected to retain and concentrate on so much dietary information at this time. An introduction to AHA dietary guidelines with a brief oral and written presentation may appropriately serve a large part of this population. Spouses and other family members may be good targets for nutrition education at this time. It is important that the patient and family be informed of the type of diet the patient needs.

Outpatient Dietary Counseling

Individual and group counseling is very helpful in Phase II to assess patients and direct them into actual application of the diet principles introduced in Phase I. Encouraging realistic behavioral changes in eating habits to fit the patient's lifestyle is crucial to long-term compliance. Regular follow-up care to reinforce the new eating habits is one of the most important functions of the registered dietitian.

In Phase III, the registered dietitian serves primarily as a resource and motivator to help patients continue to follow new eating habits. The registered dietitian is particularly useful with patients who are striving to reduce weight, because support and encouragement are very helpful. Regular nutrition newsletter distribution as well as personal contact may benefit this group.

Effective Counseling

It is when a patient appears motivated and receptive to diet information and eating habit change that nutrition counseling is the most effective. Unfortunately, patients differ as to when they reach this readiness point. In addition, nutrition counseling is more effective and more likely to change a person's eating habits when counseling is tailored to the individual's lifestyle and preferences.

To best use the skills of a registered dietitian, you must establish nutrition and diet education goals for the cardiac rehab program. Prioritize each particular patient group as to the degree and type of nutrition counseling required, as well as how much of the registered dietitian's time should be allotted. Based on such factors as patient population, department size and goals, and skills of the registered dietitian, short- and long-term nutrition education programs can be planned to meet the needs of the patients and the cardiac rehabilitation program.

References

American Heart Association. (1984a). *The American Heart Association cookbook*. New York: Random House.

American Heart Association. (1984b). *Recommendations for treatment of hyperlipidemia in adults* (American Heart Association special report 72-204A). Dallas: Author.

Blankenhorn, D.H., Johnson, R.L., Mack, W.A., El Zein, H.A., & Vailas, L.I. (1990). The influence of diet on the appearance of new lesions in human coronary arteries. *Journal of the American Medical Association*, **263**, 1646-1652.

Connor, S.L., & Connor, W.E. (1986). *The new American diet*. New York: Simon & Schuster.

Expert Panel. (1988). Report of the National Cholesterol Education Program expert panel on detection, evaluation, and treatment of high blood cholesterol in adults. *Archives of Internal Medicine*, **148**, 36-69.

Frank, G.C. (1988). Nutritional therapy for hyperlipidemia and obesity: office treatment. Integrating the roles of the physician and the registered dietitian. *Journal of the American College of Cardiology*, **12**, 1098-1101.

Gotto, A.M. (1989). Diet and cholesterol guidelines and coronary artery disease. *Journal of the American College of Cardiology*, **2**, 503-507.

Grundy, S.M., Bilheimer, D., Blackburn, H., Brown, W.V., Kwiterovich, P.O., Mattson, F., Schonfeld, G., Weidman, W.H. (1982). *Rationale of the diet-heart statement of the American Heart Association* (Report of the Nutrition Committee 65-839A). Dallas: Author.

Grundy, S.M., & Winston, M. (Eds.) (1989). *The American Heart Association low-fat, low-cholesterol cookbook*. New York: Random House.

Chapter 9

Social Work and Pastoral Care

Linda J. Walker, PhD, MSW, MPH, ACSW

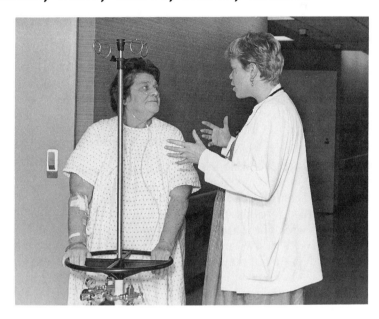

This chapter discusses the ways in which you can use social workers and pastoral care workers in the cardiac rehabilitation program. The chapter discusses professional qualifications, referral practices, areas of expertise, and contributions to be expected during the rehabilitation phases.

Learning Objectives

1. To recognize the areas in which social work can contribute to the cardiac rehabilitation program

2. To develop general guidelines for involving the social worker in the cardiac rehabilitation process

---

The author would like to express her sincere thanks to the Reverend Beth Hawkins, manager of the Department of Pastoral Care, Allegheny General Hospital, for her guidance in the area of pastoral care for this chapter.

3. To recognize the areas in which pastoral care can contribute to the cardiac rehabilitation program

4. To develop general guidelines for involving the pastoral care worker in the cardiac rehabilitation process

Cardiac rehabilitation needs to encompass the psychosocial, vocational, and quality of life concerns of the patient if the outcome of intervention is to be successful for both the patient and the health care professional (Mayou, 1986; Wenger, 1988, 1990). Both social workers and pastoral care workers can contribute to this process. This chapter will deal with the way in which both of these professionals can optimize the rehabilitative process for the patient through interaction with and on behalf of the patient and also with the patient's family members and significant loved ones.

The Social Worker

The social worker is a health care professional whose focus includes the patient, family, and community. Social work services can contribute to the care plan designed by the cardiac rehabilitation team throughout the various phases of the treatment process. The various services of the social worker or social work services department may be found in Table 9.1.

Often in health care settings there are two levels of trained social work staff. The bachelor-level worker (BSW) may be designated as a caseworker or case aide. The BSW usually provides services such as assistance with transportation, housing, and medical equipment; information and referral to programs in the community; and limited counseling. The graduate-level social worker (MSW) is trained to provide in-depth assessment of psychosocial needs, treatment planning, counseling, and case management. Both the BSW and MSW are likely to be involved in discharge planning, and their roles in this area may overlap. MSWs may belong to the Academy of Certified Social Workers (ACSW) if they have had 2 years of professional work experience under an ACSW member and have passed the ACSW examination. Many states have licensure and/or certification provisions for social workers who have met specific educational and practice requirements.

Table 9.1 Services Commonly Provided Through Social Work Services Departments

Assessment of psychosocial needs
Assessment of patient functioning
Assessment of family functioning
Assessment of the patient's perception of his or her health status and expectations for care and treatment
Intervention to reduce psychosocial stress
Counseling
Treatment planning
Discharge planning
Case management
Information and referral to community services
Information and transition to personal care, nursing home, and extended care facilities
Assistance with financial needs
Assistance with transportation
Assistance with housing
Assistance with acquisition of medical equipment and in-home help
Information about employment and vocational options
Educational and support groups
Consultation

Social Work in the Inpatient Phase

The social worker is most likely to be involved during the inpatient phase of cardiac disease. Most hospitals have a social work services program to assist patients and their families with the emotional, social, and posthospital care needs that illness can create. Hospital programs differ in the manner in which social workers become involved with patients. The procedure for social work consultation may range from automatic evaluation of every patient to referral only at the request of the physician. Ideally, you should include the social worker as a regular member of the interdisciplinary rehabilitation team.

Psychosocial Assessment

You should use the social worker to assess psychosocial needs, to help patients and families deal with the stress of illness, and to assist with discharge planning. Social work intervention in the early stages of the patient's hospitalization is preferable. The feelings and fears of the patient and family are most acute at this time and so are their needs for stress management (Levin, 1987; Yokes, 1973). The cardiac patient is confronted with the impact of a serious and possibly fatal illness, and death as a possible outcome may be a conscious or unconscious concern for both the patient and the family. The patient may also experience concerns about changes in lifestyle and self-image.

During the initial period of the patient's illness the social worker can help to reduce psychological and situational stress. Social work services can involve personal counseling and the facilitation of communication among patient, family, and hospital staff. Some families may need assistance in selecting a family spokesperson to meet family members' needs for information. Parents of young children may want suggestions about ways to deal with a child's need for information and attention when a parent is ill. Social workers can provide information and assistance in locating amenities such as food, parking, and lodging for family members. The social worker can also begin to identify patients whose special needs may make them high risk for nonparticipation in a rehabilitation program. This group may include elderly persons without family or other social supports and people from different cultural groups. Berkman, Millar, Holmes, and Bonander (1990) studied elderly cardiac patients using data from the Medicus Nursing Productivity and Quality of Patient Care Classification System. The authors found that patients who had difficulty walking without help by day 3 of hospitalization were likely to need social work services for assistance with psychosocial and environmental problems. Environmental problems frequently revolve around the inability of caretakers or other in-home service providers to adequately meet the needs of patients who are unable to function independently at home.

Evaluating Postdischarge Care

Russell (1988) noted that psychosocial assessment is one of the special contributions of the social worker to the rehabilitation team. The social worker uses this assessment to evaluate the ability of the patient and family to manage the patient's care after discharge and to participate in a rehabilitation program. Depending on the patient's condition and the availability of the family members, the social worker gathers information about the patient's living situation, family relationships, and other social support systems. Other specifics include occupational history and employment status, economic situation, recreational interests and activities, characteristic lifestyle patterns, and activities of daily living. This information provides the cardiac rehabilitation team with a measure of patient and family coping patterns, treatment expectations, and problems that might be encountered in the rehabilitation process. The rehab team can then develop strategies to encourage the patient's participation in the rehabilitation program. Additionally, the rehabilitation team can implement a daily living plan that promotes a healthy lifestyle and helps the patient to regain a sense of independence and control over personal decisions and behaviors.

Social workers are trained to deal with a variety of psychosocial and economic problems. As a result, the cardiac rehabilitation team should use social workers to assist with patient and family concerns about interpersonal relationships, financial problems, and insurance coverage. Other areas in which social workers may assist are employment and vocational training concerns (Streater & Erlandson, 1984). The goal of the social worker is to individualize the patient and identify her unique characteristics that can be employed to deal with the stress of illness and an altered lifestyle. The social worker views the patient in terms of her social system and is sensitive to the impact of the patient's illness on this system (Dhooper, 1983). Numerous researchers have reported that the impact of illness varies for the male and female as a result of gender difference. The impact of the illness is also affected by role and relationship expectations, mortality rates, and views of caregiving (Barusch & Spaid, 1989; Mayou, Foster, & Williamson, 1978; Shanfield, 1990; Young & Kahana, 1989).

Helping the Patient Deal With Recovery

During the inpatient phase the social worker and the cardiac rehabilitation team can help patients anticipate the implications and demands of the recovery phase. This may involve discussions about the normal range of emotional responses to cardiac illness, changes in daily activities and behaviors, and typical responses of family members. Sulman and Verhaeghe (1985) developed a framework for identifying the medical and psychosocial factors that may impede the recovery of hospitalized myocardial infarction patients. The authors found that the level of denial can have a critical impact on the patient's compliance with treatment and participation in a rehabilitation program. They reported that moderate levels of denial of anxiety and loss are more conducive to compliance with treatment than are high levels of denial. All members of the rehab team need to be sensitive to the symptoms of emotional distress. Patients whose emotional responses are extreme are in need of assessment to determine appropriate intervention to help them deal with their fears and feelings (Paulley & Pelser, 1989). These patients may benefit from consultation with a psychiatrist or psychologist. The cardiac rehabilitation team may also use the period of hospitalization to encourage patients to think about their future care needs and, if they have not already done so, to prepare a will, power of attorney, living will, or medical directive and attend to other legal matters. The social worker can refer patients to the appropriate agencies for these services.

During the inpatient phase the social worker can also help patients who may present special concerns related to diminished physical and mental health. Some of these patients may exhibit sensory deficits, impaired mobility, and inability to adequately perform activities of daily living. The social worker can provide these patients with the extra encouragement they may need to participate in a rehabilitation program and can also help them access appropriate social and community resources. Morro (1989) studied the mood states of older cardiac patients and found a significant incidence of depression up to 1 year after discharge. The author recommended an assessment of mood states of older patients prior to entry into a rehabilitation program, because the study demonstrated that treatment for depression increases the likelihood that these patients remain in the rehabilitation program.

Counseling the Family

After the patient's condition has stabilized, the spouse or significant other may need short-term counseling to identify and deal with behaviors that interfere with her functioning or with the patient's treatment process. Members of the cardiac rehabilitation team can use the social worker to assist the spouse whose fears may be expressed in terms of complaining and disruptive behavior. Counseling should help the spouse recognize underlying concerns and redirect feelings into more appropriate means of expression. In some situations spousal anger may be targeted at perceived life injustices, unresolved prior problems, or changes in the marital relationship. The social worker may need to address these issues in order to maximize support for the patient's treatment program.

Through the use of family meetings or support groups, the social worker and other members of the rehabilitation program can provide patients and family members an opportunity to share and validate their fears and concerns and to discuss anticipated lifestyle changes. Group intervention techniques may range from a series of sessions to a single meeting offered during the patient's hospitalization or at a later point in the recovery phase. Trelawny-Ross and Russell (1987) studied the social and psychological responses of 31 married men hospitalized with suspected myocardial infarction. They found that both the patients and their wives believed that an opportunity to receive advice and encouragement shortly after the patient's discharge would have helped the families to be more understanding and supportive rather than restrictive and protective. Brown, Glazer, and Higgins (1983) described the use of one-session educational support groups with heart surgery patients and their families during the final phase of hospitalization. The purpose of this session is to help with the transition from illness to recovery. Group meetings can also be used to give family members recognition for their roles in attending to the patient during the acute phase of illness and for carrying extra household duties and other responsibilities. Family members may need the permission and encouragement a group setting can create to attend to their own personal and business affairs and to take primary responsibility for their own physical and mental health.

Discharge Planning

Discharge planning is an opportunity for collaboration among the patient, family, and cardiac rehabilitation team to ensure that the patient will have access to services that will help him maintain or improve the level of functioning achieved in the hospital. Some patients may need to recuperate in an extended-care facility such as a nursing home, Veteran's Administration hospital, or other inpatient rehabilitation center. In these cases the social worker helps the patient and family understand the need for the placement. Additionally, the social worker can help the family locate an appropriate facility and manage the financial and other admission requirements. Along with these services, the social worker is able to provide information about community resources for financial and social assistance and to assist in arranging the transfer.

If the patient is returning home from the hospital, the social worker can help with arrangements for visiting nurses, home health care, and any medical equipment or other supplies that may be required. The social worker can also provide information about and referral to community resources that provide financial help for food and rent and state and federal programs that aid needy and disabled persons. In collaboration with the cardiac rehabilitation team, the social worker can supply patients with information about programs that promote healthy lifestyle habits, such as smoking cessation, stress management, and diet modification.

Social Work in the Outpatient Phase

The level of social work involved in outpatient cardiac rehabilitation depends on the availability of social work services to outpatient programs in general. Ideally, the social worker should be a member of the cardiac rehabilitation team with responsibility for monitoring psychosocial changes and providing treatment and services that promote the patient's well-being. The social worker may need to be involved with both the patient and the family.

Meeting Outpatient Needs

You should use the services of the social worker to deal with obstacles to the patient's participation in an outpatient rehabilitation program. Some patients may need assistance with transportation, the cost of medications, or the cost of caretakers for children or other people in the home who require special attention. Other patients may need help completing insurance forms for reimbursement, learning the extent of their coverage for health care needs, and applying for supplemental

health care coverage. Patients may need information about community agencies that offer assistance with meals, shopping, laundry, light housekeeping chores, home health care, employment, and vocational counseling. The social worker may also monitor patients with special needs, such as people with limited family supports and elderly people who exhibit mental confusion and difficulty managing daily activities. Additionally, the social worker may monitor those patients with prior histories of emotional problems or drug and alcohol abuse, as well as people who have experienced recent stressful life events.

Along with other members of the rehabilitation team, the social worker can provide education and support to promote healthy lifestyles. This may encompass education and counseling about the impact of illness in terms of identifying and coping with stress, feelings of self-esteem, changes in family relationships, and changes in sexual functioning (Levin, 1990).

Funding Social Work Services

Social work services for hospitalized patients are not generally reimbursable. Charges for services to inpatients are usually included as part of the per diem rate. Social work services for outpatients may not be routinely provided by the health care institution. The availability of social work services depends primarily on the hospital administration's philosophy. Social work is a nonbillable service provided by the hospital. If the administration chooses, social work may be included in the team concept under which the outpatient cardiac rehabilitation charge is structured. The rehabilitation program may address the needs of patients who require counseling or assistance with socioeconomic problems by referring them to community agencies, mental health clinics, or private practitioners. Fees for service vary from sliding scales to set fees. In some instances patients who use counseling services may be eligible for third-party reimbursement under some private insurance plans.

Pastoral Care

Throughout history there has been a strong relationship among the spiritual, physical, and mental health components of human existence (Mitchell, 1988; Vanderpool, 1980). One aspect of spiritual existence is religion. Most religious faiths are based on the notion of accountability to a supreme being. Additionally, religion provides guidelines for behaviors and activities that can be employed to control and resolve the problems of everyday living (Deck & Folta, 1979). Pastoral care professionals use religion as a framework for coping with stress, explaining health and illness, and exploring quality of life issues with patients and caregivers.

Providing Spiritual Care

In health care settings the provision of spiritual care is generally the responsibility of religious professionals. The cardiac rehabilitation team can use the chaplain or pastoral care staff to help patients and families deal with various spiritual, emotional, and quality of life issues generated by the crisis of a health problem. Pastoral care workers can also help the cardiac rehab team identify specific religious beliefs and activities that may complement or compete with recommended treatment. The focus of pastoral care includes the patient, the family, the staff, and the community.

The qualifications of the pastoral care professional should include theological training (preferably at the master's degree level), ordination, and ecclesiastical endorsement. Training should also include clinical pastoral education and certification by a national chaplaincy association, such as the American Protestant Hospital Association, the Association for Clinical Pastoral Education, and the National Association of Catholic Chaplains.

Holst (1985) noted that hospitals are not mandated by law or by accreditation requirements to provide pastoral care; the provision of pastoral care services depends largely on the facility's administrative philosophy. The Division of Pastoral Care sometimes provides a comprehensive ministry program 24 hr per day. If your program is based in a facility that does not have a pastoral care staff, you will need to establish contacts with clergy in the community who represent different faith groups. They may require education about cardiac rehabilitation and the special emotional needs of the cardiac patient. Educational backgrounds and counseling skills may vary widely among community clergy. The cardiac rehabilitation director needs to be sensitive to the comfort levels and skills of individual members of the clergy in the areas of pastoral counseling and spiritual assessment. Individual clergy members should also be assessed in terms of their interest in health care and their abilities to function as members of the rehab team.

Determining the Need

The referral process for pastoral care generally involves direct requests from hospital staff, patients, families, and area clergy. Pastoral care may be needed early in the patient's hospitalization to help him discuss the relationship of his illness to his beliefs about religion. The individual who views the cardiac crisis as a punishment for past sins or who expects that a supreme being will do the healing may have difficulty participating in recommended medical treatment. Pastoral care should be used to help such patients explore the roles of religion and medical science in their health care. Some patients may respond to a heart attack with acute fears of death and feelings of loss (Bickel, 1973). For other patients the stress of a cardiac problem may serve as a catalyst for an examination of their lives and values. Such patients may benefit from pastoral care intervention aimed at helping them express and cope with feelings about the illness event itself and about the need to find meaning and control in life (Pargament & Hahn, 1986). In working with heart transplant patients, the cardiac rehabilitation staff may identify people who can benefit from the opportunity to discuss various ethical and spiritual issues with pastoral care providers. Patients who have beliefs about the heart as the seat of the emotions or the home of the soul may have concerns about the meaning of a new heart in relation to their own personal senses of being. Heart transplant patients may also need to discuss feelings about the organ procurement process and the meaning of death in relation to their continued existence.

Benefits to the Patient's Rehabilitation

Pastoral care can reveal information about the patient's expectations of life and of treatment that are important in development of individualized rehabilitation strategies. The spiritual assessment is a tool that pastoral care workers use in helping patients explore questions about their existence by focusing on their beliefs and values. Other areas of the spiritual assessment pertain to the role of a supreme being in one's life, life priorities, and mortality. The spiritual assessment may enable the patient to expand her religious beliefs to include an appreciation of various quality of life and lifestyle issues. One of the goals of pastoral care is to assist patients throughout the rehabilitation process as they review and reassess values and beliefs. Another goal is to help patients confront and cope with their own vulnerabilities. Stromberg (1987) noted

> Until a person accepts the reality of his or her own mortality there will be little motivation for making any significant lifestyle changes which are vital to prolonging life. It is with this issue that the chaplain may make the most unique and significant contribution to the heart patient. (p. 130)

The cardiac rehabilitation team can collaborate with pastoral care workers to pursue the goal of active patient participation in health care. Throughout the various phases of the rehabilitation process, pastoral care workers can be consulted to help patients cope with stress and regain a sense of control over their own destinies. The hospital pastoral care staff may be more actively involved in the inpatient phase, because patients are encouraged to return to their local faith groups after discharge from the hospital. One exception is the tertiary care medical center in which pastoral care staff often provide services to out-of-town patients who reside in the area while awaiting procedures such as transplants or while completing treatment regimens. Pastoral care intervention may involve various activities with the patient or the family. Patients and families who are struggling with feelings ranging from anger and fear to uncertainty and depression may benefit from counseling and emotional support. Some patients may especially respond to intervention strategies that involve religious beliefs and activities. Most major religious groups have brief, formalized services or sacraments of healing that can be performed or arranged by pastoral care. These rituals may contribute significantly to the patient's sense of well-being (Switzer, 1989).

Age groups often vary in the role that religion plays in their lives. Koenig, George, and Siegler (1988) studied the coping strategies that older adults use to deal with stressful life experiences that include health events. The authors found that a religious behavior was most frequently mentioned as a coping strategy. The behaviors most often cited were placing trust and faith in God, praying, and obtaining help and strength from God. Bearson and Koenig (1990) studied the use of prayer by older adults. The authors found that heart palpitations, shortness of breath, and forgetfulness were symptoms that the subjects universally prayed about. Support of religious coping

behaviors such as prayer, faith in a supreme being, and participation in church activities may aid and encourage patient participation in cardiac rehabilitation. The pastoral care staff also should be used to facilitate the patient's reentry into her own faith group. Pastoral care can serve as a link to the patient's pastor and can also provide information about the patient's treatment needs. Additionally, the cardiac rehabilitation team can consult with pastoral care professionals about ethical and quality-of-life issues, emotional/spiritual resources to staff dealing with issues of death and dying, and bereavement.

Funding the Service

The acute care organization usually covers the cost of pastoral care services. The focus of service is generally the inpatient; coverage for outpatients must be arranged with the pastoral care service and the hospital administration. At the outpatient level, pastoral care costs may be included as part of the overall cardiac rehabilitation charge. Another option is to train area clergy members to meet the special needs of the program and use them as needed. The adjudicatory offices of the major faith groups can be valuable sources of information about pastors with the skills needed by your program. These offices can also provide information about church programs that engage in health education.

References

Barusch, A.S., & Spaid, W.M. (1989). Gender differences in caregiving: Why do wives report greater burden? *The Gerontologist*, **29**, 667-676.

Bearson, L.B., & Koenig, H.G. (1990). Religious cognition and use of prayer in health and illness. *The Gerontologist*, **30**, 249-253.

Berkman, B., Millar, S., Holmes, W., & Bonander, E. (1990). Screening elder cardiac patients to identify need for social work services. *Health and Social Work*, **15**, 64-72.

Bickel, A.O. (1973). Ministering to coronary patients and their families. In L.E. Holst & H.P. Kurtz (Eds.), *Toward a creative chaplaincy* (pp. 42-54). Springfield, IL: Charles C Thomas.

Brown, D.G., Glazer, H., & Higgins, M. (1983). Group intervention: A psychological and educational approach to open heart surgery patients and their families. *Social Work in Health Care*, **9**(2), 47-59.

Deck, E.S., & Folta, J.R. (1979). Problem solving: Magic, religion and science. In J.R. Folta & E. Deck (Eds.), *A sociological framework for patient care* (pp. 417-423). New York: Wiley.

Dhooper, S.S. (1983). Family coping with the crisis of heart attack. *Social Work in Health Care*, **9**(1), 15-31.

Holst, L.E. (1985). A ministry of paradox in a place of paradox. In L.E. Holst (Ed.), *Hospital ministry* (pp. 3-11). New York: Crossroads.

Koenig, H.G., George, L.K., & Siegler, I.C. (1988). The use of religion and other emotion-regulating coping strategies among older adults. *The Gerontologist*, **28**, 303-310.

Levin, R.F. (1987). *Heartmates*. New York: Pocket Books.

Levin, R.F. (1990). *The cardiac family recovery program training manual*. Minneapolis: Heartmates.

Mayou, R. (1986). The psychiatric and social consequences of coronary artery surgery. *Journal of Psychosomatic Research*, **30**, 255-271.

Mayou, R., Foster, A., & Williamson, B. (1978). The psychological and social effects of myocardial infarction on wives. *British Medical Journal*, **18**, 699-701.

Mitchell, J.A. (1988). Spiritual and emotional determinants of health. *Journal of Religion and Health*, **27**, 62-70.

Morro, B.C. (1989). Post hospital depression and the elderly cardiac patient. *Social Work in Health Care*, **14**(2), 59-66.

Pargament, K.I., & Hahn, J. (1986). God and the just world: Causal and coping attributions to God in health situations. *Journal for the Scientific Study of Religion*, **25**, 193-207.

Paulley, J.W., & Pelser, H.E. (1989). *Psychological managements for psychosomatic disorders (cardiovascular disorders)*. New York: Springer-Verlag.

Russell, M.V. (1988). Clinical social work. In J. Goodgold (Ed.), *Rehabilitation medicine* (pp. 942-950). St. Louis: Mosby.

Shanfield, S.B. (1990). Myocardial infarction and patient's wives. *Psychosomatics*, **31**, 138-145.

Streater, S.E., & Erlandson, R.J. (1984). Social and vocational considerations in cardiac rehabilitation. In L.K. Hall, G.C. Meyer, & H.K. Hellerstein (Eds.), *Cardiac rehabilitation: Exercise training and prescription* (pp. 367-392). Champaign, IL: Life Enhancement Publications.

Stromberg, R. (1987). The voices of coronary care: A confrontation with vulnerability. In L.E. Holst (Ed.), *Hospital ministry* (pp. 127-138). New York: Crossword.

Sulman, J., & Verhaeghe, G. (1985). Myocardial infarction patients in the acute care hospital: A conceptual framework for social work intervention. *Social Work in Health Care*, **11**(1), 1-20.

Switzer, D.K. (1989). *Pastoral care emergencies* (pp. 54-78). New York: Paulist Press.

Trelawny-Ross, C., & Russell, O. (1987). Social and psychological responses to myocardial infarction: Multiple determinants of outcome at six months. *Journal of Psychosomatic Research*, **31**, 125-130.

Vanderpool, H.Y. (1980). Religion and medicine: A theoretical overview. *Journal of Religion and Health*, **19**, 7-17.

Wenger, N.K. (1988). Components of a rehabilitation program for coronary patients. In J. Goodgold (Ed.), *Rehabilitation medicine* (pp. 217-226). St. Louis: Mosby.

Wenger, N.K. (1990). Quality of life in chronic cardiovascular illness. *Journal of Cardiopulmonary Rehabilitation*, **10**, 88-91.

Yokes, J.A. (1973). Family rehabilitation: An adult with a myocardial infarction. In D.P. Hymovich & M.U. Barnard (Eds.), *Family healthcare* (pp. 390-404). New York: McGraw-Hill.

Young, R.F., & Kahana, E. (1989). Specifying caregiver outcomes: Gender and relationship aspects of caregiving strain. *The Gerontologist*, **29**, 660-666.

Chapter 10

Management Principles

Linda K. Hall, PhD

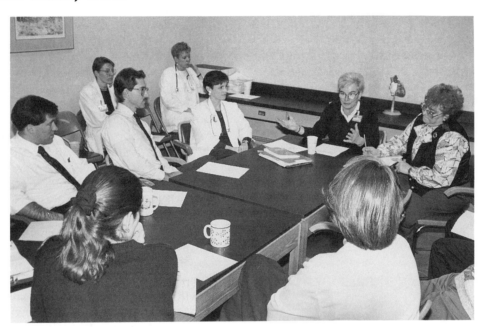

Reflect on your own day-to-day life with its deadlines, responsibilities, and have to's, need to's, and want to's that you keep adding to your "to do" list. Now, think about how you would like to be guided and managed as you work through the list. This is one of the basic principles of management: leading in the way that you would like to be managed, with the end result being a balanced budget, a happy work force, and new creative programs that are innovated without difficulty. This chapter embraces current theory on management techniques.

Learning Objectives

1. To understand the roles that you must play to be a good manager

2. To understand the skills that are necessary for management of programs

3. To understand the following methods of management:
   • total-quality management processes
   • team building
   • management by process

Management in its perfect form is an art. It is working with employees to optimize their performance; it is designing programs and products that are competitive and respond to the consumer's needs and expectations; it is responding to and administering company philosophy in product delivery; it is being a problem solver and a product salesperson. You need a number of technical as well as interpersonal skills in order to become a first-rate manager. You can learn about these skills through coursework, workshops, and reading, but applying the skills is another matter. Some people make managing people and programs look easy, whereas others have to work very hard to be average. There are several things you can do, however, whether you possess natural ability or whether you have to work very hard to be a good manager, to give yourself a positive edge as a manager of a cardiac rehabilitation program.

Assessing Your Management Qualifications

Traditionally, managers of cardiac rehabilitation programs are former nurses from the critical care unit, stepdown unit, or nursing education department who are promoted to management. These people may or may not be knowledgeable in all aspects of rehab (i.e., be "students" of rehab) and may or may not have management skills. But these are the qualities a manager needs—comprehensive knowledge and management skills—to design and manage a high-quality program. W. Edwards Deming (1982) created a theory of management based on a principle of total quality. He observed that two common problems in business and industry are the most costly in terms of productivity: these problems are people simply doing the wrong thing and people doing the right thing but doing it the wrong way. Both of these problems require corrections and rework, which Deming estimates occupies 30 to 40% of our time. Can you imagine how much larger that percentage of re-

work will be if you do not have the necessary management skills or the overall knowledge background of cardiac rehabilitation? This creates two questions that you as the potential manager need to first ask yourself and then rephrase for your administrative officer. Question 1: Do I know enough about the total concepts and programming of cardiac rehabilitation to design and implement a program? If not, where, when, and how can I get that knowledge? Question 2: Do I have the management skills, such as skills involving budget, personnel, quality assurance, cost accounting, and productivity, to be an effective manager? If not, where, when, and how can I get those skills?

Find out if the hospital has courses or access to courses to help you fill the missing pieces in your knowledge base. Additionally, establish at the outset whether the hospital views you as a manager, a clinician who will do management chores, or a manager who will do clinical chores. Every minute you spend as a clinician is a minute subtracted from management, and vice versa (see Figure 10.1). If you are expected to manage and develop programs using management techniques, then you need the time to apply the skills. Establish this with the administrative officer to whom you report before you start.

At the outset, I will briefly talk about the skills you need to manage a cardiac rehab program. I do

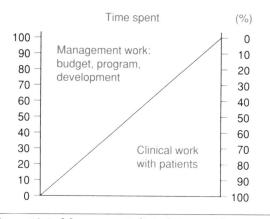

Figure 10.1 Management-clinical time grid.

not plan to discuss them thoroughly, because they are covered in more detail in other chapters in this book.

Personnel and Interpersonal Skills

In cardiac rehabilitation, working with people for people is the most important aspect of the job. Thus, managing people to work with people is the major component of a manager's job. Selecting staff members who fill the job descriptions and have the interpersonal skills to engender trust and belief in their message is critically important. The manager is responsible for the ambiance of the environment. So being a good manager is a combination of selecting and directing good staff members (chapter 7) and effectively managing the programs (chapters 1, 2, 3, and 4) that you set up. Program management is the thrust of this chapter.

Financial Acumen

In the cardiac rehabilitation program, as in any program, business, or industry, money is the major critical factor with which you will have to deal every day. You must understand the basics of line-item budgeting, zero-based budgeting, carryover, bidding processes, cost/benefit ratios, microcosting, and predicting future case load for cost/revenue projections. Chapters 13 and 14 discuss budget and productivity, but once again they serve only as the groundwork. You will also learn through experience and by meeting with other finance people in the hospital. Finally, budget and productivity will not be met without the revenue that the program receives as fees for service. Understanding reimbursement problems and achieving effective reimbursement are covered in chapter 12.

Quality Assurance and Efficacy Measures

Built into any successful program is continual evaluation. A successful program also has policies and procedures that serve as guidelines for the program, in effect outlining how the program is to be run, how procedures are to be applied, and how the application is to be documented. Once you have developed policies and procedures, you must evaluate how well your department carries them out. Quality assurance is a method of measuring what you do and how well you do it and making a plan for change when needed; this is covered in chapter 15.

A Principle of Management

Management books are available in any commercial bookstore across the country. Also, if your hospital or affiliated administrative offices are on the cutting edge of technology they will have a human resources department that features beginning and advanced principles of management courses. Usually these courses espouse the current theory of management that is considered "in" across the country. At this time the major buzzwords in management are *total quality, team building, participatory management,* and *ownership.* There has been a major turnaround in management techniques in the past couple of years, which came about because of Deming's success (1982) in bringing Japan's low-cost/high-productivity manufacturing methods to the forefront. You will need to be cognizant of these methods to manage your program and problems optimally. Some of the major management decisions you will face are dealing with the great influx of new mothers into the work force, managing job sharing, managing your product line, convincing workers that they are a part of the decision-making process, and getting people to do the right things right the first time. What I will present here is a compilation of a number of ideas, thoughts that follow modern thinking, and procedures that I have found to work. Take them, use them, change them, and certainly be continuously looking for new ways of managing people. In all cases start by asking yourself, how would I like to be managed?

Management by Objective

Set a goal or objective or visualize what you would like to achieve based on what your research tells you about the field of cardiac rehabilitation. The AACVPR (1991) guidelines ask program managers to risk stratify, case manage patients, selectively monitor patients, individualize a patient's risk factor modification, and measure efficacy of programs. Assess your program, and then make statements about the aspects of the program you would like to see grow, how you want these areas to grow, and the desired outcome. Continue to read the literature concerning these statements, and read to find more comprehensive information to provide positives and negatives. Call directors of other programs and ask what they are doing and how. Separate the problem or the desired outcome into parts that are workable, and work on only one area at a time. Organize all of your notes, thoughts, and ideas into a workable model: Include (a) what presently exists, (b) what the guidelines establish as the rule, (c) what research tells you, and (d) some ideas for a new methodology.

Staff Ownership

After you have put together a rough outline of your "vision," present it to your staff. Provide written materials, especially articles that discuss how this new program will affect what people do on the job, at least 2 to 3 days before the presentation. Staff members will read the material and discuss it (and its pros and cons) among themselves, and by the time the meeting is held you can focus on the key areas of the proposal.

Kiefer and Senge (1986) stated that a new management proposal that conflicts with current practice can create tension. They believe that this tension is resolved one of two ways: The emotional tension drives people to remain with current practice or the tension drives people to meet the new challenge.

In the example of the ECG monitors, staff members have difficulty believing that the patient will be safe. Nurses especially are concerned about missing ventricular arrhythmias and premature beats. You will need a thorough review of the literature and a review of past incidences of emergencies in your therapeutic setting to assist you in

moving the staff to the "new way" of applying therapy.

Once you have sold your department on the new idea, the next step is to create an action plan. The action plan should clarify the original proposal that you put before your staff. Remove what is questionable, or conduct research to clear up any questions; be sure all material supports the desired end point. Prioritize the proposal in a way that the first order of work is that which is most important and the second order is the next most important and so on. Keep questioning yourself, and encourage questions from the staff, until you have a very clear action plan and defined desired outcome.

Putting the Plan to Work

Now is when the really hard work begins with the new proposal. It is best to gather a working committee from your department members and do some brainstorming and investigation. The first order of business is to make two lists. The first list contains all of the reasons why this will be a good change, in essence the driving forces behind the change. The second list should be of all of the reasons that the change might not work, or the restraining forces. Type the two lists and give copies to all members of the department to discuss, add to, and delete from. This is where brainstorming and real planning come into play. Create a plan for removing the restraining forces; tackle each one and remove it as you would hurdle obstacles. Some of the restraining forces that often show up in cardiac rehabilitation are these: Physicians do not see the need for change; physicians believe they will lose control of their patients; there is a

---

PRESENTING NEW CHALLENGES

Vision: Turn the monitors around to face the exercise floor, position the staff on the floor, and put the monitors on alarm and auto-print. Take ECG strips one time per mode, or as needed.

Current Method: Monitor and printer are on a desk. A staff member, nurse, or monitor reader sits behind the monitor and takes ECG strips on a regular schedule.

Discuss the following question with your staff. Do they see the merit in the proposed change? How can they use skills that they already have? What do they see as stumbling blocks or things

that might make the proposal fail? What are the preliminary steps needed to remove the stumbling blocks? Will they buy the new process or proposal? These specific questions need to be answered, because if the staff members do not like the proposal and don't believe it will work, it won't. The staff members actually apply the therapy, so they have to believe that what they do is beneficial and is based on sound principles and research, and that they have the skills or will be taught the skills to do it well.

potential increased risk of sudden death events; there is a potential loss of revenue; and the proposal may be costly to implement.

Find ways around the restrainers: Find out how other centers implemented the proposal; read the research and present a synopsis of it, making sure to include negatives as well as positives; invite a ''star'' professional to speak to and persuade the administration, physicians, and some of your nonbelievers; and balance the lost revenue with reduced cost or increased activities. As managers, we spend a lot of time working on the driving forces behind programs or proposals, when we should spend our time removing the restraining forces, the obstacles that prevent programs and proposals from working. We should continue to strengthen the positive aspects of the program, but we should concentrate our major efforts on tempering the effect of the negatives.

Perhaps an example will help. Suppose I am working with a patient who has undergone bypass surgery and has never exercised regularly in his life. My mission is to help him increase his daily physical activity to at least 30 min of walking per day. Each of us involved in exercise physiology can list at least 100 benefits to the body garnered from exercise. So I begin by telling the patient all of those reasons, and I try to ''drive'' him into exercise because of the many benefits he will accrue from it. However, the reason that he does not exercise is that his work, family responsibilities, and lifestyle do not allow him 30 min a day to walk. Rather than spend all of my effort on touting the merits of exercise, I should spend most of my time helping him to sort out his day to find the 30 min for walking. Maybe he can combine activities, for example, talk with his wife or children while they all walk.

Building a Team and Assigning Responsibilities

Now that you have done the majority of the work, the proposal should be shaping up for implementation. Each member of the committee has done her homework, a number of the barriers to success have been removed, and the positive forces for success are in action. Bring the reshaped and perfected proposal back to the total department, ask for final approval, and set up the steps for implementation. What skills does the staff need? Who will direct the project? How can you ensure success? What method of incorporation carries the least amount of negative consequences? How will you measure the outcome to see if the change is for the better? When should you measure the outcome? Once you have answered all of these questions, set the department to work with a degree of autonomy. Let the leader you choose lead. Do not interfere, but set deadlines for reports that will let you know how things are going. This does not mean that you should never be in the area yourself; be present and be a presence, but be a positive presence.

Kiefer and Senge (1986) believe that alignment, personal ability, and personal mastery are keys to success; these elements fit into the management of vision or ideas scheme presented here. The authors suggest that the more complete the alignment of the staff to the new idea or program, the more successful the implementation will be. This is not to say that there is not creative conflict and disagreement. Kiefer and Senge (1986) believe that ''a high degree of alignment is really a necessary condition for creative disagreement, since the quality of interpersonal relationships in a highly aligned organization allows people to argue about ideas without fearing loss of acceptance or damaged relationships'' (p. 6).

Finally, the overall success of the new program will depend on the skills, knowledges, and abilities of the individuals implementing it. The staff members should have ongoing commitments to developing their own and each other's personal talents. The manager must ask, Who does what best and how can he or she help the others?

Managing People

Remember that you are not managing programs, rather you are managing people who implement and run the programs. People have feelings, need to be respected, and also need praise and constructive criticism. What is difficult for the middle manager is making two different groups of people believe you have their best interests at heart. Your boss and the upper administration want to believe that you are working hard to curb expenses, generate revenue, and run your program effectively and efficiently. Your staff members want to believe that you are working to increase their pay, lessen their work loads, and provide ideal working conditions with adequate paid time off. Sometimes the two groups' goals are mutually exclusive, but a good manager can manage and please both. You do this by getting your employees to become invested in the program, and allowing them a say in many of the decisions; you can even carry this to the point of giving a committee of employees decision-making power about such things as holiday time off. Participatory management can sometimes delay decision making because there is a "process" involved. However, the decision, once made, usually affords a quicker implementation because everyone wants it to work.

Finally, work individually with each of your staff members. Get to know them, spend time listening, and check in with them regularly. Research shows that people who are angry enough to complain will tell 10 people how angry they are and why (Albrecht & Zemke, 1985). When the problem is satisfactorily resolved, they only tell five people about the resolution. Simple arithmetic will tell you that unhappy staff members will put you in a losing situation; you can easily avoid this situation by contact, conversation, constructive criticism, and most of all praise.

Moving Toward Total Quality Management

Quality care for patients is the name of the game, and it will generally run into problems for one of three reasons: lack of knowledge, inadequate systems, and behavior and attitude problems. I shall discuss the lack of knowledge issue here because that is a management issue. Behavior and attitude problems and systems are discussed in chapters 7 and 13.

Actions that employees may take to improve knowledge are discussed in other chapters in this book but are drawn together here for cohesiveness. These actions specifically apply to staff members as they are hired and then continue to grow in their jobs.

Orientation

A new employee should go through a thorough orientation involving the hospital and all of its general policies and procedures as well as the department and all aspects of its policies and procedures. The new staff member should observe procedures, read about policies and procedures, perform procedures under supervision to a standard level of accomplishment, and then be allowed to work on his own. A new staff member should have a checklist of procedures, jobs, duties, and activities to follow. You should note when he has attended meetings, received certifications, or accomplished the level of ability desired.

In-Service Training

A monthly in-service seminar should be a part of any organization. You can use these sessions to alert staff members to new procedures, to help them learn about new equipment operation and new drugs, and also to update the staff on what's new in the field nationally.

Continuing Education

Encourage staff members to attend local meetings, regional meetings, and symposia that specialize in cardiac and pulmonary rehabilitation. Investigate whether your hospital pays for academic credits for continuing education. Encourage your staff to continue educational pursuits. An active and challenged mind is often very productive.

Provision of Reference Material

It is essential that you provide a mechanism for staff members to keep up-to-date on what is new in the literature for their fields. At The Christ Hospital I provided a list of 28 weekly, biweekly, and monthly journals. Each month one of the department members was assigned to review the journals and photocopy any article related to our fields of interest. At Allegheny General, one of our staff members reviews journals, copies articles, and then posts the articles on the staff bulletin board. Also, require anyone who attends a symposium or a national meeting to share the syllabus with the staff and also report on salient points of the meeting.

Further Reading

Berger, S., & Sudman, S. (1991, March/April). Making total quality management work. *Healthcare Executive*, 22-25.

Deming, W.E. (1982). *Quality, productivity and competitive position*. Cambridge: Massachusetts Institute of Technology, Center for Advanced Engineering Study.

Heilig, S. (1990, July/August). The team approach to change. *Healthcare Forum Journal*, **33**(4), 19-22.

Kiefer, C.F., & Senge, P.M. (1986). *Thinking and the new management style program*. Cambridge: Massachusetts Institute of Technology, Alfred P. Sloan School of Management.

Koska, M.T. (1990, July). Adopting Deming's quality improvement ideas: A case study. *Hospitals*, **64**, 58-64.

References

Albrecht, C., & Zemke, R. (1985). *Service in America*. Homewood, IL: Jones-Irwin.

American Association of Cardiovascular and Pulmonary Rehabilitation. (1991). *Guidelines for cardiac rehabilitation*. Champaign, IL: Human Kinetics.

Deming, W.E. (1982). *Quality, productivity and competitive position*. Cambridge: Massachusetts Institute of Technology, Center for Advanced Engineering Study.

Kiefer, C.F., & Senge, P.M. (1986). *Thinking and the new management style program*. Cambridge: Massachusetts Institute of Technology, Alfred P. Sloan School of Management.

Chapter 11

Marketing and Public Relations

Terri Hornbach, BS

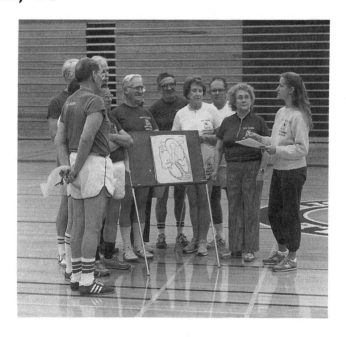

Establishing programs as outlined in chapters 1 through 4 is a beginning, and setting up policies and procedures to manage the programs is the next step. Once you are operational, how do you attract patients? That is the role of marketing and public relations. Letting the professionals, public, and patients know what you do and how well you do it is important in capturing a market share of revenues. This chapter deals with marketing your program in order to generate revenue.

Learning Objectives

1. To define your marketing audience

2. To become familiar with research tools available to assist in defining your market strategy

> 3. To become familiar with the specific marketing tools that will make your program visible to the buying public
>
> 4. To learn how to establish a marketing plan for your program

During the 1980s, when the health care environment became competitive and complex, marketing was introduced in hospitals in an attempt to recapture or stabilize declining revenue and patient bases. Unfortunately, some administrators saw marketing as little more than a glorified advertising department. Public relations (PR) activities had been in place in hospitals for some time. Until the early 1980s, however, PR departments did little more than produce a ''let's see who just had a baby'' employee newsletter and serve as a clearinghouse for an occasional media call.

It was obvious that, in the 1980s, administrators sometimes found it difficult to use either discipline to its full potential. One reason is that administrators erroneously viewed both marketing and PR as merely ''promotion,'' perhaps because promotion is the most visible function inherent to both disciplines. As a result, marketing and PR often were afterthoughts to developing or enhancing hospital programs, sought after only for promotion capabilities and not for their value in research and planning activities.

PR activities matured and diversified as administrators and practitioners saw the need and potential to influence attitudes toward their hospitals, their hospitals' services, and health care in general. Likewise, marketing grew beyond advertising efforts as administrators began to witness its value in the planning and designing of services that were attractive to potential health care consumers.

Cardiac rehabilitation programs can benefit from both marketing and PR. The planning and research capabilities of both disciplines, and their focuses on key publics, can influence opinion and attitudes toward the concept of cardiac rehabilitation and can bring buyers to your products.

Although marketing and PR function well as partners in the health care setting, each inherently works to achieve a different end. Marketing, as defined by Kotler (1975), is ''the set of human activities directed at facilitating and consummating exchanges.'' That exchange usually involves products or services traded for money or for other products or services.

Public relations, on the other hand, is concerned with opinions and attitudes. Cutlip and Center (1978) define PR as ''the planned effort to influence opinion through good character and responsible performance, based upon mutually satisfactory two-way communications.''

These two disciplines have a symbiotic relationship, interacting with and often enhancing each other. Through the understanding and cooperation created by sound public relations practices, a positive business climate is developed in which buyers willingly seek your services. A community that perceives a hospital as low-quality or uncaring, for example, will be reluctant to buy any of its services.

Likewise, marketing practices can enhance or damage an organization's image and credibility. For instance, some hospitals market wellness programs, which often stress improvement of self-image not only through better lifestyle habits such as exercise but also through acceptance of one's inherited body flaws. At the same time, some of those hospitals develop and promote cosmetic surgery services, leaving themselves wide open to public criticism and numerous PR headaches.

This chapter emphasizes the similarities between PR and marketing and discusses how they can enhance a cardiac rehabilitation effort. Those similarities include

- defining target publics,
- researching your plan, and
- the planning process.

The *marketing mix*, which typically falls under the domain of the marketing discipline but has implications for public relations as well, is also discussed.

Defining Target Publics

Determining who your buyers will be is as essential to a cardiac rehabilitation program as it is to any consumer product. But defining who the target publics are goes beyond the buyer and includes other influential figures who might dissuade or even prevent your client from getting to your services. Physicians, administrators, patients, and competitors all may affect referrals to your service.

Physicians

Although physicians are the primary source of referrals to the cardiac rehab program, you cannot assume that those referrals will come readily or eagerly: You must measure the physician's regard for the value of rehabilitation. Many physicians are trained to believe that only medical and surgical treatments are necessary to create a successful outcome. Likewise, their education often stresses the traditional view that the physician can adequately provide all of the patient's treatment needs.

Other physicians believe that treatment that emphasizes emotional and physical wellness, individual commitment, and a multidisciplinary team of care providers will lead to better quality of life and potentially greater health benefits for their patients. This philosophy holds the most promise for commitment to a cardiac rehabilitation program.

Other factors may influence a physician's interest in or commitment to a cardiac rehabilitation program. Research conducted by Miller (1988) suggests that the ability to continually monitor a patient's progress may be the primary reason physicians refer to the program, followed by psychological benefits and improvement in the patient's functional capacity. On the other hand, Miller suggested, cost and the physicians' beliefs that they can sufficiently manage a patient's rehabilitation themselves are key factors against physicians referring to a program.

Hospital Administrators

The key decision maker in establishing a cardiac rehabilitation program is the hospital administrator, whose reasons for the program can be numerous, including the following:

- Physician relations. An excellent cardiac rehabilitation program can be a factor in maintaining or improving relations with current staff physicians who seek a well-rounded practice and referral environment in heart services. Furthermore, such a program can help attract new cardiologists and cardiac surgeons to the medical staff.
- Competition. A hospital lacking tertiary services such as open heart surgery can still lure outpatients back to a cardiac rehab program that's close to home. On the other hand, a tertiary care center lacking a cardiac rehabilitation program risks losing patient base, including referrals to other related and non-

related services, to competing hospitals.
- Hospital accreditation and review measures. As government, accreditation, and review agencies look more closely at outcome factors at hospitals, programs that may enhance the quality of life and overall health of a patient may become of greater value to the administrator.
- Service enhancement. A hospital that designates heart services as a center of excellence may require cardiac rehabilitation to fully establish such a reputation.
- Financial incentive. Unfortunately, the desire to add to a hospital's bottom line may not be reason enough to add a cardiac rehabilitation program to its list of services. A survey by *Hospitals* magazine (Sabatino, 1989) found that 39.4% of all cardiac rehabilitation programs in the hospitals surveyed made a profit, with 38.4% breaking even. That left 22.2% as money losers. Wellness and health promotion programs fared even worse, with 48.9% breaking even or generating revenue.

Patients

Is the hospital's patient base, both current and potential, appropriate for a cardiac rehabilitation program? Are community attitudes toward wellness and quality of life sufficient to maintain interest in such a program?

Consider the following:

- Age, sex, and similar demographic factors that may affect need for such a program. For example, a very young or mostly female population may generate a smaller patient base for cardiac rehabilitation than an older, primarily male population.
- Interest in and commitment to the wellness philosophy.
- Convenience factors, including the distance patients are willing to travel. Also consider free time, location, and transportation.
- Understanding of health benefits from such a program. How well has the community been educated on such matters, and how accepting have people been of these ideas?

Competitors

While assessing target publics, you should examine one group that also will have a tremendous impact on the success of your program—the competition. Look closely at the failures of weak competitors to avoid making similar mistakes, and scrutinize the strengths of others. Can you compete against those? In examining your competitors, consider the following questions:

- From where are they drawing their patient bases? Are your heart patients being referred there, and if so, how many?
- Are their services more appealing or prestigious than yours?
- How sound are their relationships with referring physicians?
- Are their facilities attractive and well furbished with necessary equipment?
- Are their staffs competent, experienced, and respected?
- Are they operating at full capacity, and if not, why?
- Are there more programs in your community than the potential patient base warrants?

Researching Your Plan

Research is a key element in any marketing or public relations plan. Among other things, it helps you define the needs and motivations of your target publics, the nature of your competition, and the structure and offerings of your program.

Research begins with a hypothesis—an educated guess about what you're hoping to find. A hypothesis is simple, direct, and easily quantifiable. For instance, your hypothesis may be "Physicians see cardiac rehabilitation as essential to the quality of patients' lives" or "The greater Cincinnati health care market does not have enough Phase II cardiac rehabilitation programs to meet market demands."

After you establish your hypothesis, research can begin. There are two kinds of data obtained through research that are useful in proving or disproving your hypothesis—primary and secondary data. *Primary data* is collected directly from research subjects, specifically for the project at hand. Questionnaires, random surveys, focus groups, and interviews are examples of research used to collect primary data.

Secondary data, on the other hand, already has been gathered for another purpose and published in some form. Government documents, such as census reports, are one source of such data. Professional associations, medical and business research journals, and even competitors' promotional materials (if attainable) also can offer useful secondary data.

Primary data may lend the most insight to the development of your program, because it is collected directly from those who will most influence the program's success. Therefore, the remainder of this section focuses on primary-data collection techniques.

Data Collection Methods

The *survey* is a common, simple method of collecting data. Usually, it is administered orally, or in writing via a questionnaire. The interview subjects may be approached through the mail, via telephone, or in person.

Mail surveys usually have a low response rate. Follow-up reminders, or repeat mailings, might be necessary to provide a sufficient response rate and valid findings. Small tokens, such as $1 bills, are commonly used to elicit response.

Mail surveys should contain stamped, preaddressed return envelopes. They should not require more than 15 min to answer, should use few open-ended questions, and should be graphically appealing and easy to read. It is essential, also, to pretest your surveys in order to pinpoint flaws or misleading or confusing questions.

Telephone surveys, likewise, should be brief. Plan to make calls during a time that is most convenient for your interview group—tough to do if you're planning to interview physicians.

In-person interviews allow you to probe more deeply for information than you can in telephone or mail surveys, and the information can be more detailed. On the down side, such interviews are time consuming, both in information gathering and tabulation. The presence of the interviewer, including how she poses questions nonverbally, may bias the responses of the interviewee.

The *focus group* is another method of primary research. Focus groups allow you to gather six to eight people of specific interests together for an indepth discussion of a particular topic. The advantage of such a group is the free and open exchange of ideas, opinions, and reactions. You can probe concerns and negative reactions before a program is developed.

One disadvantage of focus groups is cost. Usually, such an activity demands a professional moderator who is skilled in posing objective questions and handling strong reactions without biasing participant input. In addition, participants are usually paid fees that can range from $25 to $150 per session, depending on their occupations and de-

Marketing and Public Relations • 147

mands on their time. Meals are often included as well, and you must consider audiovisual recording and site costs.

Sample Selection

A random sample will help eliminate bias in the selection of survey participants. A random sample simply ensures that each participant has an equal chance of being selected for the survey. Therefore, if the survey were conducted at another time, with another sample of participants, the results would be nearly the same.

One simple method of ensuring randomness is to select every "*n*th" person from an alphabetized list of all potential interview participants. Or, assign serial numbers to all potential participants, and select the group you need using a table of random numbers (available in statistics or math textbooks or from some computer programs.)

Data Tabulation and Analysis

Numerous methods are available for interpreting data collected in research, and these are beyond the scope of this chapter. For those who have not studied statistics and need assistance beyond calculating simple percentages and averages, two resources are available. One is in-hospital staff members who have expertise in data tabulation and analysis, such as the management engineering or planning personnel. Another resource is computer software packages, which will conduct calculations of data that you input; however, the interpretation of such data may be up to you.

The Marketing Mix

Key to the success of any marketing strategy is the manipulation of four important variables, known as the *marketing mix*. McCarthy and Perreault (1984) describe these four variables as the "four Ps": product, price, place, and promotion.

All four can enhance or detract from the other, and all are interdependent. For example, one Cincinnati hospital offers a credible cardiac rehabilitation facility to its heart patients, complete with state-of-the-art equipment and well-credentialed staff. However, the hospital failed to consider that the older clientele such a program would attract would be reluctant to drive to, or park in, what they perceived to be a high-crime neighborhood.

Some referrals were lost to hospitals in cleaner, safer suburban communities.

Product

Your product, or program, should be designed to meet the needs of your target publics, including the hospital's need for maximum return on investment. Your market research should indicate what those needs are. Answers found in such research may yield strategies to help you

- maintain market share in an increasingly competitive environment,
- capture an untapped portion of the health care market,
- enhance existing heart services, or
- recruit or retain physicians through the offering of quality cardiac services.

Research should indicate what product offerings are most desirable to your key buyers. For example, will Phases I and II suffice, or is there a need (or resources available) to provide Phase III on site? And what facility design, equipment, staffing, program structure, and even hours and location will be most appealing to physicians and patients?

Price

Numerous factors influence pricing decisions. The costs of staff, equipment, and space are obvious. You must also consider insurance reimbursement, consultants' fees, competitors' fees, and patients' abilities and willingness to pay (including how much) for such a service.

The hospital's objectives for the program will affect its pricing structure. Is the program to be a revenue generator, an image builder, or a physician recruitment or retention tool? Is administration willing to take a loss on such a venture in order to recruit new cardiologists, for example, or for the altruistic value of improving the quality of patients' lives?

Place

Don't underestimate the power of accessibility. As mentioned earlier, neighborhood safety, parking, transportation, convenience of location, and traffic hassles affect compliance and commitment, as well as referrals.

PROMOTION AND PRICING DECISIONS

Danada Wellness Center in Wheaton, Illinois, affiliated with Central DuPage Hospital in Winfield, Illinois, implemented a strategy to not only reduce patients' risk of heart disease but to feed clientele into other hospital programs. Danada implemented a risk reversal program targeted at individuals who knew they had heart disease or knew they were at serious risk for the disease. Danada wanted to attract individuals not currently or formerly enrolled in its cardiac rehabilitation program, thereby increasing the hospital's base of potential heart clients.

Danada used print advertising, direct mail, and a hospital-to-community publication to promote the program. Results with print advertising were disappointing, especially considering the fact that it involved a great outlay of promotional dollars. Greatest success came from direct mail, which was sent to individuals who had been hospitalized at DuPage for heart-related or risk-factor-related problems, and from the community publication, which featured the program in-depth and provided follow-up stories as well.

Promotion for the Danada Wellness Center's program was most effective when targeted at a key audience, rather than spread broadly in a hit-or-miss fashion, such as the print advertising.

The Health Care Advisory Board (1990) in Washington, DC, however, in analyzing similar plans found mass promotion through print and radio advertising, as well as publicity through the news media, to be highly effective. The content of the advertising, the placement (times aired or newspaper section used), as well as its creative value could be factors in the conflicting findings. The Danada staff also found that repeat exposures, versus one-time exposures, help maintain interest in the program. In other words, clients will pick up the phone and inquire only when exposed to promotion. If the promotion stops, interest wanes.

Danada's program was priced at $2,250 for a 2-year package. The cost reflects the high-value product the Danada staff wanted to offer prospective clients. The cost included a full range of diagnostic tests, risk assessment, behavioral counseling, monthly educational classes, and a health club membership, as well as unlimited visits with the center's staff physician, nurse, exercise physiologist, and dietitian.

Because of the emphasis on diagnostic testing, some, but not all, third-party payers covered the cost of the program. However, M. Livingston (personal communication, July 1991) reported that clients were so drawn to the program that many chose to enter despite the outlay, knowing that the benefit to their longevity was worth the risk to their wallets.

The program, which has been under way for 4 months at the time of this writing, has drawn 15 clients out of approximately 120 queries and is anticipated to generate a 50% profit.

Because such a program allowed the center to use existing staff and facilities and repackage services into a new product, start-up operational costs were low. However, the profit estimate does not take into account promotional costs, which can be quite expensive depending on media buys and the actual creation of the ads and direct mail pieces. Quite frequently, promotional costs are not considered in planning for new programs, but they should be. The cost for promotion can be quite an eye-opener, and the amount spent should be weighed against the short- and long-term objectives of the program.

Danada conducted no research prior to the program's outset to determine client interest or physician support in the program. This can be risky. However, previous case histories of other successful programs can be of help and can serve as informal research in this process.

Informational letters were sent to internal medicine physicians prior to the start of the program. Response in the form of meetings between the Danada staff and physicians was very low, as is typical with such attempts to reach the physician audience. Use of significant personnel and financial resources, in the form of multiple approaches and costly incentives, often is the only way to obtain some kind of response from this hard-to-reach group.

DuPage's hospital administration was very excited about this program, according to the Danada staff. The administration saw an opportunity to expand the existing heart product line in a manner that was not simply self-serving. The potential to increase stand-alone profits for the center and to increase incremental profits in related heart services also was very attractive.

Also consider facility issues. The attractiveness of the facility, as well as the availability of lockers, showers, and even towel service (though not as important as a qualified staff), can affect perceived image of the program's competence.

Promotion

Promotion is the most visible aspect of marketing and PR activities. However, it is only successful inasmuch as the program it serves has been well developed.

The choice of promotion activity will be influenced greatly by the desired end results. The activities of advertising and direct mail are usually, but not exclusively, under the domain of marketing, because they are usually developed to specifically bring the buyer to the product. Likewise, PR's promotion activities, such as media relations, special events, and publications, are useful in persuading or generating an understanding of an issue.

Advertising

Advertising can reach selected audiences through trade or professional publications. Or, it can be used to target broad audiences via the mass media—generally, radio, television, and mass-circulation newspapers and magazines. Ads can serve as image enhancers or can be designed to elicit a planned consumer response (e.g., a purchase or a phone call to a service).

Direct Mail

Flyers, newsletters, coupons—just about anything that can be sent via the U.S. Postal Service—are useful in communicating with very specific audiences. Response mechanisms, such as phone numbers or preaddressed reply cards, can help gauge the success of the intended message.

Media Relations

Stories in the news media, either broadcast or print, give the cardiac rehab staff an opportunity to build an image of authority or credibility. The media's appetite today for medical news, including sources who can address issues in lay terms, is nearly insatiable. Unlike advertising, however, the participant in a news interview has no control over the final outcome of the communicated message. As soon as cameras are turned off or note pads tucked away, the final message lies in the hands of reporters and editors.

Special Events

Special events attract target publics to a site, to an activity, or to individuals (e.g., speakers). Such events give staff members an opportunity to meet face to face with potential clients or referring physicians. The control of the communications effort, for the most part, lies in the hands of the events

---

PLACE AND PHYSICIAN COMMITMENT

The Health Care Advisory Board (1990), in its publication *Hospital Cardiology: Vol. 1. Major Business Strategies*, analyzed "platinum quality" rehabilitation programs.

The assessment of the Health Care Advisory Board indicates that platinum-quality rehab programs improve hospitals' potential for strong stand-alone profits and can serve as feeders into other hospital cardiology programs.

In these cases, hospitals go beyond standard programs to offer "value-added" or "VIP" programs to clientele. Often, the emphasis is on outstanding service, with individual attention and high-class facilities, as well as on a prestigious staff of therapists, physiologists, and physicians.

One such strategy implemented at the Danada Wellness Center includes a spacious facility with

individual showers and lockers; four pieces of original artwork adorn the lobby. Individualized risk factor assessment and goal setting rid the "cookbook" approach to cardiac rehab that often besets other facilities.

Other tactics suggested by the Health Care Advisory Board include convenient hours (early morning and evening hours), high staff-to-client ratios, and a full range of services (psychological counseling, a full-time nutritionist, and formal educational programs for the patient and family.)

The platinum-quality approach may satisfy the physicians' needs for personal recognition as discussed under the empirical-rational model for change and may also support the client's need for relationships and sharing according to the normative-reeducative model.

planner. On the down side, events can be expensive and time consuming.

Events relevant to cardiac rehabilitation include the following:

- Sponsorship of Continuing Medical Education (CME) programs for physicians and other key medical personnel
- Community health education programs
- Open houses
- Sponsorship of fitness activities, like walks or races
- Displays, speakers, or screenings that can travel to off-site events sponsored by other organizations

Publications

Publications can be promotional, informational, or both. The most common publication formats include newsletters and brochures. Publications that take a promotional slant can sell a buyer on your services and can encourage a response (e.g., through a hotline phone number). Informational publications can educate your audience on various aspects of disease, wellness, and rehabilitation. Publications can also enhance a program's reputation, because they establish the authors as authorities on given topics.

The Planning Process

A well-defined marketing and public relations plan is the foundation of any successful business activity. A plan not only defines where you want to go, it establishes how you intend to arrive at that destination, how you will know if your journey has been successful, and what course of action you will take if it has not.

There are four key elements of a sound plan: defining objectives, choosing strategies, implementation and control, and evaluation.

Defining Objectives

At this point in the planning process, you establish the ends you hope to achieve through your marketing and PR efforts. Your research results, including your examination of your target publics, should direct what you need or would like to accomplish. Sound objectives should be specific, measurable (through quantitative or qualitative methods), and attainable within the program's limits.

Your plan's objectives should complement those developed in the hospital's overall strategic plan.

For instance, the emphasis the hospital places on being a leader in local heart services may affect how strongly you need to target your objectives toward developing an image as a premier cardiac rehabilitation facility.

Choosing Strategies

The plan of action consists of selected strategies designed to help you achieve your objectives. Manipulation of the marketing mix factors, as well as implementation of public relations techniques, will form the basis for your strategies.

For instance, a hospital seeking to ensure physician referrals to its new cardiac rehabilitation program may send its staff out on ''calls'' to potential referring physicians. Key staff members schedule a brief meeting with each physician and arrive equipped with a packet of information outlining the program's services, staff credentials, and the program's referral process. The staff member notes negative responses, which are later examined. The program director then attempts to correct or respond to areas of concern.

The strategic portion of the plan should include budgets and timetables and should consider the demands such activities will place on the schedules of staff members.

Strategies for Creating Change

Changing attitudes is difficult. If your research indicates that any of your target publics show reluctance or negativity toward your rehabilitation efforts, your strategies may well include the process of creating change.

Bennis, Benne, Chin, and Corey (1976) discussed three strategic models of change. The first, which stresses an empirical-rational approach, suggests that people, as rational beings, are motivated by self-interest and personal gain. Individuals, under this model, are convinced through knowledgeable argument and reasoning. Miller (1988) suggested that the key to the success of such a strategy may include financial rewards, personal recognition, and convenience.

Another strategy is based upon the normative-reeducative model of change. With this model, change is brought about through personal values as well as enhanced group relationships and sharing. Development of multidisciplinary task forces and physician advisory committees, as well as a personalized approach to patient care, may be effective change strategies under this approach.

Unlike the first two strategies, the power-coercive model is likely to bring about only temporary changes. It emphasizes the use of force—

through rewards, punishments, and commands—to create change. Coercion by power holders is the key strategy here. For example, a powerful staff physician might threaten to refer patients to another hospital for open heart surgery if a cardiac rehabilitation program isn't offered. Although the program may be implemented, internal hostilities may also result. If that physician eventually withdraws support, or leaves the staff, the program will be left standing on unstable ground.

Implementation and Control

During the implementation phase, strategies are put into action. If strategies falter, corrective measures are taken. For example, what if the physicians mentioned in the strategy example refuse to meet with staff members to discuss the new program? In place of personal meetings, you can implement a direct mail campaign followed up by telephone calls. Or, you may scrap entirely strategies that appear to be failing.

Watch budgets and timetables closely during this phase. If deadlines are missed or expenses run over budget, examine the reasons why. Attempt to bring the timetable or budget back under control, if this is deemed necessary.

Evaluation

The planning process is cyclical; evaluation enables the planner to redefine objectives and develop a new plan from the results of the old.

During the evaluation phase, you will examine whether your strategies achieved the objectives set forth in your plan. For example, did you win referrals from physicians previously referring to a competitor's program? Or, did you achieve a predetermined level of compliance from your patients, based on education and communication efforts implemented prior to the program's opening?

At this point, obtain feedback from target publics, including your own staff, on the success of your objectives. Equipped with feedback, evaluation of objective results, and further research, you can begin the planning cycle again.

The Marketing and Public Relations Departments

Before embarking on any PR and marketing activity, approach your hospital's PR and marketing staffs. The professionals on these staffs have both the education and experience necessary to help you implement a successful plan. You'll find a variety of skills in these departments—not just marketing and PR generalists, but specialists in such areas as media relations, market research, physician relations, and more. Because the success of your marketing and PR plan reflects as much on these people as on you, they'll be eager to help direct your efforts and offer staff assistance.

References

Bennis, W., Benne, K., Chin, R., & Corey, K. (1976). *The planning of change* (3rd ed.). New York: Holt, Rinehart & Winston.

Cutlip, S.M., & Center, A.H. (1978). *Effective public relations* (5th ed.). Englewood Cliffs, NJ: Prentice Hall.

The Health Care Advisory Board. (1990). *Hospital cardiology: Vol. 1. Major business strategies.* Washington, DC: The Advisory Board Company.

Kotler, P. (1975). *Marketing for nonprofit organizations.* Englewood Cliffs, NJ: Prentice Hall.

McCarthy, E.J., & Perreault, W.D., Jr. (1984). *Basic marketing: A managerial approach* (8th ed.). Homewood, IL: Irwin.

Miller, M. (1988). A framework for enhancing physician involvement in the rehabilitation continuum. In L. Hall & G.C. Meyer (Eds.), *Cardiac rehabilitation: Exercise testing and prescription* (pp. 43-66). Champaign, IL: Human Kinetics.

Sabatino, F.G. (1989, January 5). The diversification success story continues: Survey. *Hospitals,* pp. 26-32.

Chapter 12

Reimbursement Issues

G. Curt Meyer, MS

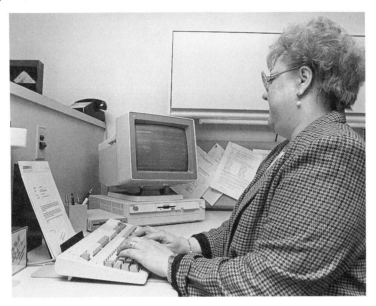

One area that can present you with more problems than any other is reimbursement from third-party payers for services rendered. This chapter presents a clear-cut road map to understanding reimbursement problems. Areas of greatest concern are recent developments and changes in coverage guidelines. This chapter presents not only answers and foundational information about reimbursement but also suggests ways you can enhance your reimbursement strategy.

Learning Objectives

---

1. To become familiar with the language of reimbursement

---

2. To gain understanding of the classification system of health insurance companies

---

3. To develop a plan for optimizing reimbursement for your program

---

4. To gain insight into marketing to third-party payers for increased reimbursement for service

---

National health care spending has increased quickly during the years since the implementation of the Medicare program. Expected spendings in 1990 were $600 billion for total health care. Of this, Medicare represented $102 billion, Medicaid $60 billion, private insurance $192 billion, and private pay $150 billion. These statistics are astounding. Further, these figures represent total health care spending in America at $68,333,000 per hour (this represents an expense 24 hr a day, 365 days a year).

Providers, third-party carriers, and government have the responsibility of attempting to bring cost increases under control. As such, during the last several years, these parties have worked at determining prospective payment, determining outcomes from a cost-effective standpoint, and attempting to evaluate the cost of quality care. Cardiac rehabilitation has been and should continue to be included in this process of evaluation. To be better able to contribute to this process, you need to understand several aspects: classification of insurances, the guidelines for coverage of cardiac rehabilitation, the appropriate mechanism for billing of services, utilization review, and ways to use program evaluation to market to third-party carriers.

Classification of Health Insurance Companies

Health insurance companies primarily can be divided into two distinct sectors:

- Private sector
- Public sector

The private sector contracts with individuals or groups and determines the benefits that will be offered through the terms of agreement between the third-party carrier and the patient or enrollee. Such contracts result in the enrollee paying a premium either directly or through an employer to the third-party carrier. Such third-party carriers who represent the private sector include independent insurance companies and a number of health maintenance organizations (HMOs).

The public sector is that group of third-party carriers that are administered under a government-sponsored program. Primarily the government's involvement is the collection of premiums through a taxing mechanism; enrollment is such that payment is made based on the coverage guidelines as published through the *Federal Register* or on worker's compensation fees. These programs include Medicare, Medicaid, Civilian Health and Medical Programs of Uniform Services (CHAMPUS), Worker's Compensation for Medical Care, and Bureau of Vocational Rehabilitation.

To more completely understand the mechanisms by which these various insurance companies or government agencies work, contact a local representative of such groups and refer to a variety of other published materials (e.g., Meyer, 1988).

In the private sector, payment for services is usually performed under a ''usual, customary, or reasonable payment'' mechanism. This payment mechanism is also referred to as Level 1 and Level 2 charges. Usual charges for a service are determined from those actual charges sent to the carrier on the provider's service report form. In the state of Pennsylvania usual charges were first determined by a confidential fee survey in 1966. Each of those charges for various procedures was reported by doctors and/or clinics on claim forms to the third-party carrier. Upon review of the span of charges, the carrier, in this case Blue Cross/Blue Shield of Pennsylvania, calculated that the usual charge would be paid at 75% of all reported charges for that procedure. Each year these charges are monitored and a usual fee for each procedure is determined for the following year.

Customary charge (sometimes referred to as Level 2 charge) is 90% of the usual charge for each procedure by doctors who have the same specialty in a given geographic location, weighted by the number of times the procedure is reported. This amount is the maximum amount of money that the carrier will pay to the physician or clinic for a given procedure (Pennsylvania Blue Shield, 1981).

The *reasonable* component of the usual, customary, and reasonable payment plan is that which accounts for complications or unusual clinical situations that require and justify a higher amount of payment for such service. When the *reasonable* component applies, a review by the medical director of the third-party carrier is often required. This review determines whether a higher payment mechanism than the Level 2 or customary fee is appropriate.

Reviewing the Coverage Plan

Payment for various services always will be determined by the benefits listed in the contract between the insurance company and the enrollee. In some cases benefits are determined by procedures that are not covered under the plan. In all cases, the provider should confirm whether the plan covers a specific service. For example, it is appropriate that a member of the cardiac rehabilitation team contact the insurance carrier and verify whether cardiac rehabilitation is a covered service under that plan. This will allow the patient, provider, and carrier to know whether the service is covered either fully or partially, and appropriate payment mechanisms can be obtained.

Cardiac rehabilitation often requires a large amount of explanation to the benefits manager for the third-party carrier. You must understand and be able to communicate the clinical intervention to the benefits manager in order to obtain the appropriate type of coverage for the patient. As well, it may be necessary for an insurance verification person from your hospital to speak to someone from the medical review section in order to clarify whether cardiac rehabilitation services are covered. In all cases, there are nurses, physicians, and other types of clinicians who are able to communicate with providers about appropriate coverage for services.

Specifically in the private sector, coverages of services are usually listed in the manual that the carrier often supplies to the providers. An example of this is the reimbursement guide for hospitals from Blue Cross/Blue Shield Association (1988). This manual includes information about admitting, coverage, billing, and BC/BS telephone numbers, addresses, programs, and services. Each carrier should have a reference book such as this for referral by the provider.

In the public sector, Medicare publishes through the *Federal Register* a copy of the coverage guidelines. Each type of provider and each type of service are covered through the *Federal Register* in the HIM 10 or HIM 15 (U.S. Department of Health, Education, and Welfare, Social Security Administration). It is extremely important that your program is on the mailing list for this publication. The intermediary mails the updates that are published from the Medicare office. In cardiac rehabilitation, Section 3525 as published on September 15, 1982, outlines the coverage for cardiac rehabilitation services through Medicare (Department of Health and Human Services, Healthcare Financing Administration, 1982).

Section 3525 is transmittal number 988, published in September 1982 from the Intermediary Manual, Part 3, Claims Process. Within this documentation, Medicare has outlined that patients who (a) have documented diagnosis of acute myocardial infarction within the preceding 12 months, (b) have had coronary bypass surgery, and/or (c) have stable angina pectoris are considered to have a clear medical need for cardio-

vascular rehabilitation. Further, the document states that cardiac rehabilitation programs must fulfill specific conditions in relation to the facility, the availability of a physician, the availability of necessary cardiopulmonary emergency diagnostic and therapeutic life-saving equipment, and the identification of the program area and staffing by qualified personnel. The document also states that a prospective candidate for cardiac rehabilitation may be evaluated for the program by means of an exercise stress test. The indications for coverage for stress testing are listed as (a) evaluation of chest pain, especially a typical chest pain; (b) development of exercise prescription for patients with known cardiac disease; and (c) pre- and postoperative evaluation of patients undergoing coronary artery bypass procedures. The document mentions other areas such as ECG rhythm strips and diagnostic and therapeutic services, each of which has its own utilization screen that you must identify before you establish specific protocols.

Section 3525 of the appendix states that it is "not normally considered reasonable and necessary to provide psychotherapy to all cardiac rehabilitation patients, or even to test all such patients to determine whether they have a mental psychoneurotic or personality disorder." However, if a patient is diagnosed with a mental neuropsychotic or personality disorder, psychotherapy furnished by a psychiatrist or psychologist rendering such services, incident to a physician's professional service, may be covered.

Further developments in outpatient billing for psychologists and social workers are presently occurring. Legislation has recently passed allowing for outpatient psychologist services to be billed directly to Part B Medicare. However, the specific coverage guidelines have not been released from the Healthcare Financing Administration (Florida Blue Cross, 1990).

Patient education services are not covered under the outline as listed in Section 3525. Such a service is considered "the same kind of information that would have been furnished to a patient and/or family member by the attending physician following the patient's acute cardiac episode." Therefore formal lectures and counseling on these subjects are not considered reasonable or necessary as separately identified services when they are provided as part of a cardiac rehabilitation exercise program.

The duration of the program is identified as reasonable and necessary for up to 36 sessions, usually 3 sessions a week in a single 12-week period. Within the document, Medicare has identified the following exit criteria as appropriate levels for terminating therapeutic outpatient treatment, exercise treatment, and rehabilitation: (a) The patient has achieved a stable level of exercise tolerance without ischemia or dysrhythmia, (b) symptoms of angina/dyspnea are stable at the patient's maximum exercise level, (c) the patient's resting blood pressure and heart rate are within normal limits, and (c) the stress test is not positive during exercise.

Recent Developments and Coverage Guidelines

In the private sector the Blue Cross/Blue Shield Association released its clinical recommendations for outpatient cardiac rehabilitation services in July 1988. The document reviewed coverage guidelines as previously outlined in Section 3525. The study was performed under the premise that cardiac rehabilitation programs were introduced before the effectiveness of these programs was completely tested (Blue Cross/Blue Shield Association, 1988). A review of current plan coverage identified that 86% of the responding plans covered cardiac rehabilitation services. Furthermore, the plans not only covered myocardial infarction, coronary artery bypass graft surgery, and angina, but some of the plans covered the following diagnoses: percutaneous transluminal coronary angioplasty, mitral valve, coronary heart disease, heart transplant, hypertension, arrhythmias, and pacemakers. The document further identified that 54% of the plans provided coverage for Phase I of cardiac rehabilitation, 43% for Phase II, and 17% for Phase III. As a result of this study, and of the Greenland and Chu paper (1988) in *Annals of Internal Medicine*, Blue Cross/Blue Shield developed a cardiac rehabilitation summary of clinical and coverage recommendations. This is found in Table 12.1, which stratifies patients as low risk, intermediate risk, high risk, and very high risk and outlines clinical recommendations and coverage recommendations. At the time of this writing, these recommendations have not been implemented by all 103 Blue Cross/Blue Shield plans in the nation. The recommendations are suggested by the Blue Cross/Blue Shield Association, but individual Blue Cross/Blue Shield plans are not required to adhere to these guidelines. However, some plans have applied these coverage guidelines.

The public sector has made some steps toward evaluating the coverage guidelines for cardiac rehabilitation. In 1987, the Healthcare Financing Administration (HCFA) requested that the Office of Health Technology Assessment (OHTA) evaluate the safety and effectiveness of cardiac rehabilitation. This evaluation took place during 1987 and was reported in a publication from the National Center for Health Services Research and Healthcare Technology (Feigenbaum & Carter, 1987). This evaluation concluded that ''cardiac rehabilitation services are considered safe and efficacious therapy to improve the cardiovascular and psychosocial status of patients with documented coronary heart disease to the extent that it improves exercise tolerance or otherwise enhances functional capacity.'' No evidence exists to indicate that cardiac rehabilitation improves prognosis in patients with coronary heart disease. Patients with a recent acute myocardial infarction, CABG surgery, and stable angina pectoris are among those that have benefited from this technology.

The heightened awareness and evaluation of the technology of cardiac rehabilitation have led to its identification as an appropriate therapeutic intervention in increasing the functional capacity of patients. Further, we need to address long-term outcomes and prognoses of patients after such intervention.

Provider Guidelines for Coverage

Cardiac rehabilitation services may be provided in a variety of settings: hospitals, physician offices, outpatient clinics, comprehensive outpatient rehabilitation facilities, physical therapy practices, and YMCAs. As a provider, you need to understand various guidelines in order to receive reimbursement through either the public or the private sector. A hospital generally receives a provider number from the regional office of the HCFA upon the successful completion of a review process. Depending upon the state in which the hospital is located, either the Department of Health and Human Services or Medicare may provide a validation survey. Other accrediting bodies such as the Joint Commission on Accreditation of Healthcare Organizations and the Commission on the Accreditation of Rehabilitation Facilities (CARF) may have input as to the hospital's ability to receive a provider number. For example, in Florida rehabilitation providers must be CARF accredited (Florida Department of Labor and Employment Security).

Physician-owned clinics primarily work through a Blue Shield, Medicare Part B, and private insurance program in which each clinic uses the physician's provider numbers to receive reimbursement

Table 12.1 Summary of Clinical Coverage Recommendations

Patient categories	Clinical recommendations	Coverage recommendation
1. Low risk • Uncomplicated MI, CABG, PTCA • Functional capacity 8 METs • Asymptomatic	Formal cardiac rehabilitation program not required	Not eligible for benefits
2. Intermediate risk • Functional capacity less than 8 METs • Symptomatic New York Heart Association Classes I, II, III	Formal cardiac rehabilitation program excluding continuous ECG monitoring	Eligible for a maximum of 6 weeks, three visits per week
3. High risk • At high risk of recurrent MI evidenced by specific symptoms or conditions	Formal cardiac rehabilitation program including continuous ECG monitoring	Eligible for 6 weeks, three visits per week If clinically indicated, eligible for an additional six visits, one visit per week
4. Very high risk • At very high risk of recurrent MI evidenced by specific symptoms or conditions	Formal cardiac rehabilitation program contraindicated	Not eligible for benefits

Note: CABG = coronary artery bypass graft; ECG = electrocardiogram; MI = myocardial infarction; PTCA = percutaneous transluminal coronary angioplasty.

From *The Reimbursement Guide for Hospitals* by Blue Cross/Blue Shield Association of Florida, 1988, Jacksonville, FL: Author. Copyright 1988 by Blue Cross/Blue Shield. Adapted by permission.

for rehabilitation services. Primarily such a clinic uses the Medicare guidelines as outlined in Section 3525 as the gold standard in providing cardiac rehabilitation. At times a representative from the fiscal intermediary may visit the facility to ensure that it follows appropriate life safety codes, emergency life support equipment, and infection control policies. Appropriate reference for this can be found in the AACVPR (1991) *Guidelines for Cardiac Rehabilitation Programs.*

Comprehensive outpatient rehabilitation facilities (CORF) are governed by the Omnibus Reconciliation Act of 1980, Section 933. Upon the successful completion of a comprehensive outpatient rehabilitation facility survey, the facility is eligible to receive a provider number (CARF, 1990). Other types of providers are governed primarily on a state-by-state basis. As such it is beyond the

scope of this chapter to address all of the criteria (with the many variables for each state) in the provision and licensure of these types of providers. Contact your state department of regulations with any questions about regulations for these types of cardiac rehabilitation providers.

Billing for Services

In many cases, billing is the most critical financial aspect of a cardiac rehabilitation program. Often the bill is the only communication tool between the provider and the payer of services. Thus you must understand the billing process to ensure the success of your cardiac rehabilitation program.

Preadmission determination of coverage is essential to the sound operation of a cardiac rehabilitation program. A staff member of the cardiac rehabilitation team should verify that payment will be made either through a third party carrier or through private pay. This process can be very complex in the cardiac rehabilitation setting. The staff member in charge of verification must have a sound understanding of the exact policy type and extent of coverage for policies in order to conduct an appropriate preadmission determination of coverage. In most cases, the preadmission review staff member requests a copy of the insurance card of the policy holder, then telephones the writer of the policy to determine coverage. Once this information is obtained, the patient is informed of the amount of copayment that she is responsible for above and beyond any payment made by the insurance company.

Almost every procedure provided within the context of medicine is listed in the *Physician's Current Procedural Terminology* (American Medical Association, 1983). The *Physician's Current Procedural Terminology*, or CPT-4 Code Book, lists all procedures and codes so the procedures can be converted to a code on the bill. In the 1990 edition of the CPT-4 Code Book, Code 93797 is the number for physician services for outpatient cardiac rehabilitation, without continuous ECG monitoring (per session). Code 93798 is physician services for outpatient cardiac rehabilitation with continuous ECG monitoring (per session). Therefore in the cardiac rehabilitation field, these two codes represent the primary procedures provided. Other codes for stress testing, rhythm ECGs, and other related services can be found in this book.

Another code book that is essential to successful billing is the *International Classification of Diseases* (9th rev.). Also called the ICD 9-CM Code Book (1990), it provides, for every possible diagnosis, a code used in the billing of a service. The primary mechanism by which insurance companies work is a matching of the diagnosis with the appropriate intervention or procedure. Therefore oftentimes the billing mechanism, via computer, matches the ICD 9 code with the corresponding CPT 4 code for a "clean claim."

Health care providers primarily use two types of bills. The first is called the HCFA 1500 Super Form Bill (see Appendix C). This is primarily used by physician offices to bill for office visits and by outpatient cardiac rehabilitation programs. You can obtain a copy of this bill from the intermediary through the HCFA. Contact the provider relations person for the fiscal intermediary that services your area for a copy of this form. The bill that is more commonly used by other types of providers is called the Uniform Bill (UB) 82 (see Appendix C). This is used not only by Medicare but also by many private insurance companies. The UB 82 has 96 "form locaters," which are the areas of the bill where information is entered.

Form locaters 1 through 14 provide the various demographic and provider-number data that are necessary for the insurance company to keep appropriate records. Form locaters 15 through 18 deal with the date, hour, type, and source of admission. Clearly these do not apply to cardiac rehab candidates; these locaters are more applicable to inpatients. Form locaters 19 through 21 deal with the accident hour, discharge hour, and patient status at discharge. Form locater 22, which applies to cardiac rehab, looks at the period that the billing covers; often in cardiac rehabilitation, this is a monthly bill that lists the number of visits from the first of the month to the end of the month. Form locaters 23 through 28 deal specifically with the number of days of coverage. This number varies depending upon the type of insurance underwritten to the individual.

Form locater 50 is the specific description of the service performed. Often this is simply listed as *cardiac rehabilitation*. The column to the direct right of the description column is for the CPT 4 codes relative to the description.

Form locater 51 identifies the revenue code, which is similar to the procedure code. Revenue codes are listed in many of the private carriers' manuals and specifically the Blue Cross/Blue Shield manual. These are the actual charge codes that are used for various procedures. Revenue codes beginning with 943 are specific to cardiac rehabilitation. Other examples of revenue codes are ECG telemetry monitoring—732, and stress testing—482. You can easily obtain a complete listing of the revenue codes for Blue Cross/Blue Shield by reading the *Reimbursement Guide for Hospitals* (Blue Cross/Blue Shield Association of Florida, 1988). Form locater 52 identifies the number of units or increments of that specific service, and 53 lists the charges. Form locater 57 identifies the payer for services; this may be entered as Blue Cross or Aetna, for example. Form locaters 58 and 59 have to do with the release of information and the benefits assigned. Form locater 60 shows the amount of deductible that the patient must pay, and form locater 61 shows the amount of co-insurance that the patient must pay. Form locaters 62 through 64 show the estimated responsibility, prior payments, and estimated amount due. Form locater 65 identifies the insured's name, 66 the insured's sex, and 67 the relationship of the patient to the insured individual. This may include husband, wife, daughter, or son.

Form locaters 68, 69, and 70 primarily provide identification data to the insurance company such as identification number, employer group name, and insurance group number. Form locater 76 is where the description of diagnosis as found in *International Classification of Diseases* (9th rev.) is listed. Form locater 77 is for the principal code as found in the ICD 9 Code Book. Often in cardiac rehabilitation, other diagnosis codes may be included, which are found in form locaters 78 through 81; these may include such diagnoses as diabetes, obesity, or depression. Form locaters 83 through 86 identify the procedures that are performed, whether they are surgical or medical intervention. In all cases the CPT 4 codes should follow the descriptions. The rest of the form identification areas are not important to you other than form locater 92, which identifies the physician. Often, the insurance company will verify whether the physician identified was the referring physician.

Overall the billing process is not extremely complex. Primarily you need to have a sound understanding of the appropriate terminology and code numbers to be applied in the proper form location area. If the form is completed correctly, the bill is usually processed as a "clean bill" and the third party carrier does not request or require further documentation.

Infrequently (you hope), you will receive a claim with a denial of payment. Along with the denial of payment may be listed a reject code, which is simply a means for insurance companies to code any reason for rejecting a claim. Therefore you should understand the reject codes as listed in each of the provider manuals. Often a reject code may be relative to patient education or exercise therapy. You can correct this with a phone call and proper documentation presented to the third party carrier identifying these services as components of the actual cardiac rehabilitation program. In both the private and public sector, patient education is often not covered by insurance companies. As well, prevention programs are often denied for payment.

Utilization Review

Utilization review can be an internal as well as an external function. By performing quarterly internal utilization review with staff members, you can possibly prevent denial of claims. When the cardi-

ac rehabilitation staff is aware of the items that must be included for payment, the staff can develop a checklist for utilization review (see Table 12.2). The key aspects of the utilization review process are the referral, plan of care, diagnosis, intervention, frequency of treatment, duration of treatment, short-term goals, long-term goals, and physician signature. Through internal utilization review and the appropriate setup of the checklist, you should be able to keep claim denial to a minimum.

Table 12.2 Cardiac Rehabilitation Checklist

1. Physician referral
2. Plan of treatment
3. Functional goals
4. Educational goals
5. Estimated number of visits _____
   a. Physician signature _____
6. One month or 30-day recertification _____
7. Daily progress notes
   a. Identify short-term gains
   b. Compliance with plan of care
   c. Educational review of learning
8. Discharge summary

External utilization review has attracted a significant amount of attention during the last 4 years. Both the public and private sectors have emphasized use of the external utilization review for appropriate determination of payment. The federal government has developed Medicare Utilization Review Forms 700 and 700a. These are presently under a pilot study and should be finalized soon. The role of the outpatient rehabilitation services form (HCFA-700/701) is to provide medical review, certification/recertification, and a plan of care form for outpatient Part B services. The form has been designed to promote national consistency in reporting and to reduce unnecessary requests for additional medical records. The form shows the relationship between the date of the diagnosis and the date of intervention as well as the specific diagnosis and intervention. More importantly, the form identifies and focuses on the short-term and long-term goals as well as the progress that is achieved relative to these goals. For any rehabilitation services, the goal of the third party carrier is to assure that the outcomes are appropriate for the time, intensity, and cost of the intervention.

Therefore if progress is not made as identified on these utilization review forms, payment likely will not be made. Of interest is the grouping of the following services as used on the HCFA-700 form. These services include occupational therapy, physical therapy, speech language pathology, outpatient cardiac rehabilitation, respiratory therapy, and psychiatric services. Regardless of the specific type of rehabilitation, there is a generic common ground in rehabilitation that the government has identified in the components in this form. This form is used by hospitals, CORFs, rehabilitation agencies, and clinics.

Future developments that may take place include identification of prospective payment for given diagnoses. For example, an uncomplicated inferior lateral MI patient may receive payment for x + number of visits. However, a complicated inferior lateral MI patient with diabetes may receive payment for x number of visits. In the areas of physical therapy and occupational therapy, these utilization screens have already been developed by diagnosis on the outpatient setting (Department of Health and Human Services, Healthcare Financing Administration, 1982).

Medicare and Medicaid also have developed audit forms for the various levels of office visits in physician clinics. These levels of office visits include *minimal, brief, limited, intermediate, extensive,* and *comprehensive.* Seventeen criteria are used to determine whether the physician is able to bill for a brief visit versus a limited or other office visit. Clearly the public sector is being more aggressive in determining the level of care associated with the payment of service. It appears that this will be a trend in the future.

Use of Program Evaluation to Market to Third-Party Payers

Program evaluation should be the cornerstone of any rehabilitation program. CARF (1990) has identified program evaluation as an essential component to rehabilitation services. Program evaluation provides you feedback about the types of patients that your program is serving, where the referrals are coming from, the diagnoses that make up the patient population, patient satisfaction with the service, and most importantly the specific functional changes that the patient achieves from the intervention provided. This is another way of identifying program evaluation—as measurement of outcomes. You must examine outcomes relative to goals, such as the goals identified through JCA-

HO (1989). In cardiac rehabilitation, specific outcomes are expected through the rehabilitation process. You must identify these outcomes both in your policy and procedure manual and in the plan of care. These expected outcomes are the first area that the third party carrier will look at to determine whether the intervention is necessary and appropriate. Outcomes may be evaluated in a variety of areas. The AACVPR *Guidelines for Cardiac Rehabilitation Programs* (1991) contains a sound explanation of outcomes.

Of major importance to the determination of outcomes is the measurement of efficiency. The patient's changes in functional, educational, and psychologic measurements during the time between admission and discharge will reveal the cost-effectiveness of the program. Clearly, a large gain in these outcomes with a relatively short intervention will cost less, showing a high efficiency factor. This is exactly what the third party carriers look for in determining payment for services. In the future, the outcomes relative to cost may become a competitive factor in determining whether a patient will attend Program A or Program B. Therefore your challenge is to focus on areas that provide the most effective intervention to result in the best possible outcome.

Furthermore, outcomes need to be measured not only at the time of the patient's discharge from the outpatient program but, more appropriately, a year later. These long-term outcomes relate to rehospitalization, work status, amount of total health care expense, and independence. You must evaluate all these factors when determining the cost-effectiveness of cardiac rehabilitation. Some studies that have looked at the cost-effectiveness of cardiac rehabilitation (Edwards et al., 1990; Huang et al., 1989)) have shown that patients participating in supervised cardiac rehabilitation programs have lower total health care expenses than do controls.

Conclusion

Overall, although few changes occurred between 1982 and 1990 in the actual writing of coverage guidelines for cardiac rehabilitation, much has occurred as a result of providers' attention to needs and cost-effective aspects of rehabilitation services. Some states have identified guidelines and have worked with the insurance companies to determine what services are appropriate for payment. Other developments have occurred with risk factor stratification, the amount of frequency and duration of telemetry monitoring, technology, and types of providers. With this constant and large-scale change that will continue to occur in health care, it becomes the responsibility of the providers, the third-party carriers, and the patients to work together to assure that payment is provided for patients who need rehab services. Furthermore, as economic pressures increase, it will be everyone's responsibility to maintain a certain level of health through lifestyle changes.

Further Reading

Blue Shield, *Policy Review and News*. This is a quarterly publication by Blue Shield. Eastern, western, and central district offices for subscription: (215) 564-2131, (412) 471-7916, and (717) 731-2045.

Chenoweth, D.H. (1988). *Health care cost management*. Indianapolis, IN: Benchmark Press.

Coddington, D.C., Keen, D.J., Moore, K.D., & Clarke, R.L. (1990). *The crisis in health care*. San Francisco: Jossey-Bass.

National Center for Health Services Research. (1986). *Private health insurance in the United States*. Rockville, MD: U.S. Department of Health and Human Services.

References

American Association of Cardiovascular and Pulmonary Rehabilitation. (1991). *Guidelines for cardiac rehabilitation programs*. Champaign, IL: Human Kinetics.

American Medical Association. (1983). *Physicians' current procedural terminology* (4th ed.). Chicago: Author.

Blue Cross/Blue Shield Association. (1988, July). *Technology evaluation and coverage clinical recommendations for outpatient cardiac rehabilitation services*. Chicago: Author.

Blue Cross/Blue Shield Association of Florida. (1988). *The reimbursement guide for hospitals*. Jacksonville, FL: Author.

Commission on Accreditation of Rehabilitation Facilities. (1990). *Standards manual for organizations that service people with disabilities*. Tucson, AZ: Author.

Department of Health and Human Services, Healthcare Financing Administration. (1982, September 15). Payment for services furnished to patients in hospital based and free standing cardiac rehabilitation clinics. *Federal Register*, **41**(934), Section 5241.

Edwards, W.W., Franks, B.D., Iyribox, Y., & Dodd, S.L. (1990, May). Physiological and expense implications of PTCA Rehabilitation. *Medicine and Science in Sports and Exercise*, Abstract: American College of Sports Medicine.

Feigenbaum, E., & Carter, E. (1987). *Health technology assessment report, #6 Cardiac Rehabilitation Services* (DHHS Publication No. 88-3427). Rockville, MD: U.S. Department of Health and Human Services.

Florida Blue Cross. (1990, July-August). *Medicare part B update*. Jacksonville, FL: Florida Blue Cross/Blue Shield.

Florida Department of Labor and Employment Security, Division of Worker's Compensation. *Facts about worker's compensation insurance for employers*. (Available from 2551 Executive Center Circle West, Tallahassee, FL 32301-5014).

Greenland, P., & Chu, J.S. (1988). Efficacy of cardiac rehabilitation services with emphasis on patients after myocardial infarction. *Annals of Internal Medicine*, **109**(8), 650-653.

Huang, D., Ades, P.A., & Weaver, S. (1989). Cardiac rehospitalizations and cost are reduced following cardiac rehabilitation. *Circulation*, **80**(2), 610.

The International Classification of Diseases. (1990). Clinical modification, 9th revision. Ann Arbor, MI: Edwards Brothers.

Joint Commission on Accreditation of Healthcare Organizations. (1989). *Accreditation manual for hospitals*. Chicago: Author.

Meyer, G.C. (1988). Overview of insurance—Obtaining and maintaining coverage in cardiovascular rehabilitation. In L.K. Hall & G.C. Meyer (Eds.), *Cardiac rehabilitation: Exercise testing and prescription*, Vol. 2, pp. 67-102. Champaign, IL: Human Kinetics.

National Association of Rehabilitation Facilities. (1990, May). Legislative bulletin. In C. Bordon (Ed.), *HCFA form 700, 701, 702 regarding requests for medical review information for Part B intermediary outpatient rehabilitation bills*. Washington, DC.

Pennsylvania Blue Shield. (1981). *Procedure, terminology and manual with fee schedule allowances*. Camp Hill, PA: Author.

Professional Health Educators, Inc. (1988). *Challenges in physical therapy: Lesson 1: Why documentation spells survival*. Bethesda, MD: handout.

St. Anthony Hospital Publications. (1988). *ICD 9.9.CM code book* (Vols. 1-3). (Available from

P.O. Box 14212, Washington, DC 20044, 800/ 632-0123.)

South Carolina Medical Society. (1987). *South Carolina cardiac rehabilitation plan certification program*. Charleston, SC: Author.

United States Department of Health, Education and Welfare, Social Security Administration HIM 10 (6-66). Reprint date: variable.

Chapter 13

Budget and Revenue: Meeting the Bottom Line

Linda K. Hall, PhD

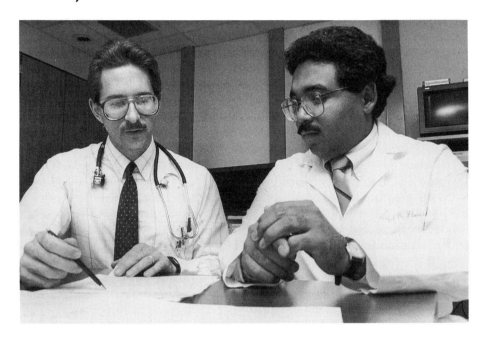

Optimum fiscal management of any program is often the difference between success and failure. Making sound expenditure decisions and managing your programs to accrue the maximum revenue are the two output/input factors of meeting a profitable bottom line. This chapter discusses many aspects of expenditure and revenue generation that are inherent in running a cardiac rehabilitation program. Included are other options for revenue generation to ensure your success in meeting cost/revenue balance.

Learning Objectives

1. To understand the basics of budgetary principles in managing a cardiac rehabilitation program

2. To have a baseline understanding of line items and line item budgetary processes

3. To understand the potential for ''other market'' revenue generators to enhance your bottom line

This chapter discusses the nuts and bolts of any program in any organization, business, or commercial venture: How much does it cost, how much do you earn, and what is your margin of profit? In an age when health care costs are rising at twice the rate of inflation, an average of 12 to 15% per year, and health care–related expenses to the nation will equal 20% of the gross national product by the year 2000, do not expect a health care agency to underwrite a losing proposition unless the secondary benefits make it profitable. Inform your administration at the outset that cardiac rehabilitation is not a big money-maker and in a lot of cases does not break even. Second, become a student of budget and finance; this is a part of your job that you should not give away. Rather, it is the part of your total management scheme that you should work on zealously. Ask other cost center managers how they manage budgets. Take courses about budgeting, and seek educational information from the hospital finance department about budgetary process.

Third, realize that after you pay the initial expense of getting a program up and running, 75 to 85% of your expenses will be for personnel, 10% will be for educational materials, and the rest will be for miscellaneous things; you will eventually spend an enormous amount of time trying to reduce the costs of this last category in order to cut your budget. There is not a lot of waste in a cardiac rehabilitation budget, so if you are asked to cut your budget it usually means laying off someone. This is why you must be fiscally prudent and responsible from the word *go*.

The Budget Process

In working on a start-up budget or even your yearly budget, you should adhere to several general principles.

1. When you are planning the staff and the staff qualifications, make sure that every job is filled by a staff member with the appropri-

ate qualifications. Nurses, exercise specialists, dietitians, and physical therapists are expensive. Across the nation salaries range from approximately $7.92/hr for an inexperienced bachelor's degree exercise specialist up to $17.50/hr for an experienced master's degree nurse/exercise physiologist. These people should not transport patients or enter data into a computer; assign these jobs to an orderly and a data entry technician, so trained medical professionals can do hands-on patient exercise and education. Streamline your job descriptions so that the people you are paying the most are doing the jobs that require the most skill; don't pay people high salaries to do menial tasks that could be done by someone earning less. This will become easier to assess as you get into productivity and its measurement standards (see chapter 14).

2. When buying equipment, consult the clinical engineering department of your hospital to determine what this department's employees have been trained to fix, service, and work with. Consider the following example: Your hospital uses Brand X monitoring equipment on all of the floors in the hospital where cardiac ECG telemetered monitoring is done. You prefer to use Brand Y in the outpatient cardiac rehabilitation lab because this brand has several capabilities that you want. However, clinical engineering can service Brand X in-house but does not stock the parts or have personnel who are trained to service Brand Y. The company that sells Brand Y wants $5,000 per year for a service contract. You buy Brand X.

3. Check around before buying your exercise equipment. Check with other programs about the service record, durability, and life expectancy of the brand of equipment you are considering. Also, see if there are bicycles, old Master's two-step benches, shoulder wheels, arm ergometers, hand weights, dumbbells, and even treadmills in physical

therapy, occupational therapy, or some other area of the hospital. Remember, program quality is judged by the quality of the personnel who manage and apply it, not by the glitz of the area and equipment.

Staffing Costs

Across the nation salaries vary for personnel depending upon qualifications, degrees, licenses, and other things such as cost of living, hospital salary grades, and program philosophy. Refer to Table 13.1 for a range of hourly wages that you may use as a reference when figuring staffing budgets. The usual number of annual work hours are figured at 2,080. Cardiac rehabilitation staff are usually salaried, not hourly, and are not paid for overtime. Quite often nurses will tell you that they

Table 13.1 Salary Ranges by Degree and Experience

Position	Degree	Experience	Salary ($/hr)
Exercise specialist	RN	None	10.88-13.50
	BS	None	7.90-8.20
	RN, BSN	CCU, step-down, no rehab	12.00-16.00
	BS	Rehab, ACLS certified	8.32-9.00
	MSN	CCU, ACLS, no rehab	12.00-16.82
	MS	Internship, no ACLS	10.90-12.50
	MSN	CCU, ACLS, rehab	12.30-17.78
	MS	Rehab, ACLS	12.30-14.50
Clinical coordinator	MS/ MSN	Yes in all phases and with management experience	13.40-17.80

Note. These are hourly wages reflecting an example of lows to highs within the regional United States. They are based on 1990 dollars; adjust yearly by adding cost-of-living increase. ACLS = advanced cardiac life support; CCU = critical care unit.

are able to earn higher wages working as a staff nurse than they can earn working in cardiac rehabilitation. However, in cardiac rehabilitation they do not work nights or evenings, do not have emergency call, and do not work weekends; they essentially have 8-hr/day jobs and are considered professional and exempt employees.

Directors are not included in Table 13.1 because I generally view directors of departments from several angles:

- Manager/clinician—this person is usually an MSN, BSN, or MS who works with patients and runs a small department. Depending upon how other manager/clinicians in the hospital or work setting are paid, the range may be anywhere from $30,000 to $40,000.
- Manager—this person is an MS or MSN with much clinical and management experience and is a full-time manager. The pay range is about $35,000 to $40,000.
- Director 1—this person is an MS or MSN with an MBA or a PhD. This person has much experience; pay will range from $40,000 to $50,000, depending upon negotiations.
- Director 2—this person has a national reputation; has done much writing, research, and national speaking; is a potential grantwriter; and is well recognized in the field. This person will earn $50,000 to $70,000, or more. These salaries are estimates and will vary according to area of the country, requirements of the hospital/agency, or cost of living indices.

Equipment

Any number of equipment companies and different types of equipment are around; some equipment is very basic, and some has microchips and computer screens. I have an old-fashioned belief that the more luxury features you tack onto an item, the more often it is in the repair shop. Be sure that your hospital clinical engineering department can calibrate and fix what you buy. The basic equipment needed for cardiac rehabilitation is a track or a treadmill where patients can walk and a monitoring system for high-risk patients. Other equipment will provide a larger variety of exercise modalities and thus a complete cardiovascular and muscular strengthening program. Bicycles (both ergometer and airdyne type), rowing machines (both wind and cylinder), stair climbers, cross-country ski machines, dumbbells, and some form of universal-type weight machines will make for a very diverse program that encompasses all the risk levels in cardiac and pulmonary rehab. Remember that you need to have an exercise station for each person in the rehabilitation class. Additionally, per AACVPR (1991) guidelines, weight training is now considered appropriate for cardiac rehabilitation programs; remember this in your equipment purchase plans.

When buying equipment consider repair, replacement, services, and initial quality of the equipment. You can also ask directors of other programs what equipment they have, why they bought it, whether it was a good deal, and whether they would purchase it again.

Budgetary Line Items

Every budget system is different; however, you should consider some general guidelines in preparing a year's budget when you set up and as you continue a cardiac rehab program. Table 13.2 provides a sample of a line item budget and the items you are most likely to use. When you are setting up your department, try to locate it in a hospital and not in a medical office building. Usually the office building is in the for-profit and the hospital is in the not-for-profit area of the health care system. Although hospital administrators may want to locate your program in the medical office building, they may forget this 2 to 3 years later and question why you have such a large budget. At The Christ Hospital, where my department was in the medical office building (rent = $56,000 per year), the program would have broken even if not for the rent.

Here is where the fun begins. Imagine that your budget is established and your department has been working for about 2 years when the hospital has a financial crisis and you have to cut your budget. I have been in this situation twice, and my department has had to cut its budget by about 6%. Based on the sample budget in Table 13.2, this cut equals about $19,000. There really is no fat in the budget in Table 13.2. You can look at the cost of electrodes, but if electrodes make up less than 4% of the budget, a cheaper electrode won't make much difference. At the most you can remove travel, meetings, and miscellaneous and save $4,000. However, you will end up with a staff that is unhappy, demoralized, and not growing. One area that you may be able to reduce is purchased services or consults. For example, my department has traditionally purchased psychological consults from a private psychologist. This began because the hospital did not have this service available when the department was formed 11 years ago. Within the last 4 years the hospital has developed a department of psychiatry and now employs a number of psychologists and psychiatrists. I can now consult that department at no charge and the hospital gains the revenue from the reimbursement for service. This reduces my budget by $20,000. It is financially more prudent to use services that are available in the hospital rather than to contract services outside the hospital.

Table 13.2 Sample Line Item Budget—Imaginary Program

Item	Estimated Expenditure ($)
Salary and wages[a]	187,000
Benefits (25%)	46,750
Laundry/linen	1,500
Contract maintenance	2,500
Property rental	60,000
Medical/surgical supplies (electrodes @ $0.41)	4,000
Printing and office supplies	2,500
Teaching supplies	4,000
Publications and subscriptions	250
Travel and meetings	2,000
Miscellaneous	1,500
	313,000

Note. Based upon 400 cardiothoracic surgery patients, 300 myocardial infarction inpatients, 150 Phase II outpatients (50% nonmonitored), and 350 stress tests per year.

[a]Staff of seven—two BS exercise specialists, two MS exercise specialists, one MSN exercise specialist, one MSN experienced manager clinician, and one secretary/receptionist.

Quality Patient Care and Budget

When working to reduce your department's costs you must be careful that you do not interfere with the very systems that ensure excellent patient care. It is critical that you do not cut back on articles and inventory items that ensure the excellent care that you are providing. Rather than eliminating the item, check to see that you are not overstocking it.

Two cost items will allow you to utilize and impact your budget to the best advantage: personnel and rent. Personnel and rent make up 85% of your budget, so this is where you must be most efficient and effective. You want revenue generating activities going on in your department area all of the time. However, if you have to hire an expensive staff to supervise the activity, examine the cost/revenue ratio before going ahead with the project. Do you have some revenue-generating activity going on in your area every hour that you are open? If not, this is where you must make your first revenue-generating effort. Remember, however, that you must accomplish the effort without increasing cost (i.e., more staff, more electrodes, or more educational materials). So the task is to increase income without increasing cost. You can introduce a number of different things into your exercise area that require little supervision and may generate some revenue: employee fitness programs, dietary education, weight management programs, and any exercise program for people without cardiovascular or pulmonary problems that operates with a minimum of supervision. One area that you should explore immediately and consider implementing is exercise and health-education programs for the well elderly. I am often reminded that these are not "cardiac rehabilitation" programs, which are what this book and my department are all about. However, these other program areas are well within the purview of a cardiac rehabilitation staff. Also, they fit very well into the program model of cardiac rehabilitation. And last, they are low-cost revenue generators.

Cutting your budget means reviewing where you spend the most money. In the sample budget in Table 13.2, employee wages equal 75% of the budget. Review your job descriptions, look at who does what, and study the application of work through productivity studies. Make sure that you are not overhiring (too many people to do the work) or that you are not hiring overqualified people (too many degrees and certifications and too much experience). I suggest that if you have a large program and staff, you hire highly qualified staff to supervise exercise and education, and hire an individual with a bachelor's degree to assist; then train the assistant to the standard you desire.

Microcosting

Once you decide the focus of your program and you have a policy and procedure manual, you will need to know the cost of your operation. Microcosting each procedure will allow you to look at all of the expenses involved in the procedure and set a charge for the procedure that is reasonable and at the same time allows a profit margin. When you microcost you figure in everything that may directly or indirectly affect the procedure. Table 13.3 provides a guideline for fixed and vari-

able expense classes you may want to consider when establishing a microcost system. A fixed cost is anything that remains constant in total, regardless of changes in patient or procedure volume. Variable costs vary proportionately with changes in the number of procedures performed or patients treated.

Table 13.3 Fixed and Variable Expense Classes

Fixed	Variable
Legal and audit fees	Postage
Nonclinical consulting services	Professional clinical fees
	Medical/surgical supplies
Travel, dues, seminars	Chemicals/reagents
Cleaning supplies (partial)	Cleaning supplies
	Pharmaceuticals
Minor equipment	Oxygen and other
Miscellaneous	medical gases
Telephone	Intravenous solutions
Office and general supplies	and administration sets
	Prostheses
Fuel and utilities	Films solutions and
Malpractice insurance	paper
	Electrodes/batteries
	Degreaser/alcohol swabs
	Purchased clinical services
	Electrocardiogram paper
	Linens/soap
	Education materials/ books
	Brochures
	Forms/paper

Fixed capital
Depreciation
Interest
Rent/lease
Equipment maintenance
Warranty contracts
Asset insurance
Property taxes
License fees

Create a chart that allows you to allocate costs, equipment, supplies, and work minutes to each procedure. Tables 13.4 and 13.5 are examples of sample worksheets for writing costs. Calculate the number of each item used per procedure, how much each costs, and so on. This is especially important when you are looking at the cost of staffing a procedure. Not only should you consider how much time each staff member spends during the procedure but also how much time is spent before and after the procedure. Multiply the number of hours times the hourly wage, and add employee benefits to the cost. Additionally, make sure that the costing for staff includes the time for the total number of staff members who are involved directly or indirectly in the procedure. I urge you to consult your finance and management engineering departments for assistance in computing a microcost account. Table 13.6 presents a rough worksheet on the microcosting for four procedures done in my area. A word of explanation is required here. There are many methods of microcosting, and you should use the same procedure that other departments in your hospital use. The method for microcosting used in Table 13.6 includes the fixed salaries (director, secretary, dietitian) that are spread over all revenue-

generating activities. Additionally, depreciation, rent, disposables, and other fixed costs are figured into the microcosting in Table 13.6. Some methods do not do this but rather deal with actual costs only.

Note in Table 13.6 the minimal difference in the cost of the Phase II monitored session ($33.71 per visit) versus the Phase II unmonitored session ($32.24 per visit). The difference is equal to the cost of the electrodes and the batteries. This proves that your greatest expenses lie not in monitoring equipment and disposables but in staff to supervise the session and in overhead.

Defending and Enhancing Your Bottom Line

In 1990 the Health Care Advisory Board presented its Red Book on strategies for enhancing hospital cardiology services and increasing revenues. This book contains some strategies for cardiac rehabilitation and also some very well-founded arguments you can use with administrators to sell the ideas. The strategies are presented as a series of 21 tactics with descriptions, conclusions, and sales points.

Two major tactics are specific to cardiac rehabilitation. Tactic 11 describes why you should create a "platinum quality" cardiac rehabilitation program. The basic reasoning is that once you have a patient in your system, you want him to like it so much that he will come back for a repeat procedure. Statistics from the *American Journal of Cardiology* (Wittels, Hay, & Gotto, 1990) support the

Table 13.4 Sample Worksheet for Disposable Supplies Microcosting

Description of supply	Stock type	Cost/ unit ($)	No. used/ procedure
Electrodes	Disposable	0.32	10
Degreaser	Bottle	0.29	1
Alcohol swabs	Box	0.001	4
Towels	Bundle	0.25	2
Electrocardio-gram paper	Pack	0.02	12

Table 13.5 Variable and Fixed Labor for Microcosting

Employee and hourly rate ($)	Exercise testing	Phase I	Phase II	Phase III	Departmental meeting	Hospital meeting	Management
Exercise specialist (13.76)	1.114	.78	.47	.38	1.0	.25	
Physician (85.00)	.25		.001		1.0	.25	
Nutritionist (14.00)			.25	.25	1.0	.25	
Clinical coordinator (17.63)	.25	.01	.01	.01	1.0	.25	

Table 13.6 Microcosting Spread Sheet (part 1)

| | 1 | 2 | 3 | 4 | 5 | 6 Direc var sal | | 7 | 8 | 9 | 10 | 11 |
Procedure	Rev/UOS	FY90 Rev	FY90 UOS	MHR/Proced	Stand MHR tot	14.582	14.92	Var sal/proced	Direct var non-sal exp	Total stand var ($)	Total variable ($)	Total var ($/proced)
Inpatient	55.00	594,495	10,809	0.78	8,431.02	–	125,79	11.638	1.900	20,537	146,328	13.538
Stress test	184.70	76,835	416	0.781	324.90	–	4,84	11.653	5.389	2,242	7,089	17.042
Monitored exercise	36.90	59,040	1,600	0.473	756.80	11,036	–	6.897	2.890	4,624	15,660	9.787
Unmonitored exercise	6.10	8,693	1,425	0.473	674.03	9,829	–	6.897	1.421	2,025	11,854	8.318

Table 13.6 Microcosting Spread Sheet (part 2)

| | 12 Fixed portion of sal and dept overhead | | 13 Gen dept overhead | | 14 Tot dept ovh | 15 Tot D ovh/proced | 16 Spec depre | 17 Other depre | 18 Hosp OVH | 19 Tot hos OVH | 20 Hos OVH/P | 21 All cost | 22 All cost/proced |
Procedure													
Inpatient	21,205	46,471	113,912	97,737	279,326	25.842		7,878	80,992	88,871	8.222	514,524	47.601
Stress test	817	1,179	4,390	37,086	44,884	105.91	2,688	384	3,121	14,694	14.694	57,286	137.707
Monitored exercise	1,903	4,171	10,225	8,773	25,073	15.671	5,222	707	7,270	8,249	8.249	53,932	33.707
Unmonitored exercise	1,695	3,715	9,107	7,814	22,331	15.671	4,650	630	6,475	8,249	8.249	45,940	32.238

Note. 1 = revenue charge per unit of service; 2 = revenue for the specific unit of service for the budget year (1990); 3 = no. of units of service applied in the budget year; 4 = standard worker-hour per procedure (from productivity data); 5 = total standard variable worker-hours (column 4 × column 3); 6 = direct standard variable labor charge; 7 = direct standard variable labor charge per procedure; 8 = direct variable nonsalary expense; 9 = total variable nonsalary per procedure; 10 = total variable cost; 11 = total variable cost per procedure; 12 = distribution of salary based on earned hours; 13 = distribution of general department overhead; 14 = total department overhead and fixed salaries distributed per procedure; 15 = department overhead and fixed salaries distributed per procedure; 16 = specific depreciation allocated to specific procedures; 17 = nonspecific depreciation allocated to all procedures based upon earned hours; 18 = hospital overhead excluding depreciation; 19 = total hospital overhead allocated per procedure; 20 = total hospital overhead allocated per procedure; 21 = total all costs; 22 = total all costs per procedure.

repeat procedure idea as a sales point. Table 13.7 presents statistics for repeat procedures in invasive cardiology and cardiovascular surgery.

This repeat information supports several salient arguments why the administration should support cardiac rehabilitation.

1. Creating a loyalty through excellent care ensures the patient's return when the repeat procedures are warranted.
2. Marketing efforts for a superior or high-quality rehabilitation program may help to capture patients from competing hospitals.
3. A superior quality program achieves patient and thus physician satisfaction.
4. A superior and comprehensive Phases I, II, and III program continuum will help you develop an ongoing relationship with patients.
5. A superior and comprehensive cardiac rehabilitation program reinforces the idea that the hospital is a showcase cardiac care hospital.
6. Because the patients who require cardiac rehabilitation have a chronic disease, they are highly likely to require further invasive treatment.

With these arguments in hand, you may wish to approach the administration with a plan for a superior quality program that features VIP treatment of patients, individually tailored treatment regimens, high-quality facilities, excellent patient-to-staff ratios, counseling, dietary services, and educational classes. These arguments support the continuation of your current program and administrative backing.

Table 13.7 Repeat Market for Invasive Cardiology and Cardiovascular Surgery Procedures

---

20% of patients have repeat angioplasty within 6 months to correct restenosis

6% of patients have bypass surgery within 6 months to correct restenosis

9% of patients have repeat angioplasty within 5 years of the initial procedure

5% of patients have bypass surgery within 5 years of the initial procedure

17% of bypass surgery patients repeat the procedure within 12 years of the initial surgery

Some bypass patients will subsequently have angioplasty (small number, percent and age unknown)

Note. Data from Wittels, Hay, & Gotto (1990).

Tactic 10 in the Health Care Advisory Board's publication fits very nicely into the idea of having a superior quality cardiac rehabilitation program. If you have developed such a program, then you have the education programs, the personnel, and the facilities to develop a special program that emphasizes halting the progression of disease. The Health Care Advisory Board calls the program the ''Heart Disease Reversal Program.'' I have difficulty with this title, because reversing heart disease is such a controversial issue; I prefer to call the program ''Progression Prevention,'' or another highly visible, catchy name that your marketing department dreams up.

The primary objective of this tactic is to establish a year-long comprehensive program designed to slow or stop the progression of heart disease. The target audience includes those people who have been diagnosed with the disease; have had angioplasty, catheterizations, heart attacks, or bypass surgery; or have a strong family history of heart disease. The target end result is to capture inpatient revenues from the substantial portion of the participants who will ultimately need in-hospital cardiac care, surgery, or testing. Quite often cardiac rehabilitation and wellness programs target many of their screenings to huge groups of people at malls, supermarkets, and health fairs. Research shows that with this method you gain only 1% of the total tested in further referrals. The risk intervention program described here involves a population with intervention and referral guarantees; these people already have the disease, or a strong potential for developing it.

The program is designed to last for 1 year. It starts with a complete risk assessment including lipid profile and other blood tests, comprehensive physical exam, stress test, pulmonary function test, body composition assessment, and flexibility and strength tests. Then the participant enters into a full-year program of exercise, education, and consultation, with the focus on nutrition, stress management, exercise, and access to physicians. Total recommended cost is $2,400 per person in advance, 90% reimbursable. The important thing about this type of program is that it must be a high-quality program and must provide comprehensive services to the participant. The primary objective of such a program is to ensure that the participants who subsequently require inpatient care, invasive tests, and surgeries will have strong allegiances to the hospital and its physicians. The estimate is that 30% of the enrollees will be admitted to the hospital in the 1st year. The revenue from those admissions will more than pay for any extra staff required to run the program. I have discussed this program with a few managers who have implemented it, and their only caution is that you must spend a great deal of money on up-front advertising and marketing to get the program going.

The Bottom Line

As I cross the country attending meetings and speaking, I am continually amazed at the number of times I am asked to help someone justify the existence of cardiac rehab because of its inability to meet the bottom line. Quite often departments count totally on reimbursement to justify their positions as hospital departments. This book points out ways to help you justify your existence even if your revenues don't. I want to encourage you to review and track every possible dollar that you may lay claim to as having been generated through cardiac rehab contact with a patient.

1. Any patient who has been through your program and reenters the hospital for any procedure has an allegiance to the hospital and its services that in part was created by your department. You may claim part of the revenue (ancillary source) for your department.

2. Cardiac rehabilitation patients undergo graded exercise tests when they enter and exit the cardiac rehabilitation program. The cardiac rehabilitation program may claim these as charges generated by the cardiac rehab department and therefore revenues credited to the department.

3. Track any emergency room admissions, catheterizations, thallium stress tests, gated blood pool studies, electrophysiological tests, ultrasounds, and other procedures that may have been instituted as a result of something discovered during cardiac rehabilitation. Claim part of the revenue generation.

4. Track all repeat bypass surgery patients who underwent rehabilitation with your department. They came back because they were pleased with your work as well as that of the surgeon and surgery department.

5. Use the most efficient management techniques in staffing, utilization, productivity, and third-party reimbursement techniques that are available.

And finally, make your department a superior quality cardiac rehabilitation program that leaves a positive mark on every patient who has contact with it.

References

American Association of Cardiovascular and Pulmonary Rehabilitation. (1991). *Guidelines for cardiac rehabilitation*. Champaign, IL: Human Kinetics.

Health Care Advisory Board. (1990). *Hospital cardiology: Vol. I. Major business strategies*. Washington, DC: The Advisory Board Company.

Wittels, E.H., Hay, J.W., & Gotto, A.M. (1990). Medical costs of coronary artery disease in the United States. *American Journal of Cardiology*, **65**, 432-440.

Chapter 14

Productivity and Utilization

Linda K. Hall, PhD

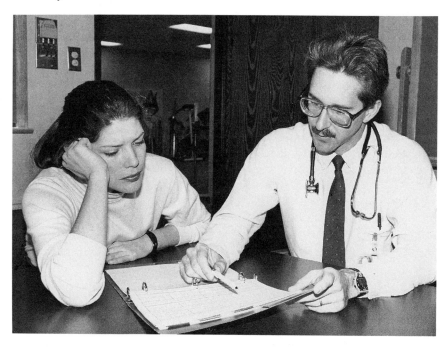

Productivity may be a new word to many cardiac rehabilitation managers because for the most part we have looked at how we work from patient consults ordered by a physician and completed by our department staff. As health care becomes more market driven, managers must consider how much it costs to do each unit of work related to how much revenue each unit of work generates coinciding with how many units of work each staff member is able to produce. This chapter describes how to measure what the previous sentence defined: productivity.

Learning Objectives

1. To understand the manner in which productivity is measured

2. To understand what the measurement of productivity means in terms of staffing, work loads, and revenue generation

3. To understand the use of productivity measurement as a management tool

A general definition that is often used for *productivity* is "working hard and working efficiently." These factors contribute to a definition of productivity; however, the true definition must be delineated more broadly. Productivity is a measure of the resources needed to produce a product, or a measure of input to a system to procure output from the system. We read and hear productivity reports every day in the newspaper and on the radio and even when we read our electricity and gas bills. Baseball batting averages in the sports pages are percentages of hits for the players' numbers of at-bats. Steel mills gauge productivity from a point of how many ingots they can produce from a ton of ore. Our electric bills are based on the number of kilowatt-hours of electricity it takes to run all of our electric appliances for a specific period of time.

Definitions of key terms will assist you as you continue in this chapter. They will be used frequently in examples and discussion.

Productivity—A measure of the system's performance, or a measure of how much input produces a certain amount of output.

Utilization—A measure of the amount of time a worker needs to perform productive work. Suppose, for example, that it takes .78 hr to complete one inpatient cardiac rehab visit, and a staff member completes seven visits in an 8-hr day. The utilization is about 78% for her work on inpatient rehab. On the same day, the employee meets with an outpatient class of 8 patients with a time standard of .473 hr per patient. Because there are two staff members per outpatient class, the employee's utilization for that class is 23%, and total utilization is 100% for the day.

Efficiency—This is a measure of the time required to perform a procedure. As a worker becomes more efficient, he can perform more procedures per time unit. For example, suppose a worker reduces the amount of time to do a stress test from 30 min to 20. This produces a positive change in efficiency of 33.3% and al-

lows three tests per hour instead of two per hour.

When we discuss productivity in the hospital setting we are mostly concerned with labor, because it equals about 65% of the total cost to run the hospital. Measuring productivity, utilization, and efficiency enables us to determine how many employees we need to operate the department, how much to charge per procedure, how much to pay the employees, and what procedures need to be developed within the department to facilitate the work.

For example, suppose that your department can complete three treadmill tests per hour for 8 hr per day at a charge of $220 per treadmill, with additional profee billing (charges for the physician's services) of $120, giving a total charge of $340 per treadmill.

Revenue = *5,520 GXT at $340 each	= $1.87 million
Expenses (from Table 13.6)	= $ .758 million
Net gain	= $1.112 million

*To estimate GXT's, multiply the number of tests (3), by the number of hours (8), by the number of days a week (5), by the number of weeks (46, which allows for holidays, etc.).

After reviewing this data you may wish to look at several possibilities in relation to this area of the program.

1. You can increase your technological status by spending some of the net gain for newer equipment. If you do that you can perhaps continue to make the same net gain, because the newer technology may be more efficient and you may be able to do more tests per hour or may need fewer staff members to do the same number of tests.

2. You can maintain the same profit level each year in order to continue to upgrade your technological status and thus remain competitive. You may be able to do this by improving staff productivity and utilization by

increasing the number of tests per hour or decreasing the number of staff members per test.

There are many different ways to establish a productivity and utilization program for your department. See if your hospital has a productivity department or a management engineering department with someone who is qualified to assist you or create the program for you. With the advent of Medicare diagnostic-related groups and the development of critical pathways, measuring efficiency, utilization, and productivity is a good way to keep costs to a minimum while maximizing revenues.

Setting Up a Productivity and Utilization Program

Chapter 15, which discusses quality assurance (QA), suggests that you keep a service record enumerating the statistics of the department (i.e., number of procedures performed, how often, by whom). If you set up your productivity and utilization program at the same time that you organize your QA program, quite often you can interchange a number of the data entries. Essentially, what you are doing in productivity and QA is measuring the efficiency and the effectiveness of your program. Efficiency is a measure of whether you are doing the job right, and effectiveness is a measure of whether you are doing the right job.

Beginning Productivity and Utilization Measures

In order to get started in either program you need to enumerate all of the basic components of your program (i.e., list all of the activities that your staff does). Then you must separate the activities into *fixed (support) activities* and *variable activities*.

Fixed (Support) Activities
These activities do not change in nature regardless of the changes in patient volume, procedures, and visits. These include such things as department meetings, in-service training, seminars, and committee meetings.

Variable Activities
These activities change as patient volume, number of procedures, and number of visits change. The activity is associated with a standard unit of measure that will determine how you count the activity.

The unit of measure is usually a time standard with a specific staff member involved. Nutrition counseling, for example, is measured by the number of minutes the nutritionist spends with patients relative to weight loss or cholesterol intervention programs. Time standards are established through a time/motion study, in which a management engineer or similar employee observes the department members doing their work over a period of a month or so. At the end of the study period, the management engineer establishes time standards for each activity within the department. See Table 14.1 for an example of the time standard assigned to each of the variable activities and fixed positions in a cardiac rehabilitation department. You should request repeat time/motion studies (two or three total) until you believe that the time standards truly reflect the amount of time that staff members are involved in each procedure. If you change a policy and thus change the way a procedure is conducted, you may have to adjust the time standard.

Once you have established what procedures you will count and how much time it takes to do them, whether they are fixed or variable, then you have to establish how you will count them. If your program is large and treats both inpatients and outpatients, it will be to your advantage to set up a data-keeping system on a computer or integrate it with your billing system. At The Christ Hospital we set up an IBM system in our office for tracking all of the patient data. At Allegheny we record all of the procedures that we perform on our Clinipac system, whether we bill for them or not. From that system, AGH's data sheets are printed at the end of each pay period. I get a series of printouts that have groupings by procedure and by staff member; thus I am able to track activity by total department productivity (see Table 14.2), individual worker productivity (see Table 14.3), and revenue generation (see Table 14.4). From these I am able to submit my QA and my productivity and utilization monthly reports.

Creating a Report

All reports at AGH are generated every 2 weeks and follow the hospital pay period time schedule. Every 2 weeks within the schedule we submit a report on the number of activities that were done and the number of productive hours that were worked. Productive hours are different from the

Table 14.1 Cardiac Rehabilitation Time Standards Per Activity

Labor charge number	Variable activities	Hours/ patient
47700059	Routine inpatient daily fee	0.780
No charge	Spouse education class	0.194
47700554	Psych therapy—brief	0.500
47700505	Psych therapy—extended	1.000
No charge	Spouse education— psychological instruction	1.000
No charge	Phase II psychological instruction	1.000
47701008	Phase II Class	0.421
47701255	Stress test & letter	1.114
47701479	Nutrition consult—15 min	0.250
47701503	Nutrition consult—60 min	1.000
47701701	ECG monitored exercise prescription	0.750
47701552	Exercise—prescription 15 min	0.250
47701800	Exercise—prescription 30 min	0.500
47701859	Exercise—prescription 45 min	0.750
47701909	Exercise—prescription 60 min	1.000
47701354	Monitored exercise	0.473
47701404	Maintenance	0.473
47701453	Unmonitored Phase II	0.473
No charge	Heart to Heart—Organized volunteer program	0.250
47701560	Phase IV class—annual	0.387
47701578	Phase IV class—monthly	0.387
47701395	Progress checks/exercise review	1.000
47701727	Lifestyle—weight class patients	0.887
47701925	Lifestyle—weight class employees	0.887
47701941	Employee fitness nuts— yearly	0.286
No charge	Exercise III—nutrition	0.415
No charge	Exercise IV—nutrition	0.191

Support activities	Standard	Hours worked per year
Director (1.0 FTE)	1.000	1851 (11.0%SHV)
Clinical coordinator (1.0 FTE)	0.800	1480 (11.0%SHV)
Senior exercise specialist (1.0 FTE)	0.250	463 (11.0%SHV)
Secretary (1.5 FTE)	1.000	2777 (11.0%SHV)
Staff meetings/in-service	1.000	

Note. ECG = electrocardiogram; FTE = full-time employee; SHV = sick, holiday, vacation.

Table 14.2 Completed Performances for Department 4770

Service	In-patient	Out-patient	Total
1. Bedside exercise	6	0	6
2. Chart review	57	0	57
3. Discharge instructions	70	0	70
4. Discharge summary	70	0	70
5. Inpatient exercise monitored	189	0	189
6. Outpatient exercise monitored	0	55	55
7. Exercise progressive	86	0	86
8. Initial consult	94	0	94
9. Initial exercise prescription	0	4	4
10. Maintenance	0	64	64
11. Nutrition assessment	36	0	36
12. Outpatient group education	0	1	1
13. Patient education	283	0	283
14. Psychological evaluation	5	0	5
15. Psychotherapy	5	0	5
16. Respiratory services	0	6	6
17. Routine daily fee	441	0	441
18. Stress testing	0	14	14
19. Supervised cardiac exercise therapy	0	4	4
20. Unmonitored exercise phase II	0	52	52
Total for patient type	1.342	198	1,540

Note. Numbers 1-5, 7, 8, 11, and 13 all comprise inpatient cardiac rehabilitation, which is then billed as Number 17—Routine daily fee. This does not mean that every patient undergoes every procedure during every visit; however, patients are seen for an average of 47 min per day. Items 14 and 15 involve consults called by our department to see inpatients with regard to psychological problems. All other items are outpatient functions and are self-explanatory. This is a summary of all department activities for a 2-week period from 12/02/90 to 12/15/90.

number of hours paid, because we may have staff on paid medical leave, on paid vacation, or on paid holiday during that time period. Productive hours are only those hours that people work. Once we submit these data to management services they are applied to the standard hours listed in Table 14.1 and are multiplied to give the total standard hours of productive work (see Table 14.5).

At the end of Table 14.5 you will see a utilization index for the specific pay period. There are several objectives that you desire from each member of your staff.

1. Each employee will be 80% efficient; this means each employee spends 6.4 hr of each 8-hr day in revenue-producing activity.
2. Your department functions at a utilization index of at least 80%.
3. Each member of your staff generates annual revenues equal to three times her annual salary. (This is not standard; it may differ among hospitals and businesses but is the kind of indicator that you may wish to establish and track.)

Using the Productivity Report

Once your productivity and utilization system has been up and running for 6 months and you have made all of the adjustments that you need to make, you can start reading and using the reports for several things:

1. Is there a balance in the work loads of varying staff members in the department?
2. Is your utilization under 80%? If it is, make sure that you are not underreporting the work. If it consistently is under 80%, then you are overstaffed or your staff is not doing enough productive work.
3. Is your utilization over 80%? If so, you are shortchanging your staff in areas such as charging, letter writing, documentation, in-

service training, seminars, and department meetings.

This documentation is the easiest way to justify the addition of staff and programs, space requirements, and internship programs. The system is objective, it gives statistical justification, and the data are hard to argue with. It is also another way of demonstrating what you have to give up if a particular staff member is not hired.

Table 14.3 Summary of Completed Performance by Employee

Employee	Procedure	Quantity
02	Routine daily fee	69
02	Initial consult	7
02	Chart review	7
02	Patient education	50
02	Exercise monitored	33
02	Exercise progressive	7
02	Nutrition assessment	2
02	Discharge instructions	9
02	Discharge summary	9
02	Total	193

Note. This is a summary of the inpatient contacts that the employee with billing code 02 made in a 2-week period, 12/02/90 to 12/15/90. One summary for each employee is printed out each 2-week period.

Table 14.4 Revenue and Usage Printout

Description		Point value constant	Total point value	- - Total - - Frequency	Revenue	- - Other - - Frequency	Revenue	- - Medicare - - Frequency	Revenue	- - Title XIX - - Frequency	Revenue	- - Blue Cross - - Frequency	Revenue
Routine daily fee	Current	.0000	.0000	961	55,738.00	97	5,626.00	510	29,580.00	66	3,828.00	288	16,704.00
	Inpatient	.0000	.0000	961	55,738.00	97	5,626.00	510	29,580.00	66	3,828.00	288	16,704.00
	Outpatient	.0000	.0000	0	.00	0	.00	0	.00	0	.00	0	.00
	Year-to-date	.0000	.0000	3,509	.00	376	21,814.00	1,896	109,965.00	184	10,672.00	1,053	61,074.00
	Inpatient	.0000	.0000	3,509	.00	376	21,814.00	1,896	109,965.00	184	10,672.00	1,053	61,074.00
	Outpatient	.0000	.0000	0	.00	0	.00	0	.00	0	.00	0	.00
Initial consult	Current	.0000	.0000	202	.00	23	.00	99	.00	19	.00	61	.00
	Inpatient	.0000	.0000	202	.00	23	.00	99	.00	19	.00	61	.00
	Outpatient	.0000	.0000	0	.00	0	.00	0	.00	0	.00	0	.00
	Year-to-date	.0000	.0000	756	.00	74	.00	399	.00	43	.00	240	.00
	Inpatient	.0000	.0000	756	.00	74	.00	399	.00	43	.00	240	.00
	Outpatient	.0000	.0000	0	.00	0	.00	0	.00	0	.00	0	.00
Chart review	Current	.0000	.0000	125	.00	12	.00	70	.00	10	.00	33	.00
	Inpatient	.0000	.0000	125	.00	12	.00	70	.00	10	.00	33	.00
	Outpatient	.0000	.0000	0	.00	0	.00	0	.00	0	.00	0	.00
	Year-to-date	.0000	.0000	490	.00	48	.00	282	.00	23	.00	137	.00
	Inpatient	.0000	.0000	490	.00	48	.00	282	.00	23	.00	137	.00
	Outpatient	.0000	.0000	0	.00	0	.00	0	.00	0	.00	0	.00
Patient education	Current	.0000	.0000	565	.00	61	.00	292	.00	42	.00	170	.00
	Inpatient	.0000	.0000	565	.00	61	.00	292	.00	42	.00	170	.00
	Outpatient	.0000	.0000	0	.00	0	.00	0	.00	0	.00	0	.00
	Year-to-date	.0000	.0000	2,066	.00	230	.00	1,085	.00	112	.00	639	.00
	Inpatient	.0000	.0000	2,066	.00	230	.00	1,085	.00	112	.00	639	.00
	Outpatient	.0000	.0000	0	.00	0	.00	0	.00	0	.00	0	.00

Table 14.5 Cardiac Rehabilitation Productivity Monitoring Information

Variable activities	Standard hours	Volume	Total
Routine inpatient daily fee	0.780	437	340.86
Spouse education class	0.194	23	4.46
Psychological therapy—brief	0.500	0	0.00
Psychological therapy—extended	1.000	21	21.00
Spouse education—psychological instruction	1.000	23	23.00
Phase II psychological instruction	1.000	8	8.00
Phase II Class	0.421	8	3.37
Stress test & letter	1.114	16	17.82
Nutrition consult—15 min	0.250	0	0.00
Nutrition consult—60 min	1.000	0	0.00
ECG monitored exercise prescription	0.750	0	0.00
Exercise—prescription 15 min	0.250	0	0.00
Exercise—prescription 30 min	0.500	1	0.50
Exercise—prescription 45 min	0.750	0	0.00
Exercise—prescription 60 min	1.000	0	0.00
Monitored exercise	0.473	44	20.81
Maintenance	0.473	33	15.61
Unmonitored Phase II	0.473	20	9.46
Heart to Heart—organized volunteer program	0.250	10	2.50
Phase IV class—annual	0.387	38	14.71
Phase IV class—monthly	0.387	0	0.00
Progress checks/exercise review	1.000	0	0.00
Lifestyle—weight class patients	0.887	6	5.32
Lifestyle—weight class employees	0.887	12	10.64
Employee fitness yearly	0.286	144	41.18
Exercise III—Nutrition	0.415	10	4.15
Exercise IV—Nutrition	0.191	0	0.00
		Total	527.13

Support activities	Standard	Activity	Total
Director (1.0 FTE)	1.000	80	80
Clinical coordinator (1.0 FTE)	0.800	80	64
Senior exercise specialist (1.0 FTE)	0.250	80	20
Secretary (1.5 FTE)	1.000	120	120
Staff meetings/In-service	1.000	14	14
		Total	298

Total standard hours (variable and support)	825.13
Productive hours worked (regular)	990.00
Utilization index (825.13/990 × 100)	83.34

Note. ECG = electrocardiogram; FTE = full-time employee.

Chapter 15

Quality Assurance in Health Care

Linda K. Hall, PhD

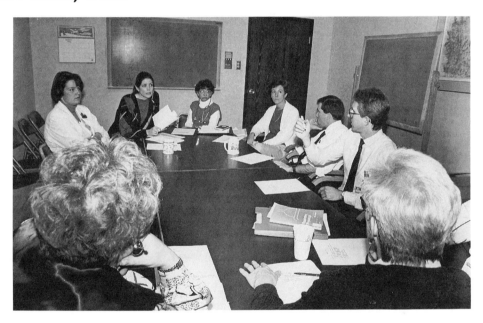

This chapter contains the tools you will need to make sure that all that you do is appropriate, from inception to delivery, and that your delivery and final outcomes are high quality. This chapter covers measurement of delivery of your product, quality assurance, and JCAHO accreditation.

Learning Objectives

1. To learn the language of JCAHO and of QA and to apply this language to your work environment

2. To learn how to implement a QA program and why

3. To answer the question, "How does my department compare in its health care delivery?"

Evaluation, assessment, and accountability in applying day-to-day care to the patient summarize the mission of the hospital, health care organization, and health care professional. As health care costs rise at an alarming rate, people have become more prudent health care shoppers, looking for the best care for their money. Almost every hospital is struggling to maintain a profitable census, maintain optimal nursing numbers, and produce a practice image that will attract patients. As few as 15 years ago, the health care industry counted on word of mouth and customer satisfaction as its public relations and advertising to ensure enough patients to maintain a healthy bottom line. Now, you only need to turn on the television or radio or open a newspaper or even a nationally syndicated magazine such as *Newsweek, Time,* and *Sports Illustrated* to learn about which hospital has the latest in lithotrypters and positron emission tomography scanners. The objective of public relations and marketing efforts is to convince the public that this center provides the best health care.

Through the ever-present media, people now have access to information not only about the fancy machines but also about the quality of the care. The potential patient is much more knowledgeable about disease, care, and outcomes and is a much more selective health care shopper than he was 5 to 15 years ago.

The standards against which one may measure health care performance are established by any number of agencies: JCAHO, the Public Health Department, and the Medicare Licensure Board, to name a few. In general a hospital will invite JCAHO once every 3 years to survey the hospital and measure its performance. The hospital pays JCAHO for the accreditation process, and an appointed team of surveyors usually made up of physicians and nurses spend 3 to 5 days in the hospital reviewing all aspects of care provided by the hospital. The standards of care to which the hospital are held deal with all aspects, including record keeping, laundry, kitchens, food, boilers, shelving, job descriptions, and nursing.

The regulations are written up in several manuals that may be purchased from the headquarters of JCAHO and are listed in the reference section of this chapter (JCAHO, 1990a, 1990b, 1990c, 1990d). This chapter addresses issues of preparing your department from its inception to practice within the guidelines of JCAHO. In essence it is better to assure quality care from the beginning rather than redevelop or revise programs and paperwork.

Setting Up Your Department to Assure Quality

There are some very specific guidelines that you should follow to set up a department. If you set up the department following these guidelines you will be setting up the quality assurance factors to meet the JCAHO accreditation process.

Physical Setting

Guidelines for the physical setting of your facility include the amount of space between exercise equipment, distance of shelving and shelved contents from the ceiling, doors and door frames (including the way doors open), toilet access, fire safety, patient privacy, chart confidentiality, and valuables protection. You may seek assistance from management engineering, or from the hospital construction and architectural consultants if you are building a new facility. Finally, you may consult several sections in the JCAHO manual (1990a); refer to the sections on plant, technology, and safety management as well as the hospital-sponsored ambulatory care services. The primary objective is to build the facility right the first time.

Program Management and Structure

As you have read this book I hope that you have followed all of the suggested procedures, such as writing job descriptions and establishing policies and procedures. Several guidelines are very important from a JCAHO point of view and are also good management techniques:

1. Every job that is a part of the program should have a job description that outlines the duties of the job and the credentials required of the person filling the job. (See chapter 7 for samples of job descriptions.) You should review these annually and any time someone is hired for the position.
2. You should have a résumé for each person who is employed in your department. The credentials of each employee should match the essential credentials listed in the job description (see chapter 7).
3. The department should have an up-to-date written set of policies and procedures, which you review annually or update each time you make a change in any aspect of your programming. These policies and proce-

dures should define all of the aspects of care: how, when, and by whom procedures should be performed. Each aspect of what goes on with a patient, from how he is referred into your department to how he is discharged, must be delineated in the policy and procedure manual.

4. For each policy and procedure that you write, you must have a way to document that it has been done, measured, or implemented.
5. There must be evidence that the patient is made aware of her rights in the treatment process and also her responsibilities.
6. There should be guidelines delineating staff scheduling and patient scheduling.

Now that the nuts and bolts of structure for the building and the program are defined, we can progress to the essence of setting up the quality assurance indicators for the actual process of practicing cardiac rehabilitation.

Quality Assurance Application

Before looking at the process of applying cardiac rehab, you must understand some basic principles about quality assurance application. Read through these principles, which will help you structure a plan to set up your department's QA program.

Characteristics of Quality Assurance

The quality assurance plan is made up of four factors: the quality of the service/care, the appropriateness of care, the identification of problems, and the resolution and follow-up of problems. You should monitor quality and appropriateness through routine data collection about the relevant aspects of the care that is applied, such as how many visits a week, what is the intensity of the work, and what are the results. This is a service record, and may look like those shown in Table 15.1. Periodically you are expected to review the numbers to see if there are problems, such as equipment breakdowns, or physicians failing to make proper referrals. The review of data should also determine if you are applying the right care and are achieving the appropriate and expected outcomes. When you identify problems, you should investigate them to determine if they are natural occurrences or if they indicate flaws in the program. For example, suppose that less than 75%

of your patients in Phase II complete the program, yet the national average shows that 75 to 80% of Phase II patients should complete the program. What is causing so many people to drop out of your program? You should return to the patient records to discover why people left the program early and any other pertinent data. Once you have assessed why they left, you may then decide whether you and your department need to make changes in the program. You must document the process of review and the action taken. You should also revisit the problem in 3 to 6 months to see if the action taken changed the outcome.

And finally, the program is evaluated annually by the department staff, the consumers, the medical staff, a quality assurance committee, and ultimately the board of trustees. This route of evaluation is the route that all information takes in JCAHO's quality assurance plan. The ultimate body responsible for quality assurance in the hospital is the board of trustees.

Principles of Quality Assurance

The QA program in your department will follow the same schematic as the QA program for the whole hospital.

1. The program should be planned and systematic. One person in your department should be in charge of QA data collection. The QA plan defines the scope of your cardiac rehabilitation program and delineates the types of patients you care for and how you care for them. The plan enumerates specific aspects of care, such as those patients who are considered high risk or areas where there may be high volumes of patients, and it targets possible problem areas. Here is where the plan begins to target the indicators that the department will measure to determine appropriateness and quality of care. Measurement must be objective yet effective, efficient, and pertinent.
2. The manner in which the data are collected is very important. Computers can make your data collection interactive with other aspects of care, billing, productivity management, and budget management. At The Christ Hospital in Cincinnati, Ohio, we developed a computer program which when used during the initial interview with the patient collected incredible amounts of data relative to the aspects of care. See Table 15.2 for an

Table 15.1 Quality of Care/Service Report

Indicators	January	February	March	April	May	June
I. Volume indices						
A. No. of admissions						
B. No. of discharges						
1. DNF						
Medical reason						
Time factor						
Financial						
Other						
C. No. of patient visits						
1. No. cancelled						
2. No. unkept						
3. No. staff cancellations						
D. No. of at-home patients						
1. No. of bikes out						
E. No. CABG						
F. No. valve						
G. No. transplants						
H. No. angina						
I. No. MI						
J. No. PTCA						
K. No. COPD						
L. No. PVD						
M. No. diabetes						
N. No. inpatient						
O. No. other						
II. Quality indices						
A. Equipment down >3 days						
1. No. equipment service calls						
B. No. of patient complaints						
No. of family complaints						
No. of MD complaints						
C. Patient origin						
Primary physician						
Cardiologist						
Surgeon						
Other						
D. No. lipid profiles						
E. No. dietary consults						
F. Untoward events						
1. No. arrests unsuccessful						

184

Indicators	January	February	March	April	May	June

    2. No. complications requir-
       ing MD consultation

       Sustained CP

       MI during exercise

       Arrhythmias

       Other

    3. No. ER transport

  G. Time hospital discharge to GXT
     >4 weeks

  H. Time GXT to 1st appointment
     >2 weeks

   I. No. LOS 8-12 weeks

   J. No. LOS >12 weeks

  K. No. MD reports not done
     >3 weeks

   L. No. final reports not done
     >4 weeks

  M. No. defibrillation checks not done

  N. No. drug box not done

  O. No. 6-month follow-up missing/
     sent

   P. No. student observation days/
     internship

Note. CABG = coronary artery bypass graft; COPD = chronic obstructive pulmonary disease; CP = chest pain; DNF = did not finish; ER = emergency room; GXT = graded exercise test; LOS = length of stay; MI = myocardial infarction; PTCA = percutaneous transluminal coronary angioplasty; PVD = peripheral vascular disease.

example of this data collection. When you inaugurate a computer program there are other things you should establish, such as a computerized billing system, which measures billable visits and what you did during the visit. You should establish standards of achievement against which you measure your data. The standards may be national norms or criteria set by your hospital's QA program. If you do not meet the goals, you have a basis upon which to begin your investigation and correction.

3. The program should be comprehensive in that it evaluates and measures all of the aspects of care, including equipment service, downtime, practice drills, canceled appointments, and anything that influences the delivery of appropriate care.

4. The QA plan should be coordinated with all other departments with which your department interacts. This is especially important when services cross through other departments. For example, cardiac rehabilitation uses dietary services, social work, vocational rehab, physical therapy, and nursing services, to name but a few. Data collection should be integrated relative to all aspects of care to enable you to evaluate the total team picture.

Guidelines and Examples

Now that the principles of QA are established, you will want to see and develop the actual tools that you are going to use to measure your program. Remember, the actual mechanics and structural things are already done. The building, shelving,

Table 15.2 Cardiac Rehabilitation Patient Profile

Patient: Heart, Joe S.

Spouse:	Jane S.
Address:	1234 Rhythm Court
City/State/Zip:	Anytown, OH 98765
Home phone:	321-555-1234	Work phone: 321-555-6789
Birthdate:	01/01/40	Age: 51 Sex: M

Admitting MD: T
Patient no.:   1234567

Last GXT prior to Phase II:
06/01/90

Diagnosis:

CABG	04/01/90	CABG 5×
MI	04/01/90	Anterolat
Hyperlipidemia	12/31/85	

Phase II admission: 06/02/90   Phase II completion: 08/02/90

Occupational history:	
Current employment:	Full-time
Working hours:	Days
Where employed:	General Power Inc.
Occupation:	Rocket scientist
Physical description of work:	Sedentary
Mental description of work:	Hard

Medications:

Aspirin (Ascriptin)   Atenolol (Tenormin)
Cimetidine (Tagamet)

Past history:

01/31/66	Appendectomy
04/30/83	Right knee arthroscopy
10/31/89	Chest pain
Other:	Arthritis, migraines

Family history:	Kinship:	Personal history:
Hypertension	Father/brother	10/83
Non-insulin-dependent diabetes	Mother	
Premature heart attack (pre-60)		04/90
Angina		11/89
High cholesterol—lipids	Mother/father	06/87

Risk factors:

A. Diet:
   Present weight: 185   One year ago: 200   Weight at age 21: 169
   Special diet:
   Last-known cholesterol level: 218.0

B. Smoking status:
   What do you (or did you) smoke? Cigarettes
   Used to smoke 1.5 packs a day. Smoked for 13.0 years. Quit 0.5 years ago.

C. Drinking status:
   How often do you drink alcoholic beverages? Weekly.
   How many drinks per session? 1

Psychological background:

How do you (did you) feel about your medical status?
   Frequently accepting   Sometimes angry
   Seldom depressed   Sometimes scared

How does your family feel about your medical status?
   Always supportive   Sometimes angry
   Never depressed   Sometimes scared

How have you responded to your heart disease?
   I need more assistance.

How has your family responded to your heart disease?
   Will assist in making changes.

Do you have trouble with adjusting to or with the ability to perform these routines?
   Eating—sometimes
   Sleeping at night—frequently
   Low energy level—frequently
   Return to sexual activities—sometimes
   Return to work—sometimes
   Return to recreational activities—frequently
   Return to household responsibilities—rarely

Phase III admission: 08/03/90   Phase III completion: 12/31/90

Last GXT: 08/10/90
Last lipid: 07/15/90

Note. CABG = coronary artery bypass surgery; GXT = graded exercise test; MI = myocardial infarction.

electricity, equipment placement, locked valuables area, and patient confidentiality are all appropriately set up or assured. You have a set of department policies and procedures as well as up-to-date job descriptions that match the jobs and the programs as they are applied. (Remember, these need to be reviewed at least annually and initialed by the appropriate supervising officer.) Additionally, the résumés of your current employees match their job descriptions both in experience and in degrees and certifications. Once all of those things are taken care of, you may actually set up what it is you are going to measure.

Each hospital is different and each hospital QA program varies from others, dependent upon the hospital's global objectives. At The Christ Hospital in Cincinnati the department reviewed and measured all objectives quarterly, and we set up our own objectives to be a part of the whole hospital program (see Table 15.3). At Allegheny General Hospital my department operates on two different sets of QA objectives. The global hospital objectives are related to the following areas: mortality, untoward drug reactions, readmission focus, medication errors, nosocomial infection control, and pressure sores. Our department has set up objectives that measure the quality of care and service that the patient receives (see Table 15.4) better than that of global hospital objectives.

Outcome Measures

One of the critical issues that JCAHO brought forth as a 1990 objective is the measurement of outcomes. No matter what you measure, it is essential that you establish what is an acceptable level of achievement; when you finish applying the program, treatment, or procedure, you then measure the end result to see if you have achieved the expected outcome. The new AACVPR (1991) guidelines are set up perfectly to facilitate outcome measures and expectations. Refer to Table 15.5, which enumerates the guidelines for patient assessment, recommended program, and outcomes. This table, which is reprinted from the AACVPR (1991) *Guidelines for Cardiac Rehabilitation*, will serve as a guide for establishing an assessment, program, and outcome plan for each patient who enters your

programs. Once again, setting up the paperwork to enable you to record this information on a patient chart is critical.

Figure 15.1 and Table 15.6 provide examples of such record keeping; also see Figure 3.1 on page 59. You may use these forms as guides or create your own. The objective is for your department to produce these data during JCAHO inspections and demonstrate that you follow up cases for which expected outcomes are not achieved. Figure 15.1 is set up so that you chart patient education on the front, then flip the chart over and continue the exercise charting on the back. Note that Figure 15.1 has steps for an inpatient program, yet AACVPR (1991) guidelines indicate an individualized case management approach with no steps. You can use this step concept by writing a general description of six to seven steps that include generalized exercise and walking components. Thus you can use a less formalized yet individualized step program and still meet AACVPR guidelines.

Table 15.6 is part of a computer program developed for outpatient exercise. This is a practical type of record keeping and data file, because you can run an incredible amount of information from this data base for JCAHO standards and later on for pre/post studies to determine if your program is working. Refer to Figure 3.1 on page 59 for an example of a day-to-day data sheet used to track the Phase II outpatient's daily exercise progress.

Patient evaluation of the program is important. The hospital evaluates you by its standards, but, quite often the patients have their own standards.

Table 15.3 Quality Assurance Indicators, Measures, and Outcomes

Monitoring indicator	Measure	Applied to	Outcome standard
Goal attainment	Lifestyle; mental, emotional, and physical capacities	All patients	75% of all patients should improve in all parameters to satisfactory
Program indicators	Cumulative statistics	Patients, physicians, staff	Applied weekly, monthly, and annually
Program evaluation	Patient evaluation of program	Each patient	Achieve an average of 3.5 out of possible 5 on Likert Scale
Emergency procedures readiness	Practice mock codes Quizzes, certifications, licenses	All staff	Continue working until performance is 100%
Staff evaluation	Evaluation form	All staff	Achieve a level of *meets expectations* in all areas

Table 15.4 Quality Assurance Objectives

Performance will be monitored in general by the clinical department chairman, the division director, and the department director/manager, who will specifically examine performance relative to the following criteria. It is the goal of the institution that there will be no avoidable deviation from the stated criteria. Whenever a deviation from one of these criteria occurs, a detailed review will be undertaken to determine the cause. The review process will assist the staff in minimizing avoidable deviations. Whenever it is determined that a deviation was avoidable, appropriate corrective action will be initiated.

1. All inpatients with appropriate physician orders will exhibit functional improvement and become fully ambulatory as established by their cardiac rehabilitation treatment plans, unless precluded by medical conditions.
2. All outpatients will achieve or make progress toward expected outcomes as established by their cardiac rehabilitation treatment plans, unless precluded by medical conditions or patients' abilities to comply.
3. All cardiac rehabilitation staff members who are medically responsible for patients during dynamic activities will review emergency treatment procedures monthly.
4. No evaluation of inpatient and outpatient programs by the patient shall score lower than satisfactory (biannual review).
5. All cardiac rehabilitation staff members will participate in professional education enhancement activities (e.g., in-service education programs, professional meetings, grand rounds, and staff development).
6. A quarterly random review of each staff member's charting in inpatient and outpatient programs will demonstrate compliance to program charting guidelines.

The patient is the consumer, and the consumer chooses where to take her business. I am always reminded of the following statistics from the White House Office of Consumer Affairs (Albrecht & Zemke, 1985):

1. The average business never hears from 96% of its unhappy customers. For every complaint you do hear about there are 26 other consumers who are unhappy and have problems—6 of which are very serious problems.
2. Of the customers who do register complaints, about 54 to 70% will come back again

if their complaints are resolved; if complaints are resolved in what the customers believe is a rapid manner, the return business rises to 95%.
3. The average consumer who has difficulty with a business will tell 10 people about the problem; 13% of consumers will tell 20 people.
4. If the complaint is satisfactorily resolved, the consumer will tell just 5 people about the resolution.

These statistics should answer any questions you have about why you should conduct a customer satisfaction survey. Additionally, about 30 to 40% of your patients will have repeat catheterizations, repeat angioplasty, or repeat CABG surgery within the next 1 to 12 years. If patients are pleased with their treatment for the first procedure and feel that they had an "excellent outcome," they will return to the same hospital for the second procedure. Tables 15.7 and 15.8 provide a long form of evaluation and a short form of both inpatient and outpatient program evaluation.

If you want to know what repeat business is worth, go to the revenues-over-cost column under cardiology and cardiovascular surgery for the last fiscal year in your hospital. Multiply this figure by .35, and that will be additional revenue spread over the next 10 years, and this occurs each year. For example, suppose we do 2,500 bypass surgeries a year. One-third of that is 833, and 83 of those will return for the next 10 years. Next year, another 833 will fall into the repeat category. So, potentially, each year 833 patients will be repeat.

Emergency Procedures

Although a great deal of the emergency procedures protocols and equipment are taken care of under the facilities management and structural design areas, there are some procedures that you will need to address in a data-keeping and outcome measures section. Once again the AACVPR (1991) guidelines address this in the emergency procedures chapter and also in Appendix A, which includes samples of the forms that you should use to document emergency protocols for equipment checks, drug box upkeep, and standing orders. Additionally, the AACVPR (1991) guidelines state, "Regularly scheduled 'mock' codes should be held for all staff related to patient care. . . . All staff who have direct or supervisorial contact with patients should participate in these mock codes and review

Table 15.5 Design for Patient Assessment, Recommended Program, and Expected Outcome Measures

Patient assessment and profile	Program	Expected outcome
Recent open chest or heart surgery (CABG, valve, AICD, pacemaker, etc.) as determined by patient medical records	Patient education program including information on the disease process, treatment and risk-factor education, activity guidelines, sexual activity, medications, and return to work	Self-care; increased understanding of surgically related concerns and improved quality of life
Recent diagnosis of CAD/MI or its treatment or sequelae (e.g., cath, PTCA, arrhythmia, CHF) as determined by patient medical records	Patient education program including information on the disease process, signs and symptoms, treatment options, risk factors, activity guidelines, sexual activity, medications, and return to work	Self-care; increased understanding of CAD and related concerns; improved quality of life
Reduced activity level, decreased functional capacity, or sedentary lifestyle as determined by a medical history or a graded exercise test, with or without oxygen-consumption measurements	Individualized exercise program based on risk stratification: • Monitored • Unmonitored, supervised • Home exercise program and education	Increase in activity level and functional capacity, attainment of an improved level of fitness and/or regular exercise participation
Tobacco use or abuse as determined by patient or family report, CO monitoring, or isothiocyanide saliva testing	Smoking cessation program	Reduction or cessation of smoking
Any abnormality in blood lipids and/or lipoproteins as manifested by increased total cholesterol or LDL-C, and/or triglycerides, and/or reduced HDL-cholesterol as determined by fasting draw (for LDL-C, TG, HDL-C) and confirmed by repeat measurement	Dietary lipid/modification and medical intervention program in accordance with National Cholesterol Education Program (NCEP) guidelines; weight reduction program and/or exercise program when appropriate	Alteration toward or attainment of appropriate blood lipid and lipoprotein levels as set forth in the NCEP guidelines
Hypertension as determined by blood pressure sphygmomanometry	Hypertension management program including medical intervention and education in accordance with the National High Blood Pressure Education Program (NHBPEP) guidelines; weight reduction, stress management, dietary modification, and/or exercise programs when appropriate	Decreased blood pressure or attainment of appropriate blood pressure as set forth in the NHBPEP guidelines, and reduction or elimination of blood pressure medication
Excess body weight or relative fatness as determined by scale, body mass index, skinfold calipers, or hydrostatic weighing	Dietary weight reduction program and/or exercise program in accordance with the American Dietetic Association guidelines	Reduction in body weight and fat stores and attainment of desirable body weight
High stress levels and/or inappropriate response to stress as determined by patient or family report, stress assessment tools, or psychological evaluation	Stress management program	Reduction in stress and/or inappropriate response to stress

Patient assessment and profile	Program	Expected outcome
Recent onset of elevated or poorly controlled blood glucose levels as determined by fasting blood draw	Diabetes education and medical intervention program in accordance with the American Diabetes Association guidelines; dietary modification, exercise, and/or weight reduction programs when appropriate	Controlled blood glucose levels
Limitation in work status due to cardiovascular medical conditions	Work hardening program and vocational rehabilitation counseling with a return to work assessment; stress management and/or exercise program when appropriate	Return to work if appropriate
Alcohol abuse as determined by patient or family report or by psychological evaluation	Alcohol abuse program including spouse and family therapy	Appropriate alcohol use or abstinence and appropriate family interaction
Psychological disorders (anxiety, depression, phobias, aggressive behavior, etc.) as determined by patient or family report or psychological/psychiatric evaluation	Individualized and/or group therapy	Improved psychological profile and functioning
Neuropsychological disorders (memory loss, confusion, etc.) as determined by patient or family report or by neuropsychological evaluation	Neurological or neuropsychological referral and intervention and therapy	Improved neuropsychological profile and functioning

Note. AICD = automatic implantable cardioverter defibrillator; CABG = coronary artery bypass graft; CAD = coronary artery disease; CHF = congestive heart failure; CO = carbon monoxide monitoring; HDL = high-density lipoprotein; HDL-C = high-density lipoprotein fraction; LDL-C = low-density lipoprotein fraction; MI = myocardial infarction; PTCA = percutaneous transluminal coronary angioplasty; TG = triglycerides.

Note. From *Guidelines for Cardiac Rehabilitation Programs* (pp. 19-20) by the American Association of Cardiovascular and Pulmonary Rehabilitation, 1991, Champaign, IL: Human Kinetics. Copyright 1991 by AACVPR. Reprinted by permission.

of emergency medications, equipment and supplies" (p. 48). A member of your department should design monthly practice codes, education classes, lectures, quizzes, and emergency equipment utilization checks for all the staff members who meet this definition from the AACVPR guidelines. With this program of emergency procedures practice codes and education, you should maintain documentation of each of the activities, an attendance list of department members, a grading of each department member's performance, and also a record of current certifications and licenses of each department member.

Staff Evaluation

JCAHO and you too should be very interested in evaluation and education of the staff members with whom you work. The areas of staff management that are a part of the department structure are addressed elsewhere (see chapter 7, and the beginning of this chapter). However, you should be aware of and provide for some areas of staff tracking and documentation. Quality care of the patient can run into problems for any one of three reasons: lack of knowledge, inadequate delivery systems, and behavior and attitude problems with

Cardiac Rehabilitation and Wellness Programs

Patient/family response to teaching program

1 = Needs complete review
2 = Needs reinforcement/repetition
3 = Needs no further instruction
NA = Not applicable
# = Unable to complete training

Phase I—Cardiac Rehabilitation

Patient teaching book	Assessed need	Date presented	Patient response	Evaluation/comments	Signature
Anatomy/physiology					
Diagnostic tests					
Cardiac procedures					
Coronary bypass surgery					
Recovery: heart attack surgery					
Risk factors					
Exercise/cardiac rehab					
Living with pacemakers					
Home care					
Other					

Teaching program	Assessed need	Date presented	Patient/family response	Comments	Signature
Orientation class					
Discharge class					
Nutrition class					
Diabetic video class					
Family/patient support class					
Phase II cardiac rehab consult					
Other					

Problems:

Plan:

Evaluation:

Phase I—Exercise Component

Date	Step number	Resting HR	Resting BP	Exercise HR	Exercise BP	Rate of perceived exertion	Evaluation comments	Signature
						1 2 3 4 5 6 7 8 9 10		
						1 2 3 4 5 6 7 8 9 10		
						1 2 3 4 5 6 7 8 9 10		
						1 2 3 4 5 6 7 8 9 10		
						1 2 3 4 5 6 7 8 9 10		
						1 2 3 4 5 6 7 8 9 10		
						1 2 3 4 5 6 7 8 9 10		
						1 2 3 4 5 6 7 8 9 10		

Figure 15.1 Cardiac rehabilitation and wellness program form. BP = blood pressure; HR = heart rate.

Table 15.6 Phase II Final Report

Heart, Joe S.
Phase II admission: 06/02

Target rate: 136-142 (70% Karvonen)
Completion: 08/02

GXTs:	Maximum time	Resting HR (bpm)	Resting BP (mmHg)	Protocol	Maximum rate	Maximum speed	Maximum grade	Maximum METs	Nuclear medicine
06/01	14.00	60	128/80	N	117	2.0	17.5	7	Thallium stress
08/10	13.50	56	150/88	B	150	5.0	18.0	15	test

Lipids:	Total cholesterol	Triglycerides	HDL-C	LDL-C	TC/HDL ratio	LDL/HDL ratio	Appear	Glucose
07/15	165	98	53	101	3.11	1.91	Clear	87

Treadmill:	Time	Maximum HR (bpm)	Maximum BP (mmHg)	RPE	Resistance speed	Resistance elevation	METs	Weight (lb)
06/05	5.00	122	173/84	13	2.5	0.0	2.5	185
06/15	7.50	132	170/82	12	2.5	2.5	3.3	184
07/01	10.00	134	168/86	12	3.0	5.0	5.0	181
07/15	10.00	138	174/86	10	3.0	10.0	7.9	182
08/01	12.00	136	152/76	11	3.5	10.0	8.3	179

Bike:	Time	Maximum HR (bpm)	Maximum BP (mmHg)	RPE	Resistance (W)	Resistance (kpm)	METs
06/05	10.00	118	162/60	11	62.5	375.0	3.4
06/15	12.00	121	152/64	11	62.5	375.0	3.4
07/01	12.00	133	148/68	9	62.5	375.0	3.4
07/15	12.00	144	168/70	13	125.0	750.0	6.6
08/01	15.00	140	156/76	12	125.0	750.0	6.6

Land rower:	Time	Maximum HR (bpm)	Maximum BP (mmHg)	RPE	Resistance	Distance (m)
06/05	6.00	128	178/78	13	1.0	1154
06/15	10.00	128	170/64	12	1.0	1205
07/01	10.00	134	168/76	12	1.0	1400
07/15	11.00	135	166/74	12	1.5	1592

Arm ergometer:	Time	Maximum HR (bpm)	Maximum BP (mmHg)	RPE	Resistance (W)	Resistance (kpm)	RPM	METs
06/05	2.50	138	186/74	13	6.2	0.0	45	3.8
06/15	3.50	128	156/72	12	6.5	0.0	45	3.8
07/01	5.00	134	158/78	12	12.5	0.0	50	4.7
07/15	5.50	128	154/76	12	12.5	0.0	60	5.2
08/01	5.50	126	154/70	13	18.7	0.0	60	6.1

(continued)

Table 15.6 *(continued)*

Notes:	Patient type	ECG	Comments
06/01	C	Sinus rhythm at rest; no PVCs observed	Fair exercise tolerance; states some incisional soreness; is walking at home up to 1/2 mi; leg incision draining
06/15	C	Sinus tach at rest 06/11; states some palpitations	States no problem with exercise; leg incision healing well; will see MD on 06/23
07/01	C	Sinus rhythm at rest; has occasional isolated PVCs	Tolerating increased exercise well; offers no complaints; continues slight weight loss
07/15	C	Sinus rhythm; no ectopy observed	Continues to tolerate exercise well; asking good questions in classes; continues good weight management; return to work soon
08/01	C	Sinus rhythm; no ectopy observed	Tolerating exercise well at 9.0 METs; scheduled for follow-up in 3 months; has returned to work; discharged from Phase 2

Goals:	Smoking cessation	Weight loss	Salt/cholesterol control	Exercise 5 days/week	Return to work	Psychological coping	BP management	Risk F education
This patient:	X	X	X	X	X	X	X	X
Level achieved:	4	5	3	2	5	3	1	5

Note. 1 = denial; antagonistic; 2 = 25% adherence; 3 = 51% adherence; 4 = 75% adherence; 5 = excellent adherence.

Entry weight: 185 lb	Exit weight: 178 lb
Physician letters: 06/01 07/01 08/01	Attendance: Satisfactorily completed Phase II.
Additional comments:	

Admitting MD:	T		
Diagnosis:	CABG	04/01	CABG 5x
	MI	04/01	Anterolat
	Hyperlipidemia	12/31	

Program:	Date or NA:
1) Anatomy & physiology	06/05
2) Atherosclerosis: Signs & symptoms	06/12
3) Cholesterol & fats	06/19
4) Behavior, change, & relapse	06/26
5) Exercise & fitness	07/03
6) Stress management	07/10
7) Risk factors	07/17
8) Orientation	06/05

Focus:	Smoking cessation	NA
	Exercise consult	08/01
	Stress consult	07/13

Note. Family has been to most of the sessions. Seems to be good rapport with members. Mr. Heart seems to be in control of his life and environment.

BP = blood pressure; CABG = coronary artery bypass graft; ECG = electrocardiogram; GXT = graded exercise test; HDL = high-density lipoprotein; HDL-C = high-density lipoprotein fraction; HR = heart rate; LDL = low-density lipoprotein; LDL-C = low-density lipoprotein fraction; MI = myocardial infarction; PVC = premature ventricular contractions; RPE = rate of perceived exertion; TC = total cholesterol; THR = target heart rate.

Table 15.7 Phase II: Patient Assessment

This questionnaire has several purposes. (1) We are interested in evaluating our program on a continuous basis so that we may make changes where needed and constantly upgrade the unit services. (2) We cannot continue to serve our patients' needs unless we evaluate the provision of services. (3) The Joint Commission on Accreditation of Health Care Organizations requires that we provide evidence of program evaluation. Because of these factors we would appreciate it if you would answer the following as completely and concisely as possible.

Length of time you were in the program: _____ Number of visits per week: _____

Intake information—orientation

Rate the following elements of the intake and orientation process:

	Very poor	Poor	Fair	Good	Excellent	Not Applicable
1. The initial intake interview	1	2	3	4	5	6
2. The staff explanation of the planned program	1	2	3	4	5	6
3. The explanation of the goals and objectives of your care	1	2	3	4	5	6
4. Encouragement to include family and significant others in the program	1	2	3	4	5	6
5. Encouragement to participate in the program	1	2	3	4	5	6
6. The staff knowledge and understanding of your problems	1	2	3	4	5	6
7. The intake interview organization and process	1	2	3	4	5	6

Suggestions/comments _____

Exercise information

Rate the quality of educational and practical information provided by the staff relative to the following areas:

8. The need for exercise during the rest of your life	1	2	3	4	5	6
9. Your exercise prescription	1	2	3	4	5	6
10. Your use of a variety of modes of exercise	1	2	3	4	5	6
11. Your progress on a daily, weekly basis	1	2	3	4	5	6
12. Your prescription for exercise at home on off-days	1	2	3	4	5	6

Suggestions/comments _____

Rate the staff explanation and demonstration regarding your use or application of the following:

13. Electrodes and transmitter	1	2	3	4	5	6
14. Exercise bicycle	1	2	3	4	5	6
15. Treadmill	1	2	3	4	5	6
16. Rowing machine	1	2	3	4	5	6
17. Arm crank machine	1	2	3	4	5	6
18. Wall pulley	1	2	3	4	5	6
19. Other equipment pertinent to your program	1	2	3	4	5	6

Suggestions/comments _____

(continued)

Table 15.7 *(continued)*

	Very poor	Poor	Fair	Good	Excel- lent	Not Ap- plicable

Rate the staff's knowledge and willingness to share that knowledge relevant to your questions about the following:

20. Your blood pressure and blood pressure response	1	2	3	4	5	6
21. Your electrocardiogram and heart rate	1	2	3	4	5	6
22. Your medications and responses to them	1	2	3	4	5	6
23. Your arrhythmias (funny heart rhythms)	1	2	3	4	5	6
24. Your risk factors and changes you need to make	1	2	3	4	5	6
25. Your responsibilities in the recovery process	1	2	3	4	5	6

Rate the level of competence demonstrated by the staff in performance of the following:

26. Education relevant to risk factors	1	2	3	4	5	6
27. Education relevant to exercise	1	2	3	4	5	6
28. Discussing risk factor modification	1	2	3	4	5	6
29. Explaining how to exercise	1	2	3	4	5	6
30. Explaining the function of exercise and heart health	1	2	3	4	5	6
31. Explaining the process of disease progression	1	2	3	4	5	6
32. Understanding and relating to you and your disease problem	1	2	3	4	5	6

Suggestions/comments _____

Rate the staff on the following characteristics:

33. Courtesy of the staff	1	2	3	4	5	6
34. Degree of professionalism demonstrated by the staff	1	2	3	4	5	6
35. Level of cheerfulness and optimism of the staff	1	2	3	4	5	6
36. Positive atmosphere in the rehab area	1	2	3	4	5	6

Evaluate your progress and changes from the beginning of the program to the end relative to the following:

37. Energy level	1	2	3	4	5	6
38. Smoking cessation	1	2	3	4	5	6
39. Dietary changes (lowering cholesterol)	1	2	3	4	5	6
40. Loss of weight	1	2	3	4	5	6
41. Ability to perform daily living activities	1	2	3	4	5	6
42. Sleeping at night	1	2	3	4	5	6
43. Feelings or sensations of depression	1	2	3	4	5	6
44. Feelings of self-worth and positive lifestyle	1	2	3	4	5	6
45. Feeling that you are in control of your life	1	2	3	4	5	6

46. If you could change the Phase II program, what would you do?

a. _____

b. _____

c. _____

Table 15.8 Outpatient Survey

Directions: Please evaluate how satisfied you were with your visit to this department today by checking the most appropriate box. If a question does not apply to your visit today, check NA (not applicable).

	Very satisfied	Somewhat satisfied	Not satisfied	NA
Patient care staff				
1. The courtesy and helpfulness of the staff	☐	☐	☐	☐
2. The staff's ability to answer questions and keep you informed	☐	☐	☐	☐
3. The instructions for follow-up care at home	☐	☐	☐	☐
4. Your overall confidence in the skill of the staff	☐	☐	☐	☐
5. The staff's willingness to let you participate in your treatment	☐	☐	☐	☐
Other staff				
6. The courtesy and helpfulness of the registration staff	☐	☐	☐	☐
7. The courtesy and helpfulness of the office receptionist	☐	☐	☐	☐
General				
8. The availability of appointment times	☐	☐	☐	☐
9. The availability of convenient parking	☐	☐	☐	☐
10. The overall care and treatment you received	☐	☐	☐	☐

11. How did you find out about this service?

_____

12. Will you return to this facility if you require further treatment?

____ Yes ____ No ____ Uncertain

13. Approximately how many miles do you live from this facility?

____ Within 20 ____ 20 to 50 ____ 50 to 100 ____ over 100

14. Patient sex

____ Male ____ Female

15. Patient age

____ under 21   ____ 45 - 54
____ 21 - 34   ____ 55 - 64
____ 35 - 44   ____ 65 - 74
                   ____ 75 +

16. Additional comments:

_____

_____

_____

Thank you for completing this survey.

staff, all of which depend upon your staff and how they function individually and together as a team. You need to build into your total program those areas found in chapter 7; the areas you should document are evaluation of the staff, in-service training, continuing education, and any actions taken to change specific behavior or attitudes.

Conclusion

After you have read through all of the material contained in this chapter, form a grid to see if your program covers all of the areas inherent in a comprehensive quality assurance program. First, list all of those things that you are using as your monitoring indicators, how you are measuring, to whom measurements are applied, and the desired outcome you are applying as a standard. For the examples used in this chapter, the grids and lists will be similar to those found in Tables 15.3 and 15.4, pages 188-189.

Doing the right things the right way the first time should be your aim in setting up a really excellent program. Quality assurance is one way to assure that you set up your program correctly, because policies, procedures, and job descriptions are all part of QA. The main function of quality assurance is to ask, ''How are we doing and how did we do?''

References

Albrecht, C., & Zemke, R. (1985). *Service in America*. Homewood, IL: Dow Jones-Irwin.

American Association of Cardiovascular and Pulmonary Rehabilitation. (1991). *Guidelines for cardiac rehabilitation*. Champaign, IL: Human Kinetics.

Joint Commission on Accreditation of Healthcare Organizations. (1990a). *Accreditation manual for hospitals*. Oakbrook Terrace, IL: Author.

Joint Commission on Accreditation of Healthcare Organizations. (1990b). *Ambulatory health care standards manual*. Oakbrook Terrace, IL: Author.

Joint Commission on Accreditation of Healthcare Organizations. (1990c). *A guide to JCAHO nursing services standards* (3rd ed.). Oakbrook Terrace, IL: Author.

Joint Commission on Accreditation of Healthcare Organizations. (1990d). *Quality assurance in ambulatory care* (2nd ed.). Oakbrook Terrace, IL: Author.

Discharge Instructions for the Patient With Myocardial Infarction (Heart Attack) I

Diagnosis: _____

Date: _____

Physician: _____

Cardiovascular risk factor analysis:

Risk factors are characteristics or behaviors that increase a person's chances of developing coronary artery disease (blocked arteries) or enhance its progression. Most risk factors can be controlled with lifestyle changes, which will reduce your risk of further heart attacks. The three major risk factors are smoking, high blood pressure, and elevated blood-fat levels.

Your identified risk factors include (circled)

Smoking	Diabetes
High blood pressure	Sedentary lifestyle
High blood lipids (fat)	Family history
Stress	Obesity/overweight
Cholesterol—ideal is less than 200	Triglycerides—ideal is less than 160

Guidelines for resuming normal activities:

Carefully observe these guidelines. They should also be observed by family and friends who want to help you return safely to your optimal level of health and physical activity.

1. **Physical activity:** A slow, progressive approach to resuming your previous activity level places less strain on your heart. You eventually may be able to perform many household tasks, participate in recreational activities, and return to work. Complete resumption of normal activities, however, usually occurs after the 6-week healing period. Don't expect an instant recovery, and don't resume activities at your previous levels. Alternate your activities throughout the day with rest periods. Remember, any significant period of enforced bed rest or inactivity (2 weeks or more) results in a decrease in your previous activity level. Returning to normal activity will take at least as much time as you were inactive. Before returning to full-time work, resuming major household tasks, participating in recreational activities, or driving, check with your physician.

2. **Activity guidelines:**

   * Alternate difficult tasks with easy ones and rest for 15 to 30 min between.
   * Don't rush. Allow plenty of time for everything.
   * Get sufficient sleep each night, so that you feel rested in the morning. Don't stay up late and then try to catch up on sleep the next night.

3. **Activities to avoid:** Activities involving excessive pulling, pushing, straining, or lifting generally should be avoided. These activities require more work from the heart and may impair the healing of the heart muscle. Limit excessive upper body and arm activity.

4. **Angina:** Angina is a serious warning sign—a message from your heart that it is not getting enough blood and oxygen. Although angina affects people differently, common symptoms include chest, throat, jaw, or arm discomfort, described as pain, tightness, pressure, heaviness, squeezing, or burning. If angina occurs, stop your activity, sit down, and relax. If the discomfort does not subside immediately, take nitroglycerin (NTG) as prescribed by your physician. Take an NTG tablet or use the NTG spray every 5 min until the discomfort is gone or you have taken three tablets/sprays. If the angina lasts longer than 15 min or gets worse, call your doctor or go to the nearest emergency room. Notify your physician if these symptoms occur or increase in frequency or severity.

   • Nitroglycerin tablets become ineffective once the container has been open for approximately 3 months.
   • Nitroglycerin in spray canisters remains effective until the expiration date.
   • The tablets should be placed, and the spray applied, under your tongue.
   • Do not shake the spray canister, and avoid swallowing immediately after using the spray.

5. **Body weight:** Weigh yourself daily and record your weight. Weight should be taken at the same time each day (usually morning). If you notice a sudden weight gain of 2 to 3 lb in one day of normal eating, or an unusual swelling of the legs, ankles, or abdomen, notify your physician.

6. **Stairs:** Begin slowly climbing stairs, at first only when necessary. Pace yourself: walk one to two steps (both feet on each step), pause, then continue.

7. **Bathing:** You may take a warm bath or shower, but avoid extreme temperatures, such as steam baths, saunas, spas, or whirlpools. Don't tire yourself while caring for personal hygiene.

8. **Temperature extremes:** Do not perform activities outdoors when temperatures are cold (below 32 °F) or hot (above 80 to 85 °F) or when humidity is high.

9. **Constipation:** Maintain good bowel habits by eating a well-balanced diet. When constipation occurs, avoid straining and use a mild laxative or stool softener.

10. **Emotions:** Sadness is normal during the recovery period. Feeling "blue," being "down in the dumps," or having "cabin fever" is a normal part of the recovery period. Just as your sleep cycle returns to normal, so will your moods. Occasionally, however, normal sadness will become a more serious depression. Symptoms of depression may include not wanting to return to normally enjoyable activities; continued fatigue or lethargy, even with continuing medical improvement; and a feeling of not being lovable, worthy, or competent. Again, depression is not unusual and should be brought to the attention of your physician. It is important to control your emotional stress at home and at work. Don't try to carry all the emotional responsibilities yourself; share them with members of your family and business associates. Become aware of emotionally upsetting situations and try to avoid them. If they are unavoidable, concentrate on relaxing when these situations arise.

11. **Driving:** You may resume driving your automobile at your physician's discretion. Remember to wear your seat belt.

12. **Sexual activity:** How soon you resume sexual activity after leaving the hospital depends on your progress and how you feel when returning home. A general recommendation is to wait several weeks following hospital discharge. You should speak with your physician about your situation. Some basic guidelines include the following:

   • Discuss with your partner any fears or anxieties you might have regarding sex.
   • Use a nonstrenuous position in a comfortable room temperature.
   • Because alcohol decreases the heart's ability to function, do not consume alcoholic beverages for approximately 3 hr before sexual activity.
   • If you begin to have chest discomfort or severe shortness of breath during sexual activity, discontinue the activity and follow the guidelines for relieving those symptoms.

13. **Warning signs:** Notify your physician if the following symptoms frequently occur, even though they are relieved by rest or medication. In an emergency, do not hesitate to call the paramedics.

   • Chest pain (angina)—sudden onset of chest pain not relieved by rest or nitroglycerin
   • Shortness of breath not relieved by rest

- Dizziness, confusion, or fainting
- Episode of rapid heartbeats

Medications:

You will receive a list of medications, including prescriptions for new medications. Do not take other medications, including over-the-counter remedies, without checking with your physician.

Appointments for checkup:

It is important that you receive regular examinations by a physician. Contact your local physician (family doctor or cardiologist) to make an appointment within 1 week of hospital discharge.

Discharge Instructions for the Patient With Myocardial Infarction (Heart Attack) II

Diagnosis: _____

Date: _____

Physician: _____

Cardiovascular risk factor analysis:

Risk factors are characteristics or behaviors that increase a person's chances of developing coronary artery disease (blocked arteries) or enhance its progression. Most risk factors can be controlled with lifestyle changes, which will reduce your risk of further heart attacks. The three major risk factors are smoking, high blood pressure, and elevated blood-fat levels.

Your identified risk factors include (circled)

Smoking	Diabetes
High blood pressure	Sedentary lifestyle
High blood lipids (fat)	Family history
Stress	Obesity/overweight
Cholesterol—ideal is less than 200	Triglycerides—ideal is less than 160

Guidelines for resuming normal activities:

Carefully observe these guidelines. They should also be observed by family and friends who want to help you return safely to your optimal level of health and physical activity.

1. **Physical activity:** A slow, progressive approach to resuming your previous activity level places less strain on your heart. You eventually may be able to perform many household tasks and participate in recreational activities. Don't expect an instant recovery, and don't resume activities at your previous levels. Your body may give you signals indicating the need for rest. Signals include shortness of breath, fatigue, dizziness, or chest discomfort/pain.

    Alternate your activities throughout the day with rest periods, so that you can regain strength for each activity. Remember, any significant period of enforced bed rest or inactivity (2 weeks or more) results in a loss of strength. Returning to normal activity will take at least as much time as you were inactive. Check with your physician if you have questions about specific activities.

2. **Activities to avoid:** Activities involving excessive pulling, pushing, or lifting generally should be avoided. These activities require more work from the heart and may impair its healing. Limited upper body and arm exercise (5 to 20 lb of effort) is recommended for 6 weeks or until your physician approves increased activity level.

3. **Angina:** Angina is a serious warning sign—a message from your heart that it is not getting enough blood and oxygen. Although angina affects people differently, common symptoms include chest, throat, jaw, or arm discomfort, described as pain, tightness, pressure, heaviness, squeezing, or burning. If angina occurs, stop your activity. Sit down and relax. If the discomfort does not subside immediately, take nitroglycerin (NTG) as prescribed by your physician. Take an NTG tablet or use the NTG spray every 5 min until the discomfort is gone or you have taken three tablets/sprays. If the angina lasts longer than 15 min or gets worse, call your doctor or go to

the nearest emergency room. Notify your physician if these symptoms occur or increase in frequency or severity.

- Nitroglycerin tablets become ineffective once the container has been open for approximately 3 months.
- The tablets should be placed, and the spray applied, under your tongue.
- Do not shake the spray canister, and avoid swallowing immediately after using the spray.

4. **Stairs:** Begin slowly climbing stairs, at first only when necessary. Pace yourself: Walk three to four steps (both feet on each step), pause, then continue. After 1 or 2 weeks, you may eliminate the pauses and climb stairs normally, alternating steps in the usual pattern. Continue to pace yourself.

5. **Bathing:** You may take a warm bath or shower, but avoid extreme temperatures, such as steam baths, saunas, spas, or whirlpools. Pace yourself when taking care of your personal hygiene.

6. **Temperature extremes:** Initially limit activity outdoors when temperatures are cold (below 32 °F) or hot (above 80 to 85 °F) or when the humidity is high. Allow time for your body to gradually adapt to temperature extremes.

7. **Constipation:** Maintain good bowel habits by eating a well-balanced diet. When constipation occurs, avoid straining and use a mild laxative or stool softener. If constipation continues, check with your physician.

8. **Emotions:** Sadness is normal during the postdischarge recovery period. Feeling "blue," being "down in the dumps," or having "cabin fever" is a normal part of the recovery period. Just as your sleep cycle returns to normal, so will your moods. On some occasions, normal sadness will become a more serious depression. Symptoms of depression may include not wanting to return to normally enjoyable activities; continued fatigue or lethargy, even with continuing medical improvement; and a feeling of not being lovable, worthy, or competent. Again, depression is not unusual and should be brought to the attention of your physician.

   It is important to control your emotional stress at home and at work. Don't try to carry all the emotional responsibilities yourself; share them with members of your family and business associates. Become aware of emotionally upsetting situations and try to avoid them. If they are unavoidable, concentrate on relaxing when these situations arise.

9. **Driving:** You may resume driving your automobile at your physician's discretion—usually within a few weeks, depending on your situation. Remember to wear your seat belt.

10. **Sexual activity:** How soon you resume sexual activity after leaving the hospital depends on your progress and how you feel when returning home. A general recommendation is to wait several weeks following hospital discharge. You may wish to speak with your physician about your situation. Some basic guidelines include the following:

    - Discuss with your partner any fears or anxieties you might have regarding sex.
    - Use a nonstrenuous position in a comfortable room temperature.
    - Because alcohol decreases the heart's ability to function, do not consume alcoholic beverages for approximately 3 hr before sexual activity.
    - If you begin to have chest discomfort or severe shortness of breath during sexual activity, discontinue the activity and follow the guidelines for relieving those symptoms.

11. **Warning signs:** If any of these signs or symptoms occur, notify your physician immediately:

    - Chest discomfort (angina)—sudden onset of chest pain not relieved by rest or prescribed medication
    - Shortness of breath not relieved by rest
    - Leg pain or unusual swelling of legs or ankles
    - Dizziness, confusion, or fainting
    - Irregular heartbeats
    - Episode of rapid heartbeats

Medications:

You will receive a list of medications, including prescriptions for new medications. Do not take other medications, including over-the-counter remedies, without checking with your physician.

Appointments for checkup:

It is important that you receive regular examinations by a physician. Contact your local physician (family doctor or cardiologist) within 1 week of hospital discharge to make an appointment.

Discharge Instructions for the Patient With Coronary Artery Bypass Surgery

Date of surgery: _____

Surgeon: _____

Procedure: _____

Physician's phone number: _____

Cardiovascular risk factor analysis:

Risk factors are characteristics or behaviors that increase a person's chances of developing coronary artery disease (blocked arteries) or enhance its progression. Most risk factors can be controlled with lifestyle changes, which will reduce your risk of further heart attacks. The three major risk factors are smoking, high blood pressure, and elevated blood-fat levels.

Your identified risk factors include (circled)

Smoking	Diabetes
High blood pressure	Sedentary lifestyle
High blood lipids (fats)	Family history
Stress	Obesity/overweight
Cholesterol—ideal is less than 200	Triglycerides—ideal is less than 160

Guidelines for resuming normal activities:

Carefully observe these guidelines. They should also be observed by family and friends who wish to help you return safely to your optimal level of health and physical activity.

1. **Physical activity:** Generally, a slow, progressive approach to resuming your previous activity level is best for your heart. You should eventually be able to perform many household tasks, participate in recreational activities, and return to work. Complete resumption of normal activities, however, usually occurs after the 6-week healing period. Don't expect an instant recovery, and don't resume activities at your previous levels. Alternate your activities throughout the day with rest periods. Remember, any significant period of enforced bed rest or inactivity (2 weeks or more) results in a decrease in your previous activity level. It takes at least as much time to return to your regular activity level as the amount of time you were inactive. Before returning to full-time work, resuming major household tasks, participating in recreational activities, or driving, check with your physician.
2. **Activities to avoid:** Activities involving excessive pulling, pushing, lifting, or breath holding should generally be avoided. These activities require more work from the heart muscle and may impair the healing process of the sternal incision. Limited upper body and arm activity (5 to 20 lb of effort) is recommended for 6 weeks until you see your cardiac surgeon.
3. **Stairs:** Begin slowly. Climb stairs, at first, only when necessary. Pace yourself: Walk three to four steps (both feet on each step), pause, then continue. If you have a leg incision, lead going up with the leg that doesn't have the incision. Lead down the stairs with the leg that does have the incision. After 1 or 2 weeks, you may eliminate the pauses and climb stairs normally, alternating steps in the usual pattern.
4. **Sexual activity:** How soon you resume sexual activity after leaving the hospital depends on your progress and how you feel when returning home. A general recommendation is to wait several

weeks following hospital discharge. You may wish to talk with your physician regarding your specific situation. Some basic guidelines include the following:

- Discuss with your partner any fears or anxieties you might have regarding sex.
- Use a nonstrenuous position at a comfortable room temperature.
- Do not consume alcoholic beverages for approximately 3 hr before sexual activity.
- If you begin to have chest discomfort or severe shortness of breath during sexual activity, discontinue the activity and follow the guidelines for relieving those symptoms.

5. **Constipation:** Maintain good bowel habits by eating a well-balanced diet, drinking fluids, and engaging in light physical activity such as walking. When constipation occurs, avoid straining and use a mild laxative such as Milk of Magnesia® or a stool softener. If constipation continues, check with your physician.

6. **Angina:** Angina is a serious warning sign. It is a message from your heart telling you it is not getting enough blood and oxygen. Angina can feel different to various people. Common symptoms include chest, throat, jaw, or arm discomfort, described as pain, tightness, pressure, heaviness, squeezing, or burning. If angina occurs, stop your activity, sit down, and relax. If the discomfort does not subside within 5 to 10 min, seek immediate medical assistance. Report any angina occurring before your 6-week surgical checkup to your surgeon.

7. **Emotions:** Sadness is normal during the postdischarge recovery period. Feeling ''blue,'' being ''down in the dumps,'' or having ''cabin fever'' is a normal part of the recovery period. Just as your sleep cycle returns to normal, so too will your moods. On some occasions, normal sadness will become a more serious depression. Symptoms of depression include not wanting to return to normally enjoyable activities; continued fatigue or lethargy, even with continuing medical improvement; and a feeling of not being lovable, worthy, or competent. Again, depression is not unusual and should be brought to the attention of your physician.

It is important to control your emotional stress both at home and at work. Don't try to carry all the emotional responsibilities yourself; share them with members of your family and business associates. Become aware of emotionally upsetting situations and try to avoid them. If they are unavoidable, concentrate on relaxing when these situations arise.

8. **Temperature extremes:** Initially avoid activity outdoors when temperatures are cold (below 32 °F) or hot (above 80 to 85 °F) or when the humidity is high. Avoid extreme temperatures such as steam baths, saunas, spas, and whirlpools.

9. **Bathing:** You may take a warm bath or shower. Wash your incision gently with soap and water; pat dry (don't rub).

10. **Wound care:** Bathe regularly and do not use creams or lotions on incisions until they are healed. Do not wear constrictive clothing around the areas of incision. Women may, however, wear bras. If incisions do not appear to be healing (i.e., redness, drainage, swelling, or tenderness is present), inform your cardiac surgeon.

11. **Body temperature:** Take your temperature every morning for 1 week after discharge. Notify your cardiac surgeon if your temperature stays above 100 °F for more than a day. If you feel ill as if from a cold or the flu, check with your physician.

12. **Body weight:** Check your weight every day, in the morning, for the first 2 weeks. If you notice a sudden weight gain, notify your cardiac surgeon.

13. **Driving:** You may resume driving at your surgeon's discretion—usually in 6 weeks. Avoid sitting for long periods of time. When sitting, do not cross your legs. When riding in a car, limit trips to 1 to 2 hr. If longer trips are necessary, stop and take a 5- to 10-min stretch-and-walk break every 1 to 2 hr. Wear your seat belt.

Warning signs:

If any of the symptoms listed below occur before your 6-week postdischarge appointment, please notify your cardiac surgeon promptly. If they occur after that appointment, contact your local physician.

1. Chest discomfort (angina)—sudden onset of chest pain not relieved by rest or prescribed medication. The pain of the incision should subside gradually.

2. Redness, swelling, or drainage from your incisions.
3. Instability of breastbone—excessive movement or clicking sounds.
4. Leg pain or unusual swelling of legs or ankles.
5. Body temperature above 100 °F.
6. Shortness of breath not relieved by rest.
7. Coughing up blood.
8. Dizziness, confusion, or fainting.
9. More than 10 irregular heartbeats per minute.
10. Episode of rapid heartbeat.

Medications:

Your nurse has given you a list of all the medications you are to take once you are discharged from the hospital. Take only these medications. Prescriptions have been provided for new medications. Never take medications unless your physician has prescribed them. Your physician should be made aware of all your current medicines, including over-the-counter remedies such as antacids and sinus preparations. You should never omit, increase, or decrease dosages without contacting your doctor. Some medications may slow or speed your heart rate. Any time you are placed on a new medication, check with your physician to determine its effect on your heart rate. If you have any questions about your medications, be sure to ask your nurse before leaving the hospital.

Appointments for checkup:

It is important that you are examined regularly by a physician. Contact your local physician (family doctor or cardiologist) within 1 week of hospital discharge to make an appointment.

Your cardiac surgeon will need to see you in 6 weeks following discharge. Be sure to make an appointment as soon as possible. Take a list of your current medications with you to that appointment.

Activity Guidelines

+ **Permitted activities**	– **Activities to avoid**
Weeks 1 and 2 after discharge:	
+ Personal hygiene (bathing, dressing)	– Straining or lifting activities requiring more than 5 to 10 lb of effort
+ Basic food preparation	– Walking grades or hills
+ Desk work (reading, typing, writing)	– Activities performed in extreme temperatures
+ Riding in a car (wearing a seat belt)	– Sweeping, shoveling, digging, or grass or hedge cutting
+ Board or card games	– Competitive activities
+ Craft work (sewing, knitting)	– Walking medium or large dog
+ Level walking	– Carpentry, painting
	– Driving
Weeks 3 and 4 after discharge:	
+ All activities of Weeks 1 and 2	– Straining or lifting activities requiring more than 10 to 15 lb of effort
+ Light housework (dusting, dishwashing)	– Walking steep grades or hills
+ Grocery shopping and errands	– Activities performed in extreme temperatures
+ Playing musical instruments	– Sweeping, shoveling, digging, or grass or hedge cutting
+ Using light hand and power tools	– Walking medium or large dog
+ Walking slight grades	– Competitive activities
+ Sexual intercourse	– Carpentry, painting
+ Ballroom dancing (slow paced)	– Driving
+ Pumping gas	
+ Light garden work (weeding, planting small plants, no digging)	
+ Golf (putting only)	
Weeks 5 and 6 after discharge:	
+ All activities of Weeks 3 and 4	– Straining or lifting activities requiring more than 20 lb of effort
+ Medium housework (sweeping, laundry, windows)	– Walking steep hills
+ Light carpentry and painting (no ceiling or high ladder work)	– Activities performed in extreme temperatures
+ Light auto maintenance	– Shoveling, digging, grass or hedge cutting
+ Golf (pitch and putt, no driving)	– Driving
+ Catching and tossing baseball or softball (no football, basketball, or bowling)	
+ Garden work (no digging)	
+ Walking dog	

6-Week Walking Program

When to walk:

Any time of the day is fine, but be sure to space your sessions evenly throughout the entire day (e.g., do not do all your walking in the morning). In addition, wait at least 1 hr after meals, 1/2 hr after bathing, and 1/2 hr after taking an Isordil® before you walk or engage in other physical activity.

Signs and symptoms:

Be alert for dizziness, shortness of breath, spreading (anginalike) chest pain, and excess fatigue before, during, or after exercise.

Warm-up:

Do ____ repetitions of your sitting/standing range-of-motion (ROM) exercises before each walk.

Pace:

Walk at a brisk pace that does not leave you breathless. You should be able to carry on a conversation while you walk. Try to walk continuously for the prescribed amount of time on a level grade. Do not hesitate to pause and rest if necessary.

Week 1: Walk _____ min continuously, _____ times a day.

Week 2: Walk _____ min continuously, _____ times a day.

Week 3: Walk _____ min continuously, _____ times a day.

Week 4: Walk _____ min continuously, _____ times a day.

Week 5: Walk _____ min continuously, _____ times a day.

Week 6: Walk _____ min continuously, _____ times a day.

After 6 weeks:

Continue to increase the duration of each walk by

_____ min each week until you are walking

_____ min continuously _____ times a day.

At this time, it is not necessary to walk every day. Four to five days per week are enough. In addition, you should consult with your physician for further instructions concerning your exercise program and general physical activities.

Introduction to the American Heart Association Diet

The American Heart Association diet is recommended to promote healthy, nutritious eating habits by limiting amounts of the following:

- Cholesterol
- Saturated fat
- Total fat
- Simple carbohydrates (sugars)
- Sodium
- Alcohol
- Calories (to maintain ideal body weight)

The goal of this diet is to allow you to achieve and maintain a low level of fat (cholesterol, triglycerides) in your blood in order to decrease your chance of developing atherosclerosis, or the accumulation of fatty deposits within the arterial walls. Atherosclerosis is the principal cause of coronary artery disease, which can lead to heart failure, heart attack, stroke, and death.

You and your family should adopt the following nutritional recommendations to stay healthy and prevent heart disease. Use these recommendations in conjunction with the advice from your physician. Follow your physician's instructions if there is any conflict in information.

Cholesterol:

Reduce your cholesterol intake to 300 mg or less by limiting high cholesterol food sources such as these:

- Any food of animal origin: beef, lamb, pork, veal
- Liver and other organ meats
- Egg yolks
- Whole milk, ice cream, cream, cheese, butter
- Beef fat, lard, bacon, sausage, lunch meats

Saturated fat:

Reduce the saturated fat content of your diet so that it contributes 10% or less of your total calories. Sources of saturated fat include the following:

- Any food of animal origin: beef, lamb, pork, veal
- Beef fat, lard, bacon, sausage, lunch meats
- Egg yolks
- Whole milk, ice cream, cream, cheese,
- Butter
- Salad dressings, cream sauces, fried foods, gravy
- Some nuts, coconut
- Any product containing hardened or saturated fats, hydrogenated or partially hydrogenated oils, or shortening.

Total fat:

By reducing your cholesterol and saturated fat intake, you also will reduce your total fat intake. Your goal is to reduce your total fat intake to below 30% of your total daily calories by eating low-fat foods. Choosing polyunsaturated and monounsaturated fats is desirable because they may decrease cholesterol levels in the blood.

- Polyunsaturated fat is primarily found in foods from vegetable sources: safflower oil, sunflower oil, corn oil, and soybean oil. The two exceptions are coconut and palm oils, which are saturated.
- Use the lowest amounts possible of high-fat sources, such as margarine, mayonnaise, oil, salad dressing, or cream.

- Choose margarine with liquid vegetable oil (safflower, sunflower, soybean, corn) as the first ingredient. Read the label to be sure there are at least twice as many grams of polyunsaturated fat as grams of saturated fat.
- Sources of monounsaturated fat include olive oil, peanut oil, and canola oil (Puritan®).

Carbohydrates:

Reduce and limit your intake of simple carbohydrates, which may cause your triglyceride level and body weight to rise. Examples include sweets, sugar, cake, candy, cookies, and jellies.

Increase the amount of complex carbohydrates in your diet by consuming more fresh fruits, vegetables, and whole-grain breads and cereals. These foods are also high in fiber.

Sodium:

Excessive sodium in your diet may contribute to high blood pressure and cause unnecessary fluid retention. Read package labels to discover the exact amount of sodium per serving. Aiming for 300 mg or less of sodium per serving is a conservative guideline.

- Limit sodium to 3,000 mg or less each day.
- Keep the salt shaker in the cupboard and off the table.
- Use little, if any, salt in cooking. Substitute natural herbs and spices for flavoring.

High sources of sodium include the following:

- Any canned or processed foods, such as canned vegetables, soup, sauerkraut or pickled foods
- Milk, cheese, lunch meats

Alcohol:

Use alcoholic beverages in moderation, if at all. Because you should avoid alcohol when you take certain medications, check with your physician first. Alcohol, taken in moderation or excess, may raise the levels of triglycerides and cholesterol in your blood and may raise blood pressure. Alcohol consumption should not exceed 1 oz of ethanol per day. One oz of ethanol is equal to 2 oz of 100-proof whiskey, 8 oz of wine, or 24 oz of beer.

Caffeine:

Limit your consumption of caffeine to two to three cups or less a day of coffee, tea, or soda pop. Keep in mind that chocolate and some over-the-counter medications (Anacin®, Excedrin®, Sinarest®) contain caffeine.

Calories:

Regulate your calories to maintain or achieve your ideal body weight. Consult a registered dietitian if you need assistance with weight loss.

Nutritious eating:

To maintain a well-balanced, nutritious diet, include the following foods every day:

- Protein, meat—two servings or a total of 4 to 6 oz of low-fat protein foods such as fish, poultry (skin removed), lean red meat with fat trimmed, or legumes (beans, dried peas, lentils)
- Grains, starches, complex carbohydrates—at least four servings of whole-grain, high-fiber cereals, breads, potatoes, rice, and starchy vegetables

- Vegetables—at least two servings of deep green and orange vegetables
- Fruit, juice—at least two servings, including one citrus source
- Skim milk, low-fat milk products—two servings of skim milk, part skim cheese, nonfat yogurt, or ice milk

Know your blood fat (serum lipid) levels:

Date _____
Cholesterol
Desired level: 200 mg/dl or below
Your level _____

Date _____
HDL-cholesterol
Desired level: 45 mg/dl or above
Your level _____

Date _____
Triglyceride
Desired level: 160 mg/dl or below
Your level _____

Date _____
LDL-cholesterol
Desired level: 130 to 140 mg/dl or below
Your level _____

Tips:

- Remember that decreasing the total amount of fat (any kind, any form) is the most important dietary change you can make.
- Minimize portions of and the frequency that you eat foods containing saturated fat.
- Choose lean cuts of meat and limit meat, seafood, and poultry to no more than 6 oz per day.
- Use no more than a total of 5 to 8 tsp of fat and oils per day for cooking, baking, and salad dressing.
- Substitute 0 to 1% milk, evaporated skim milk, or nonfat dry milk for beverages, in coffee, and for cooking.
- Read the ingredient list on all foods.

Label reading:

Use the ingredient listing on food labels to identify hidden sources of fat. Avoid the following high-fat/cholesterol ingredients:

- Palm or palm kernel oil
- Coconut oil
- Shortening
- Hydrogenated or partially hydrogenated oil
- Lard, beef tallow
- Butter, cream, whole milk
- Cocoa butter, milk chocolate, or malted milk
- Eggs, egg-yolk solids

Although a label may correctly say "no cholesterol," the product may contain a high level of saturated fat or excessive total fat. To determine the percentage of fat-related calories in a food, perform the following calculations:

1. Multiply the number of grams of fat by 9.
2. Multiply this answer by 100.
3. Divide the outcome of Step 2 by the total number of calories in the product.

Avoid foods containing more than 30% fat or consume them only in small portions.

Recipe substitutions:

Instead of	Use
1 c butter or shortening	7/8 c canola or safflower oil, or 1 c tub margarine, or 2 sticks margarine

1 c cream or whole milk	1 c evaporated skim milk
1 whole egg	2 egg whites, or 1/4 c egg substitute
1 c sour cream	1 c nonfat plain yogurt
1 c sugar	3/4 c sugar
1 oz baking chocolate	3 tbsp cocoa powder, plus 1 tbsp canola or safflower oil
whole-milk, natural, hard cheese	part skim, fat-reduced cheese

APPENDIX B

Job Description: Director, Cardiac Rehabilitation Department

Purpose

The cardiac rehabilitation director is responsible for all day-to-day operations, quality of patient care, and long-range planning of the Cardiac Rehabilitation Department, including all existing programs (exercise, education, behavior modification, assessment, and research) and future programs. In conjunction with hospital administration and the cardiac rehabilitation medical director, the cardiac rehabilitation director is administratively responsible for the personnel and functions of the Cardiac Rehabilitation Department.

Major activities

1. Supervise and administer the following cardiac rehabilitation program components servicing medical and surgical cardiovascular patients:

   - Inpatient cardiac rehabilitation services
   - Phases II, III, and IV outpatient monitored exercise training programs
   - Lifestyle modification programs (Lite Life Weight Control, smoking cessation, stress management, Culinary Heart Kitchen, and diabetes education) including lifestyle programs offered as part of the occupational medicine program
   - Student internship program and development of clinical affiliations agreements
   - Employee fitness
   - Corporate contracts
   - Phase II outpatient and family education
   - Outpatient psychological counseling services

   Clinical assessments, teaching/counseling skills, and exercise prescription abilities may be required with select patients.

2. Develop, implement, and revise all program protocols and operating policies for the Cardiac Rehabilitation Department not specifically identified. Monitor departmental budgetary expenditures and revenues and provide monthly variance reports.

3. Develop and expand cardiac rehabilitation services to other patient populations and employees, as well as to outside agencies, including corporations and community medical and educational facilities.

4. Coordinate services between the Cardiac Rehabilitation Department and hospital by interfacing the program with hospital administration, physicians, and other health-related personnel.

5. Supervise the cardiac rehabilitation team consisting of a clinical psychologist, clinical specialists, dietitian, exercise specialists, clerical staff, and student interns. Authorize and negotiate hiring, firing, and periodic evaluation of all personnel working within the Cardiac Rehabilitation Department. Approve all staff assignments.

6. Provide continued professional development of the cardiac rehabilitation staff through regular educational opportunities.

7. Develop and control the annual Cardiac Rehabilitation Department budget. Direct capital investments with hospital administration and board approval.

8. Direct facility planning, expansion, and renovation in consultation with the Cardiac Rehabilitation Department's medical consultant and medical director and the hospital administration.
9. Coordinate and approve all public relations endeavors, advertising, and marketing plans for services or programs provided by the Cardiac Rehabilitation Department.
10. Recommend and carry out policies to limit the legal liability of the Cardiac Rehabilitation Department.
11. Initiate and coordinate the Cardiac Rehabilitation Department's research efforts.

Nature and scope

The director must possess the following qualifications: Specialized or technical knowledge. Minimum of PhD with emphasis in exercise physiology or cardiac rehabilitation. A minimum of 3 years of experience in cardiac rehabilitation including inpatient, outpatient, and exercise testing services. Minimum of 2 years of experience in program administration and exercise testing supervision/interpretation. Current American College of Sports Medicine certification as a program director. Current or demonstrated ability to obtain American Heart Association certification in advanced cardiac life support. Background in epidemiology/behavior modification/patient education is highly desired.

Job Description: Exercise Specialist

Reports to

Clinical coordinator and/or director, medical director, Cardiac Rehabilitation Department

Purpose

The exercise specialist is responsible for performing day-to-day implementation and follow-up case management for all patients in the Cardiac Rehabilitation continuum. This involves an inpatient case load covered independently, with team support as needed to provide an individualized rehabilitation program meeting the personal and family needs of 8 to 12 patients. The exercise specialist is assigned an outpatient class or classes as additional responsibility in the Cardiac Rehabilitation Department. This work requires a general understanding of cardiovascular diseases as well as knowledge and abilities in exercise prescription, exercise physiology, behavior change, risk factor assessment and management, cardiovascular emergency procedures, nutrition, and adult education.

Major activities

1. Is directly responsible by case management assignment for patients in the inpatient program.
   - Assess and evaluate patient functional and risk factor status.
   - Assess psychosocial and economic factors.
   - Develop a program to meet the goals, objectives, and needs of the patient and family for optimal return to ADL within the limitations imposed by the disease.
   - Utilize adjunct services and the clinical coordinator to assist in crisis intervention, education, counseling, behavior modification, and exercise programming.
   - Assess and educate in discharge planning for the patient and family.
2. Is responsible for rotating assignments in spouse education and outpatient family education classes or as otherwise directed.
3. Is directly responsible by case management assignment for a class or classes in the outpatient cardiac rehabilitation continuum.
   - Assess and evaluate patient functional status.
   - Assess risk factor stratification.
   - Assess socioeconomic and work status.
   - Assist the patient in designing an exercise, education, and lifestyle modification program to meet ADL, recreational, and vocational needs.
   - Evaluate patient progress and create or modify goals and objectives with patient.
   - Discharge with appropriate program to maintain and continue optimal lifestyle function.
   - Learn and use the HBO and computer billing service.
4. Is responsible for maintaining emergency preparedness through department in-services and annual and biannual recertification.
5. Maintains patient records, progress reports to physicians, and documentation per policy and procedure manual.
6. Is a member of department committees as assigned and participates in department activities, special events, and programs as desired or directed.
7. Participates in research, staff development projects, in-service education classes, and other activities as desired or directed.
8. Maintains professional knowledge base by professional organization membership and regular attendance at in-service programs, workshops, symposia, and university classes.
9. Performs other duties as assigned by the director, medical director, or clinical coordinator.

Nature and scope of position

A. Within the parameters defined, the exercise specialist works autonomously with patients using case management techniques. Additional responsibilities may be assigned or self-generated.
B. The exercise specialist functions as a member of the Cardiac Rehabilitation Department, participating in department meetings and the development and implementation of policy and procedure and programmatic and management goals. Day-to-day care planning and rehabilitation treatment of patients is the direct responsibility of the exercise specialist. Questions, concerns, and medical decisions regarding treatment must be reported to and discussed with the physician, cardiac rehabilitation medical director and/or clinical coordinator.
C. The exercise specialist may coordinate activities with adjunct services within the hospital as needed for optimum patient care (e.g., social service, dietary, psychiatry).
D. *Minimum Qualifications:* Current knowledge and/or experience in cardiovascular disease, cardiovascular nursing, emergency procedures, nutrition, exercise physiology, health education, psychology, and medical and education strategies for CAD risk factor management. One of four sets of credentials is needed:
   1. Registered nurse required, MS preferred, with exercise physiology background
       a. BLS and ACLS certification
       b. Two years critical care nursing preferred
       c. Current state license
   2. MS in exercise physiology or related field, with 3- to 6-month hands-on internship in cardiac rehabilitation
   3. BS required, MS preferred, in physical therapy, with a current state license
   4. BS in a health-related field with 3 to 5 years direct cardiac rehabilitation experience

Job Description: Clinical Nutritionist

Reports to

Clinical specialist or director, Cardiac Rehabilitation Department

Purpose

The clinical nutritionist for the Cardiac Rehabilitation Department will be responsible for nutritional care and education of patients with coronary artery disease and valvular heart disease, patients at high risk for coronary heart disease, as well as all other individuals serviced by the department. Duties include individualized consultation and assessment of present patient nutritional status and recommendations for diet modifications. The clinical nutritionist works in conjunction with other cardiac rehabilitation team members to provide special programs in nutrition (e.g., Culinary Heart Kitchen, lipid reduction program, and weight control).

Major activities

1. Provides outpatient nutrition services, both group and individualized, to approximately 300 patients per year. This involves consultation and individualized dietary assessments based on the American Heart Association and American Dietetics Association recommendations, patient preference, and lifestyle demands. Also provides recommendations for modifying lipids, controlling blood pressure, and achieving/maintaining ideal body weight.
2. In conjunction with other rehabilitation specialist, provides nutrition education for individuals, small groups of outpatients, spouses, families, and employees. Such programs can include, but are not limited to, Phase II, Phase III, and spouse education programs.
3. In conjunction with other team members, provides ongoing nutrition education services to participants enrolled in outpatient cardiac rehabilitation. Provides documentation in patient's chart of dietary counseling and progress, as well as a quarterly summary to the director.
4. Administers and directs nutrition programs sponsored by the Cardiac Rehabilitation Department, such as weight control/weight maintenance programs.
5. Provides individual nutrition counseling to patients referred by physicians for specific dietary instruction. Reports on the patient's progress to referring physician.
6. Participates in staff developmental projects; collects and publishes research data.

APPENDIX C

Health Insurance Claim Form

HEALTH INSURANCE CLAIM FORM

(CHECK APPLICABLE PROGRAM BLOCK BELOW)

FORM APPROVED
OMB NO. 0938-0008

| ☐ MEDICARE (MEDICARE NO.) | ☐ MEDICAID (MEDICAID NO.) | ☐ CHAMPUS (SPONSOR'S SSN) | ☐ CHAMPVA (VA FILE NO.) | ☐ FECA BLACK LUNG (SSN) | ☐ OTHER (CERTIFICATE SSN) |

PATIENT AND INSURED (SUBSCRIBER) INFORMATION

1. PATIENT'S NAME (LAST NAME, FIRST NAME, MIDDLE INITIAL)

2. PATIENT'S DATE OF BIRTH

3. INSURED'S NAME (LAST NAME, FIRST NAME, MIDDLE INITIAL)

4. PATIENT'S ADDRESS (STREET, CITY, STATE, ZIP CODE)

5. PATIENT'S SEX

MALE ☐   FEMALE ☐

6. INSURED'S ID NO. (FOR PROGRAM CHECKED ABOVE, INCLUDE ALL LETTERS)

7. PATIENT'S RELATIONSHIP TO INSURED

SELF ☐   SPOUSE ☐   CHILD ☐   OTHER ☐

8. INSURED'S GROUP NO. (OR GROUP NAME OR FECA CLAIM NO.)

☐ INSURED IS EMPLOYED AND COVERED BY EMPLOYER HEALTH PLAN

9. OTHER HEALTH INSURANCE COVERAGE (ENTER NAME OR POLICYHOLDER AND PLAN NAME AND ADDRESS AND POLICY OR MEDICAL ASSISTANCE NUMBER)

10. WAS CONDITION RELATED TO

A. PATIENT'S EMPLOYMENT

YES ☐   NO ☐

B. ACCIDENT

AUTO ☐   OTHER ☐

11. INSURED'S ADDRESS (STREET, CITY, STATE, ZIP CODE)

TELEPHONE NO.

11.a.   CHAMPUS SPONSOR'S

STATUS   ☐ ACTIVE DUTY   ☐ DECEASED   BRANCH OF SERVICE
☐ RETIRED

12. PATIENT'S OR AUTHORIZED PERSON'S SIGNATURE (READ BACK BEFORE SIGNING)

I AUTHORIZE THE RELEASE OF ANY MEDICAL INFORMATION NECESSARY TO PROCESS THIS CLAIM I ALSO REQUEST PAYMENT OF GOVERNMENT BENEFITS EITHER TO MYSELF OR TO THE PARTY WHO ACCEPTS ASSIGNMENT BELOW

SIGNED _____   DATE _____

13. I AUTHORIZE PAYMENT OF MEDICAL BENEFITS TO UNDERSIGNED PHYSICIAN OR SUPPLIER FOR SERVICE DESCRIBED BELOW

SIGNED (INSURED OR AUTHORIZED PERSON) _____

PHYSICIAN OR SUPPLIER INFORMATION

14. DATE OF:

ILLNESS (FIRST SYMPTOM) OR INJURY (ACCIDENT) OR PREGNANCY (LMP)

15. DATE FIRST CONSULTED YOU FOR THIS CONDITION

16. IF PATIENT HAS HAD SAME OR SIMILAR ILLNESS OR INJURY, GIVE DATES

16.a. IF EMERGENCY CHECK HERE ☐

17. DATE PATIENT ABLE TO RETURN TO WORK

18. DATES OF TOTAL DISABILITY

FROM _____   THROUGH _____

DATES OF PARTIAL DISABILITY

FROM _____   THROUGH _____

19. NAME OF REFERRING PHYSICIAN OR OTHER SOURCE (e.g., PUBLIC HEALTH AGENCY)

20. FOR SERVICES RELATED TO HOSPITALIZATION GIVE HOSPITALIZATION DATES

ADMITTED _____   DISCHARGED _____

21. NAME & ADDRESS OF FACILITY WHERE SERVICES RENDERED (IF OTHER THAN HOME OR OFFICE)

22. WAS LABORATORY WORK PERFORMED OUTSIDE YOUR OFFICE?

YES ☐   NO   CHARGES

23. DIAGNOSIS OR NATURE OF ILLNESS OR INJURY. RELATE DIAGNOSIS TO PROCEDURE IN COLUMN D BY REFERENCE NUMBERS 1, 2, 3, ETC. OR DX CODE

1.
2.
3.
4.

B.

EPSDT   YES ☐   NO ☐

FAMILY PLANNING   YES ☐   NO ☐

PRIOR AUTHORIZATION NO.

24. A DATE OF SERVICE FROM — TO	B* PLACE OF SERVICE	C FULLY DESCRIBE PROCEDURES, MEDICAL SERVICES OR SUPPLIES FURNISHED FOR EACH DATE GIVEN — PROCEDURE CODE (IDENTIFY)	(EXPLAIN UNUSUAL SERVICES OR CIRCUMSTANCES)	D DIAGNOSIS CODE	E CHARGES	F DAYS OR UNITS	G* T.O.S	H LEAVE BLANK

25. SIGNATURE OF PHYSICIAN OR SUPPLIER (INCLUDING DEGREE(S) OR CREDENTIALS) (I CERTIFY THAT THE STATEMENTS ON THE REVERSE APPLY TO THIS BILL AND ARE MADE A PART THEREOF)

26. ACCEPT ASSIGNMENT (GOVERNMENT CLAIMS ONLY) (SEE BACK)

YES ☐   NO ☐

30. YOUR SOCIAL SECURITY NO.

27. TOTAL CHARGE

28. AMOUNT PAID

29. BALANCE DUE

31. PHYSICIAN'S SUPPLIERS AND OR GROUP NAME, ADDRESS, ZIP CODE AND TELEPHONE NO

32. YOUR PATIENT'S ACCOUNT NO.

33. YOUR EMPLOYER ID NO.

ID NO

*PLACE OF SERVICE AND TYPE OF SERVICE (T.O.S) CODES ON BACK
REMARKS

APPROVED BY AMA COUNCIL ON MEDICAL SERVICE 8/83

FORM HCFA-1500 (1-84) FORM OWCP-1500
FORM CHAMPUS-501 (1-84) FORM RRB-1500

FORM AMA OP-503

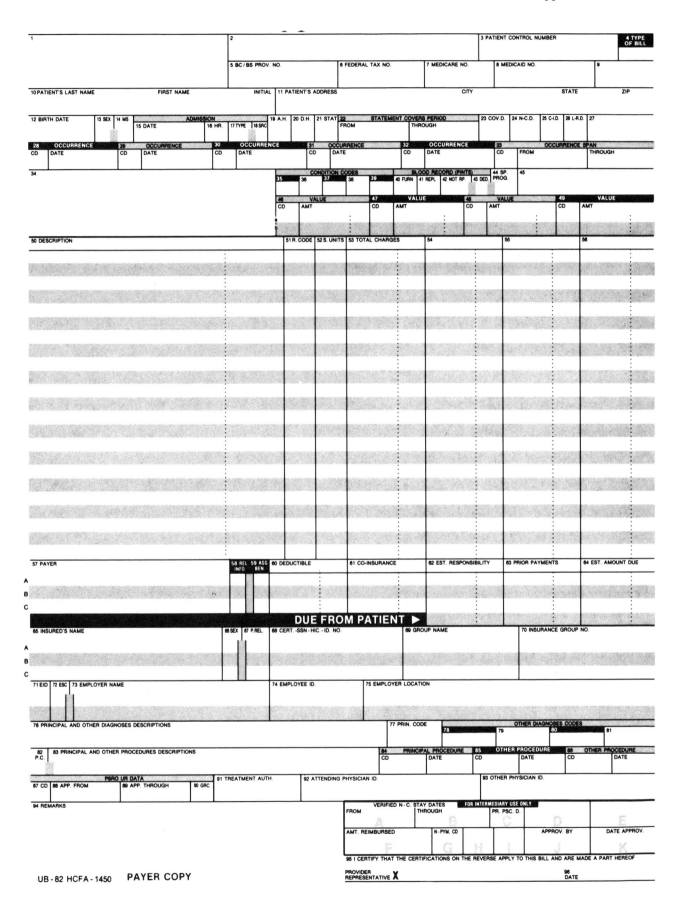

Index

Page numbers in *italics* refer to figures or tables.

225